Pediatric Headache

Pediatric Headache

Edited by

Jack Gladstein
Professor of Pediatrics and Neurology,
University of Maryland School of Medicine,
Baltimore, MD, United States

Christina L. Szperka
Assistant Professor of Neurology & Pediatrics,
Perelman School of Medicine at the University of Pennsylvania,
Philadelphia, PA, United States
Director, Pediatric Headache Program,
Children's Hospital of Philadelphia,
Philadelphia, PA, United States

Amy A. Gelfand
Director of Pediatric Headache, Associate Professor of Neurology & Pediatrics,
UCSF Benioff Children's Hospital, San Francisco, CA, United States

ELSEVIER

Elsevier
Radarweg 29, PO Box 211, 1000 AE Amsterdam, Netherlands
The Boulevard, Langford Lane, Kidlington, Oxford OX5 1GB, United Kingdom
50 Hampshire Street, 5th Floor, Cambridge, MA 02139, United States

Notices

Knowledge and best practice in this field are constantly changing. As new research and experience broaden our understanding, changes in research methods, professional practices, or medical treatment may become necessary.

Practitioners and researchers must always rely on their own experience and knowledge in evaluating and using any information, methods, compounds, or experiments described herein. In using such information or methods they should be mindful of their own safety and the safety of others, including parties for whom they have a professional responsibility.

To the fullest extent of the law, neither the Publisher nor the authors, contributors, or editors, assume any liability for any injury and/or damage to persons or property as a matter of products liability, negligence or otherwise, or from any use or operation of any methods, products, instructions, or ideas contained in the material herein.

Library of Congress Cataloging-in-Publication Data
A catalog record for this book is available from the Library of Congress

British Library Cataloguing-in-Publication Data
A catalogue record for this book is available from the British Library

ISBN: 978-0-323-83005-8

For information on all Elsevier publications
visit our website at https://www.elsevier.com/books-and-journals

Publisher: Sarah Barth
Acquisitions Editor: Melanie Tucker
Editorial Project Manager: Kristi Anderson
Production Project Manager: Sreejith Viswanathan
Cover Designer: Alan Studholme

Typeset by STRAIVE, India

Working together
to grow libraries in
developing countries

www.elsevier.com • www.bookaid.org

Contents

List of contributors xvii

Preface xxi

About the editors xxiii

Acknowledgments xxv

Dedication xxvii

PART I My headache story

CHAPTER 1   My headache story: A guide for families, primary care, and specialists 3

Jack Gladstein, MD

For families.. 3

For primary care clinicians.. 4

For specialists 5

Barriers to effective headache visits 6

Further readings 7

PART II Why does my head hurt?

CHAPTER 2   Why does my head hurt? You're not the only one: Epidemiology 11

Rebecca Barmherzig, MD

Epidemiology: For families... 11

Epidemiology: For primary care and specialists 12

Migraine.. 13

Tension-type headache 15

Trigeminal autonomic cephalalgias 15

Other primary headache disorders 15

New daily persistent headache 16

Secondary headache 16

References.. 16

CHAPTER 3   Pathophysiology of migraine 21

Carlyn Patterson Gentile, MD, PhD and Ana Recober, MD

For patients and families 21

    The migraine cycle 21

    Chronic migraine 22

    The effect of puberty and sex hormones 22

For general practitioners...23
   Migraine cycle 23
   Chronic migraine 24
   Sex differences 24
For specialists 25
   Migraine cycle 25
   Therapies developed for migraine.................................... 27
   Chronic migraine 28
   Sex differences 28
References...28

CHAPTER 4   **Genetics of migraine** **35**
Andrew D. Hershey, MD, PhD

General practitioners..38
Specialists 38
Families..39
Conclusions..39
References..39

PART III   How did it get so bad?

CHAPTER 5   **The "episodic syndromes": I.e., what migraine looks like before it "looks like" migraine**...........................**43**
Amy A. Gelfand, MD

Introduction..43
Infant colic 44
   Key points for families.. 44
   Key points for the primary care provider 45
   Key points for the headache specialist............................. 45
Benign paroxysmal torticollis (BPT) 45
   Key points for families.. 46
   Key points for the primary care provider 46
   Key points for the headache specialist............................. 46
Benign paroxysmal vertigo (BPV)..46
   Key points for families.. 47
   Key points for the primary care provider 47
   Key points for the headache specialist............................. 47
Abdominal migraine 47
   Key points for families.. 48
   Key points for the primary care provider 48
   Key points for the headache specialist............................. 48

Cyclical vomiting syndrome (CVS)..48
   Key points for families.. 49
   Key points for the primary care provider 50
   Key points for headache specialists 50
Conclusions..50
References..50

CHAPTER 6   **Effect of hormones**..**55**
Ann Pakalnis, MD and Kevin Weber, MD

Effect of hormones: What a headache specialist
   needs to know 55
The relationship between migraine and hormones:
   Information to help children and families...........................57
References..59

CHAPTER 7   **Chronic migraine and other types of primary**
chronic daily headache...**61**
Serena L. Orr, MD, MSc and Reena Rastogi, MD

Section A: What health care professionals need to know about
   chronic daily headache in children and adolescents...............61
   Introduction.. 61
   Epidemiology of chronic migraine in children and
       adolescents 62
   Burden of disease associated with chronic migraine
       in children and adolescents 64
   Risk factors for migraine chronification in children
       and adolescents 65
   Prevention of migraine chronification in children and
       adolescents 66
Other chronic headaches in children and adolescents.................67
   Chronic tension-type headache 67
   Chronic cluster headache... 68
   Chronic paroxysmal hemicrania.. 71
   Chronic SUNCT (short-lasting unilateral neuralgiform
       headaches with conjunctival injection and tearing)
       and SUNA (short-lasting unilateral neuralgiform
       headaches with cranial autonomic symptoms..................... 71
   Hemicrania continua... 71
Section B: What patients and their families need to know
   about chronic daily headache in children and adolescents......72
References..74

CHAPTER 8   Comorbidities in children and adolescents **79**
Jason L. Ziplow, MD and Dawn C. Buse, PhD

Introduction 79
For general providers and headache specialists 85
   Psychological disorders 85
   Obesity 86
   Epilepsy 87
   Atopic disorders 88
   Neurodevelopmental and neurobehavioral issues 88
   Nocturnal/sleep disorders 89
   Celiac disease 90
For patients and families 91
Disclosures 92
References 93

CHAPTER 9   New daily persistent headache **101**
Rachel Neely, MSHS, PA-C and Frank R. Berenson, MD

Epidemiology 103
Pathogenesis 103
Workup 104
Treatment 105
Prognosis 106
NDPH: What families need to know 106
References 108

CHAPTER 10 Posttraumatic headaches in youth **111**
Shannon Babineau, MD and Heidi K. Blume, MD

Introduction 111
Information about posttraumatic headache for families 111
Information for primary care clinicians 114
   What is "posttraumatic headache"? 114
   Pathophysiology of PTH 115
Information for the headache specialist 118
References 121

CHAPTER 11 POTS and dysautonomia **125**
Juliana VanderPluym, MD, Madeline Chadehumbe, MD,
and Nicholas Pietris, MD

Postural orthostatic tachycardia syndrome (POTS) and
   headache 125
   Introduction 125

Epidemiology...125
Pathophysiology..126
Clinical features common to headache disorders and POTS 127
Evaluation 128
Treatment 132
Volume expansion 133
Physical activity..133
Sleep..134
Identifying and managing triggers 134
Medical therapy 134
Prognosis..135
References...135

PART IV Ways other people can help me get better

SECTION 1 Treatments for when symptoms are acting up

CHAPTER 12 Acute medications 143
Irene Patniyot, MD and William Qubty, MD

Treatments for when symptoms are acting up...........................143
   What patients and families need to know about
     acute treatments 143
What primary care providers need to know about
   acute medication treatments 144
Acute treatment options...145
What a headache specialist needs to know about
   acute medication treatments 146
   Triptans 146
   Dopamine receptor antagonists 148
   Gepants 149
References...149

CHAPTER 13 Acute behavioral headache management 153
Dina Karvounides, PsyD, Maya Marzouk, MA,
Alexandra C. Ross, PhD, Scott Powers, PhD,
and Elizabeth Seng, PhD

Distraction..153
Efficacy of distraction in pediatric acute pain...........................154
How to support your patients with distraction...........................154
Clinical hypnosis 155
Efficacy of hypnosis in pediatric acute pain............................155
How to support your patients with clinical hypnosis 156

Relaxation strategies, mindfulness, and biofeedback 156
Cognitive reframing 156
Efficacy of cognitive reframing in acute pain episodes 156
How to support your patients with cognitive reframing 157
Parent education and family interactions 157
Efficacy of parental education 157
How to support families helping their child 158
Conclusion 158
References 158

**CHAPTER 14 What should I expect when home therapy
does not work** **161**

Sharoon Qaiser, MD and Marielle Kabbouche, MD

Introduction to intravenous headache treatments for patients
and families 161
What to do when the headache does not respond to an
infusion in the emergency room 163
Advice for the primary care clinician and headache
specialist 163
Intravenous dihydroergotamine (DHE) 165
References 167

**SECTION 2 Treatments for trying to settle
down frequency**

CHAPTER 15 Preventive treatments: Oral **171**

M. Cristina Victorio, MD

Introduction to preventive therapy 171
Information for clinicians 171
Indications for preventive treatment 171
Goals of preventive therapy 172
Pharmacologic preventive migraine treatment 172
Antiepileptic medications 174
Antidepressants 175
Antihypertensives 175
Antihistamine 176
How to implement preventive treatment in the
clinical setting 177
References 179

CHAPTER 16 Preventive injections: onabotulinum toxin A and nerve blocks 181
Rebecca Barmherzig, MD and Christina L. Szperka, MD, MSCE

Onabotulinum toxin A 181
    Information for families 181
    Information for primary care clinicians 182
    Information for headache specialists 183
Nerve blocks including sphenopalatine ganglion blocks 184
    Information for families 184
    Information for primary care clinicians 186
    Information for headache specialists 187
References 188

CHAPTER 17 Preventive behavioral headache management 191
Alexandra C. Ross, PhD, Maya Marzouk, MA, Dina Karvounides, PsyD, Elizabeth Seng, PhD, and Scott Powers, PhD

Describing behavioral headache intervention to families 192
Summary of evidence-base 193
Cognitive behavioral therapy (CBT) 194
    Cognitive CBT strategies 195
    Behavioral CBT strategies 195
    Efficacy of CBT in pediatric headache 195
    How to support your patients in accessing CBT 196
Relaxation strategies 196
    Diaphragmatic breathing 197
    Progressive muscle relaxation 198
    Guided imagery 198
    Efficacy of relaxation in pediatric headache 199
    How to support your patients in accessing relaxation training 199
Biofeedback 199
    Efficacy of biofeedback in pediatric headache 200
    How to support your patients in accessing biofeedback 200
Mindfulness 200
    Efficacy of mindfulness in pediatric headache 200

How to support your patients in accessing mindfulness
training 201

Books for interested families 201

Parental role in preventive behavioral headache
management 201

Conclusion 202

References.. 202

SECTION 3 Treatments that can act both acutely and preventively

CHAPTER 18 Devices...**207**

Samantha Lee Irwin, MB BCh, MS

Neuromodulation for migraine treatment 207

Transmagnetic stimulation (TMS) 207

For patients and families 208

For providers.. 208

Transcranial supraorbital nerve stimulator 209

For patients and families 209

For providers.. 209

Vagal nerve stimulation..210

For patients and families 210

For providers.. 210

Remote electrical neuromodulation device..............................211

For patients and families 211

For providers.. 211

References..212

CHAPTER 19 CGRP pathway treatments..**215**

Amy A. Gelfand, MD

Introduction...215

CGRP pathway monoclonal antibodies for migraine
prevention 215

For patients and families 215

For primary care providers.. 216

For headache specialists 216

Gepants 219

For patients and families 219

For primary care providers.. 219

For headache specialists 219

References..220

CHAPTER 20 Nonpharmaceutical options for pediatric headache: Nutraceuticals, manual therapies, and acupuncture **223**

Amanda Hall, MSN, FNP-C, Andrea Brand, MAc LAc, and Sita Kedia, MD, MPH

Nutraceuticals 223
    What patients and families need to know 223
    What a PCP and headache specialist needs to know 224
Manual therapies 243
    What patients and families need to know? 243
    What a PCP and headache specialist needs to know 243
Acupuncture 247
    What patients and families need to know 247
    What a PCP and headache specialist needs to know 251
References 254

PART V How can I get better? Things I can do for myself/my child

CHAPTER 21 Sleep and headache in children and adolescents **269**

Ana Marissa Lagman-Bartolome, MD, and Kaitlin Greene, MD

For patient and family 269
    What should you know about you/your child's sleep and
        headaches? 269
    How much sleep is recommended? 269
    What do you need to tell the clinician about sleep? 270
    What can you do to improve sleep and headache? 270
    What are the treatments available to improve sleep and
        headache? 270
For the primary care clinician 271
    Treatment 271
For the headache specialist 272
    Prevalence of sleep disturbance among children and
        adolescents with headache 272
    Headache as a symptom of primary sleep disorders 273
    Sleep disturbance as a trigger in headache and migraine 273
    Headache as a provoking factor for poor sleep 274
    Physiology and mechanism of relationship between
        sleep and headache 274
References 275

CHAPTER 22 Meals/food/diet/caffeine/hydration 279
Jennifer Bickel, MD and Trevor Gerson, MD

Meals 279
Food/diet 280
    Obesity 281
    Specific diets 281
Hydration 282
Caffeine 282
Conclusion 284
References 285

CHAPTER 23 Activity/exercise including yoga 287
Samantha Lee Irwin, MB BCh, MS

Exercise and headache 287
Yoga and headache 291
References 292

CHAPTER 24 Managing migraine at school 297
Elizabeth K. Rende, DNP, FAANP and
Scott B. Turner, DNP, FNP-C

Myth busters 297
After the school bell rings… 298
Empowering your child 298
The perfect scenario… 299
A word about homebound, home-schooled, and online
    education 299
School health plans and 504 accommodations 300
Pace yourself 301
A message to kids about returning to school… 302
Summary 302
For primary care and specialty providers 302
Appendix: Supplementary material 303
References 304

CHAPTER 25 Advocacy for children with migraine 305
William Young, MD and Shirley Kessel, BS

Headache expert perspective 305
Family perspective 307
Advocacy plan of action 308
Advocacy organizations 309
    Alliance for headaches advocacy 309
    American migraine foundation 309
    Association of migraines 310

CHAMP (coalition for headache and migraine patients) 310
Chronic migraine awareness 310
Global healthy living foundation 310
Headache relief guide 311
Migraine research foundation... 311
Miles for migraine 311
The migraine world summit 311
National headache foundation 312
US pain foundation 312
References... 312

CHAPTER 26 Growing up: Transitioning to adult care 315
Maggie Waung, MD, PhD, Ana Marissa Lagman-Bartolome,
MD, Jennifer Hranilovich, MD, and Hope O'Brien, MD

Headache specialist.. 315
Six T's of transitioning health care of headache patients 316
Primary care providers 320
    Pediatrician 320
    Adult care provider.. 320
Patient and families 321
References... 323

PART VI Next steps

CHAPTER 27 How to set up a headache clinic 327
Serena L. Orr, MD, MSc and Marcy Yonker, MD

Introduction... 327
The societal impact of pediatric headache............................. 327
The importance of evidence-based pediatric
    headache care... 328
The structure of multidisciplinary headache care in the
    clinic setting.. 329
The structure of headache care in the acute setting 332
Chronic headache care... 333
    Biofeedback/CBT 334
    Chemodenervation for chronic migraine 334
The evidence for multidisciplinary headache care 335
How to advocate for resources in a multidisciplinary
    headache clinic... 335
Summary and recommendations 336
References... 337

CHAPTER 28 Where can I learn more? A listing of resources **341**
Meghan S. Candee, MD Jessica R. Gautreaux, MD, and
Carrie O. Dougherty, MD

Websites 341
Seminal articles 342
AAN/AHS pediatric migraine treatment guidelines 343

Index 345

List of contributors

Shannon Babineau, MD
Goryeb Children's Hospital, Morristown, NJ; Sidney Kimmel Medical College, Thomas Jefferson University, Philadelphia, PA, United States

Rebecca Barmherzig, MD
Division of Neurology, Children's Hospital of Philadelphia, Philadelphia, PA, United States

Frank R. Berenson, MD
Atlanta Headache Specialists, Atlanta, GA, United States

Jennifer Bickel, MD
Children's Mercy Kansas City and University of Missouri-Kansas City, Kansas City, MO, United States

Heidi K. Blume, MD
Seattle Children's Hospital, Seattle, WA; Division of Pediatric Neurology, University of Washington, Washington, DC, United States

Andrea Brand, MAc LAc
A.Brand of Acupuncture, Hearts Gate Wellness, Towson, MD, United States

Dawn C. Buse, PhD
Department of Neurology, Albert Einstein College of Medicine, Bronx, NY, United States

Meghan S. Candee, MD
University of Utah/Primary Children's Hospital, Salt Lake City, UT, United States

Madeline Chadehumbe, MD
University of Pennsylvania Perelman School of Medicine, Children's Hospital of Philadelphia, Philadelphia, PA, United States

Carrie O. Dougherty, MD
University of Utah/Primary Children's Hospital, Salt Lake City, UT, United States

Jessica R. Gautreaux, MD
University of Utah/Primary Children's Hospital, Salt Lake City, UT, United States

Amy A. Gelfand, MD
Child & Adolescent Headache Program, Department of Neurology, UCSF, San Francisco, CA, United States

Trevor Gerson, MD
Children's Mercy Kansas City and University of Missouri-Kansas City, Kansas City, MO, United States

Jack Gladstein, MD
Professor of Pediatrics and Neurology, University of Maryland School of Medicine, Baltimore, MD, United States

Kaitlin Greene, MD
Child and Adolescent Headache Program, Division of Pediatric Neurology, Department of Pediatrics, Oregon Health and Sciences University, Portland, OR, United States

Amanda Hall, MSN, FNP-C
Yale University, Yale Health, New Haven, CT, United States

Andrew D. Hershey, MD, PhD
Departments of Neurology and Pediatrics, Cincinnati Children's Hospital Medical Center, University of Cincinnati College of Medicine, Cincinnati, OH, United States

Jennifer Hranilovich, MD
Assistant Professor, Division of Pediatric Neurology, Headache Program, University of Colorado, Denver; Children's Hospital Colorado, Aurora, CO, United States

Samantha Lee Irwin, MB BCh, MS
Child and Adolescent Headache Program, Department of Neurology, UCSF Weill Institute for Neurosciences, University of California, San Francisco (UCSF), UCSF Benioff Children's Hospitals, San Francisco, CA, United States

Marielle Kabbouche, MD
Neurology Department, Cincinnati Children's Hospital Medical Center and University of Cincinnati; University of Cincinnati of Cincinnati College of Medicine, Cincinnati, OH, United States

Dina Karvounides, PsyD
Children's Hospital of Philadelphia, Philadelphia, PA, United States

Sita Kedia, MD, MPH
PALM Health, Ladue, MO, United States

Shirley Kessel, BS
Executive Director, Miles for Migraine

Ana Marissa Lagman-Bartolome, MD
Pediatric and Adolescent Headache Program, Division of Neurology, Hospital for Sick Children and Women's College Hospital, University of Toronto, Toronto, ON, Canada

Maya Marzouk, MA
Ferkauf Graduate School of Psychology, Yeshiva University, New York City, NY, United States

Rachel Neely, MSHS, PA-C
Atlanta Headache Specialists, Atlanta, GA, United States

Hope O'Brien, MD
Associate Professor of Neurology, Co-Director, Young Adult Headache Clinic, Cincinnati Children's Hospital, Cincinnati, OH, United States

Serena L. Orr, MD, MSc
Department of Pediatrics, Community Health Sciences and Clinical
Neurosciences, University of Calgary, Calgary, AB, Canada

Ann Pakalnis, MD
Section of Pediatric Neurology, Nationwide Childrens Hospital, Columbus, OH,
United States

Irene Patniyot, MD
Texas Children's Hospital Pediatric Headache Clinic, Section of Neurology and
Developmental Neuroscience, Department of Pediatrics, Baylor College of
Medicine, Houston, TX, United States

Carlyn Patterson Gentile, MD, PhD
Children's Hospital of Philadelphia; University of Pennsylvania, Philadelphia, PA,
United States

Nicholas Pietris, MD
Children's Heart Program, Department of Pediatrics, University of Maryland
School of Medicine, Baltimore, MD, United States

Scott Powers, PhD
Division of Behavioral Medicine and Clinical Psychology, Cincinnati Children's
Hospital Medical Center, Cinncinati; Cincinnati Children's Hospital, University of
Cincinnati College of Medicine, Cincinnati, OH, United States

Sharoon Qaiser, MD
Neurology Department, Cincinnati Children's Hospital Medical Center and
University of Cincinnati; University of Cincinnati of Cincinnati College of Medicine,
Cincinnati, OH, United States

William Qubty, MD
Pediatric Headache Program, Minneapolis Clinic of Neurology, Minneapolis, MN,
United States

Reena Rastogi, MD
Department of Neurology, Barrow Neurological Institute at Phoenix Children's
Hospital, Phoenix, AZ, United States

Ana Recober, MD
Main Line Health, Wynnewood, PA, United States

Elizabeth K. Rende, DNP, FAANP
CentraCare Neurosciences Headache Center, St. Cloud, MN, United States

Alexandra C. Ross, PhD
UCSF Benioff Children's Hospital Child & Adolescent Headache Clinic, University
of California San Francisco, San Francisco, CA, United States

Elizabeth Seng, PhD
Ferkauf Graduate School of Psychology, Yeshiva University; Department of
Neurology, Albert Einstein College of Medicine, New York City, NY, United States

Christina L. Szperka, MD, MSCE
Division of Neurology, Children's Hospital of Philadelphia, Philadelphia, PA, United States

Scott B. Turner, DNP, FNP-C
Department of Pediatrics, Section of Neurology, University of Alabama at Birmingham, Birmingham, AL, United States

Juliana VanderPluym, MD
Mayo Clinic, Scottsdale, AZ, United States

M. Cristina Victorio, MD
NeuroDevelopmental Science Center, Akron Children's Hospital, Akron, OH, United States

Maggie Waung, MD, PhD
Assistant Professor of Neurology, Director, Young Adult Headache Transitions Clinic, University of California, San Francisco, CA, United States

Kevin Weber, MD
Department of Neurology, Ohio State University Wexner Medical Center, Columbus, OH, United States

Marcy Yonker, MD
Department of Pediatrics, Division of Child Neurology, Children's Hospital Colorado, University of Colorado, Aurora, CO, United States

William Young, MD
Professor of Neurology, Thomas Jefferson University, Philadelphia, PA, United States

Jason L. Ziplow, MD
Department of Neurology, Children's Hospital of Philadelphia, Philadelphia, PA, United States

Preface

We were asked to put together the next iteration of a textbook on pediatric headache. There has not been an updated version since the excellent works by Hershey and Powers in 2009 and, before that, by Winner and Rothner in 2001. Since then, some things have stayed the same, but some things have changed. Kids are kids, families are families, and health care is health care, but life has gotten more complex on many levels. Social media and technology have affected the way we relate to each other, view the world, and share information. New advances in medical treatment are now available. Youngsters and their families have access to good and not so good information that can both positively and negatively affect a visit for headache management. The current COVID epidemic, economic crisis, and enhanced sensitivity to racial inequities have forced us all to examine our vulnerability and learn more about ourselves and our families, and challenged us to all be better health care providers and people.

In this book, we take an approach that reflects our new reality. We have asked our contributors to address issues in pediatric headache from the perspectives of families, primary care providers, and specialists. We have asked that special materials, websites, and patient handouts be available through the book's website. This will be a valuable supplement to the text. There will be practical examples of documents that can help families get help for school accommodations, summer camps, IEP meetings, and college dorms. Samples of headache action plans can help the primary care physician explain "what if" scenarios that will prevent needless emergency department visits.

Part I of the book begins with a chapter titled "My headache story," where we cover the basics of what needs to be addressed in the primary care office and in the specialist suite. We hope that families and children will be best prepared for such a visit if they know what to expect. We acknowledge the time constraints of a busy primary care environment and offer suggestions of how to make a quick diagnosis, a reasonable plan of action, and when to refer. For the specialist, we tackle more weighty issues such as measuring disability and addressing comorbidities. Decisions about work up and imaging are addressed as well.

Part II, titled "Why does my head hurt," explores the literature of epidemiology, classification, pathophysiology, and genetics. The chapters in this part include some visual aids to help both the primary care provider and specialist explain physiology in terms that families and teens can grasp and repeat. The hope from these chapters is to avoid the stigma that youngsters with migraine carry. Knowing that there is science related to their condition may help alleviate that feeling.

All involved in headache care wonder how did someone's headache progress. In Part III, titled "How did it get so bad," we address migraine variants, the effects of hormones, chronic daily headache comorbidities, new daily persistent headache, posttraumatic headache, and dysautonomia. We hope to dispel myths, offer practical tips for clinicians, and give families reasonable expectations for disease progression. We explore what can be done in an inpatient headache unit when all else fails.

At this point, we move the focus to recovery. Part IV is titled "Ways other people can help me get better." We first move into acute treatments with medicines, devices, behavioral interventions, and acupuncture. We then delve into treatments to try to settle down frequency. These include preventive medicines, neuromodulatory techniques and devices, behavioral training, and nonmedicinal approaches. Part V describes "Things I can do for myself/my child," including sleep, diet, and exercise. These are crucial self-efficacy tools that must be applied as part of any comprehensive plan to get better. We then think beyond the health care visit. As part of getting better, families need to know how to set up a good working relationship with school. Families and teens need to become advocates. So do health professionals. We offer some suggestions about how to get involved.

Finally, we talk about transition of care to the adult world. Some of us keep our patients through college and some don't. Adolescent medicine physicians write about starting transition discussions at age 12 to start empowering youngsters to gradually assume more responsibility as they get older. Newest medications and treatments get approved in adults and eventually get studied in teens, then children. Practitioners in the adult world will welcome youngsters more freely if the youngsters and their families have successfully transitioned responsibility to their emerging adults and not allowed their families to take over.

We end the book with a resource guide. Some may skip there first, but we don't encourage it. Enjoy the wisdom of our contributors and try to see things from other perspectives. If you are a primary care provider, take a peek at what the specialists are doing and vice versa. Use the handouts and preprinted letters to make your visits more efficient and productive. Most of all, take pride in caring for children and adolescents with headache. It is a field of promise and hope.

Christina L. Szperka
Amy A. Gelfand
Jack Gladstein

References

1. Winner P, Rothner AD. Headache in Children and Adolescents. BC Decker, Hamilton, Ontario, 2001.
2. Hershey AD, Powers SW, et al. Pediatric Headache in Clinical Practice. Wiley-Blackwell, Chichester, UK, 2009.

About the editors

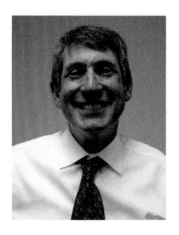

Jack Gladstein, MD is Professor of pediatrics and neurology at the University of Maryland School of Medicine. Jack graduated from the Albert Einstein College of Medicine in 1983. He completed his pediatrics residency and chief residency at Einstein in 1987. He then went on to complete a fellowship in adolescent medicine at the University of Maryland Hospital in 1989. He has remained as faculty at the university ever since. He established the Pediatric Headache Clinic in 1989, which at that time was the second pediatric headache clinic in the United States. Along with his busy pediatric headache practice, he is Director of inpatient pediatrics at Maryland and has served as Associate Dean for student affairs for many years. He was recently appointed as Vice Chair for faculty affairs. He is a proud son, husband, father, and grandfather.

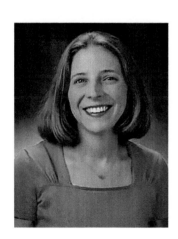

Christina L. Szperka, MD, MSCE has been interested in the treatment of chronic pain since she was an undergraduate at Amherst College, Amherst, MA, and focused on pediatric pain while pursuing her medical degree at Yale University School of Medicine, New Haven, CT. Dr. Szperka completed residencies in pediatrics and child neurology at The Children's Hospital of Philadelphia, Philadelphia, PA, and a fellowship in headache medicine at The Jefferson Headache Center at Thomas Jefferson University Hospital. She is board certified in headache medicine. She divides her time between patient care and projects aimed at improving the treatment of children with headaches. In 2013, she was named Director of the newly formed Pediatric Headache Program. She has received grants to improve clinical care of and treatment options for headache.

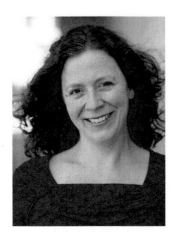

Amy A. Gelfand, MD is an associate professor of neurology and pediatrics at the University of California, San Francisco. She directs the Child & Adolescent Headache Program at the UCSF Benioff Children's Hospitals. Her research interests include examining the role of melatonin in the treatment of pediatric migraine and the relationship between childhood periodic syndromes (such as infant colic, cyclic vomiting syndrome, benign paroxysmal torti-collis) and migraine in children and adolescents.

Acknowledgments

There are many people who believed in me and allowed me to pursue *Pediatric Headache*, a field that was barely born when I opened the clinic in 1989. I want to thank Dr. Bob Woody who invited me to start the clinic with him. He recognized that someone with adolescent medicine training could help with the psychosocial and physiologic challenges of a teen with headache. Paul Winner and I had coffee at the AHS meeting a while back and we launched the AHS pediatric headache interest group which has helped many aspiring headache doctors with research and networking. Dr. Seymour Diamond always believed that pediatrics has a seat at the table and gave me the opportunity to speak about pediatric headache at Diamond Headache courses. Dr. Mike Berman and Steve Czinn have been supportive Chairs of Pediatrics who have allowed the program to grow and have trusted me to provide care to youngsters with headache. Finally, my family has always given me courage to reach and grow and pursue my dreams while being supportive in the background. My wife Bette, and our three children Aeli, Ari, and Penina and two daughters in law, Sonia and Rachel have been wonderful and a reason to come home as early as I can. I want to echo Christina and Amy in thanking all the contributors for their hard work in meeting deadlines and presenting excellent chapters that will help all of us take care of children in our care.

Jack Gladstein

I thank the authors and coeditors who took the time to research and write these chapters. I am grateful to be your colleague. I also thank my parents, mentors, colleagues, and patients who have taught me to be a doctor. From you, I learned to look beyond illness to see each person. I thank my husband and children who have taught me to be a parent of children with chronic illness. From you, I have learned humility and patience and have also drawn strength. Thank you for your understanding and support.

Christina L. Szperka

I thank my husband, Jeff, and our three children—Adam, Ethan, and Abby—for their patience and understanding while I was editing this book. Their kindness and support allowed this book to become a reality.

Amy A. Gelfand

Special thanks

Ms. Alicia Perry has been instrumental in getting this project accomplished. She hounded the authors and editors, kept all the correspondence in order, and made sure that the newest edits were always included in the updates. Without her, the book would not be as organized and cohesive.

Dedication

We dedicate this volume to three outstanding pediatric headache physicians who are no longer with us.

Steven Linder practiced in Dallas. He was an expert in the vagaries of the physical examination and taught us at regional and national meetings how to examine youngsters properly.

Don Lewis practiced in Norfolk. He combined research and practice and led by example. He was the lead author in topiramate trials and always insisted on scientific rigor. He rose to be chair of pediatrics at Norfolk and started every working day with a headache visit.

Howard Jacobs was a practicing pediatrician who took up headache medicine toward the end of his career in Columbus. He brought his general skills and applied them to headache practice in a way that looked at the whole youngster. He was great at alleviating parents' concerns while acknowledging the needs of teenagers.

My headache story

My headache story: A guide for families, primary care, and specialists ☆

Jack Gladstein, MD

For families

Having a visit with your child with headaches can be daunting. On the one hand, you see your child suffering with pain. Will the provider listen? Will she make the right diagnosis? Will she offer help that is concordant with your views?

Most probably you will start out with your primary care provider. Hopefully, she will have gotten to know both you and your youngster. Introductions may not be necessary. The purpose of this visit is to arrive at the right diagnosis, come up with a doable plan and figure out if more work up or the expertise of a specialist is necessary.

She will start out with simple questions to determine pattern, severity, family history, and impact on your child's life. She may interview your child alone, if time permits.

The hidden agendas must be addressed. You probably know of a family member or friend who had a brain tumor. If the story and exam are reassuring, you want confident reassurance that migraine or tension headache is the issue, and not brain tumor.

After careful assessment, the primary care practitioner should give you an action plan including rescue medicine and nonmedication treatments, and instructions about when to get in contact. If the problem is beyond the practice's ability, referral to a specialist should be expected. Some primary care doctors are better at headache than others, and some have good community resources while others are more on their own.

If one sees the specialist, there are some subtle differences. Of course, this person does not know you or your family. She must gather information from the start including getting an idea about coping skills and your preferences. Similar to the primary care doctor, she must get a careful history, dig deep into what has been tried and come

---

☆ Editor's note: The key to headache diagnosis is history taking. Here practitioners' styles may differ—with some preferring to use open-ended questions while others utilize a structured interview. At the end, the process was successful if two things were accomplished—a specific diagnosis was reached, and the patient and family's trust was earned.

Pediatric Headache. https://doi.org/10.1016/B978-0-323-83005-8.00027-6

to a diagnosis and a treatment plan. She is a headache expert with knowledge of the latest advances in headache treatment. She may have handouts or websites to enhance education. She has experience with addressing school issues and accommodations. You should leave the office with a lot of information, various plans for rescue, and an approach that includes the school and the family as well as addressing the youngsters' needs.

In summary, one should expect similar but different outcomes from your primary care and specialist. For both you should expect good listening skills, and a plan that includes your child's and your family needs and wishes. You will know by the end of the session whether those needs were met. The primary care doctor can often be the last stop if the problem is simple or the practitioner knows headache well. If referral is needed, it may take longer to establish trust, but the expertise acquired should help you get your child what she needs.

For primary care clinicians

In a busy office setting the most common feeling for a primary care provider who sees a patient with a chief complaint of headache is helplessness. How can I gather the information needed to help this family in such a short time? Will I overlook the patient with brain tumor? How can I find out what is wrong, assess disability, and reassure this family in a 15 or 30 minute's visit?

We feel that this all can be done with alacrity and skill. To make the diagnosis focus on pattern. Is the headache continuous or intermittent? If intermittent, are there autonomic symptoms? Most patients will fit into this pattern. If there are autonomic symptoms like nausea, vomiting, light or sound sensitivity, and there are days of normal function in between headache days, rest assured that the diagnosis is most likely migraine. To cement the diagnosis, a family history of headache with need to rest, will be helpful. Often these youngsters have car sickness. Please remember that the younger the child at initial presentation, the less likely she will have a classic presentation. In the little ones, it is ok to ask them to draw a picture of what they feel like when having a headache. Also, ask the parent it they can tell just by looking that the child has a headache. A migraine is a bad headache, where it is hard to exercise or read. On the other hand, further work up may be indicated if the child reports other systematic symptoms that point to a serious infection or inflammatory condition, sudden onset of the headache like a thunderclap, neurologic signs/ symptoms like seizure, daily or continuous headache, headache waking the child from sleep or occurring first thing in the morning, headache frequency or severity becoming progressively worse over time, positional headache, headache triggered by valsalva, a lack of family history of headache, or very young age, That workup could include labs, imaging (usually MRI), referral, or other tests depending on the circumstances.

Once a diagnosis of migraine is established by pattern and autonomic symptoms in just a few short moments, next we assess disability as measured in days of school and work missed. For those parents who must send even sick children to school, we can ask about disability as measured by number of days when their child goes to school but keeps her head on the desk and can't learn. The more the disability, the more intense the intervention.

Physical examination and neurologic examination in the primary care office tends to be perfunctory, but should be attempted to reassure parents who are worried about brain tumor. The presence of new abnormalities on exam or papilledema should prompt imaging. One approach is to pause after the history and reassure if the pattern and symptoms are consistent with migraine. Then reassure again after your physical exam, then reassure during the wrap up portion.

For youngsters with migraine, the primary care practitioner can suggest healthy habits, early intervention, and involvement of school staff and initiation of prevention medication (if comfortable). Healthy habits include regular sleep, exercise, meals, and water. Early intervention with acute medications (as covered later) will need the youngster to recognize early warning signs and first twinges. She will also need the help of the teacher and school nurse in getting medicine immediately. Some physicians will initiate a prevention medication but will have to get into comorbidities to pick the right one. Many will refer if disability causes significant school absence or drop in school performance.

Parents will consider their visit to the primary care doctor to be a good one if they were listened to, reassured, and offered a starting plan with good follow up. Referral to a specialist should be considered if diagnosis is not clear and there is concern for tumor, disability is significant, or the patient is refractory to your interventions.

For specialists

Parents and youngsters expect more from the specialist. Time for a new visit is not infinite, and there is no previous history with the family. Their level of worry, social issues, and ways of dealing with pain need to be assessed quickly and thoughtfully. Diagnoses may be rare or complicated with other concomitant illnesses. Comorbid conditions may crop up and make treatment options more complicated. Other attempts at treatment by competent professionals may not have worked optimally.

The specialist visit starts with a recap of records sent to make sure that there are no other outstanding documents. It should quickly move to making sure that the right diagnosis has been established. Often, that means asking the family to start from the beginning in their own words. Even if the specialist has pored over previous documents, this gives the parents and the youngster the feeling that they will be heard. It gives the specialist a chance to see how the parent and youngster interact, affording valuable information about their level of understanding and family dynamics. If the patient is a teenager, letting him/her take the reins here is crucial. Disability assessment and coping skills along with comorbidities must be addressed and confirmed.

If migraine is the diagnosis but treatment needs to be tweaked, the headache specialist is uniquely equipped to optimize old remedies and teach about exciting new therapies. The backbone still lies with reinforcing healthy habits, treating migraines at first twinge and offering prevention strategies based upon coping skills and disability. Proper use of medications need to be stressed and employment of prevention medications may be prescribed. Thorough knowledge of community resources for complementary medicine is a must. Developing an action plan together with the family that incorporates baseline activities (green zone), initial treatment (yellow zone) and rescue treatment (red zone) should be accomplished towards the end of the visit. Websites and additional reading material can be presented as a take home assignment.

If the diagnosis is chronic daily headache, more focus needs to be spent on the psychosocial aspects of the visits. Questions like "Who lives at home, how does everyone get along, how do you cope, are you being bullied, do you have trouble learning, Is anyone making you uncomfortable" need to be asked along with all the myriad of other questions. Co-morbidities that need inquiry include insomnia, depressed mood, anxiety, dizziness, freezing cold extremities. Again, involvement of community colleagues may be helpful in building a toolbox that may include counseling, yoga, CBT, acupuncture, and massage. Psychiatry, Cardiology, and Gastroenterology colleagues may need to help build a plan to address the comorbidities. If there are migraine spikes along with the Chronic Headache, a migraine action plan will need to be incorporated into the plan.

For rare diagnoses the headache specialist may alleviate suffering by coming up with a proper diagnosis and treatment plan. The Trigeminal Autonomic Cephalgias come to mind where introduction of Indomethacin may take the pain away that may have been present for years.

For the specialist, follow up with the youngster and family is crucial. The first visit is an initial attempt to diagnose, assess, and make a plan. It is during subsequent interactions that the plan is incrementally changed to accommodate side effects, work on adherence, and make sure that all members of the team have been informed and have had a chance to contribute to the plan. Build your after visit summary together, to make sure everyone understood.

Barriers to effective headache visits

Since the initial draft of this chapter, the world has been turned upside down by three interrelated societal issues. Covid-19, unemployment, and a heightened focus on racial inequality have brought new layers of complexity to all our interactions whether they be in the clinic or in our delay dealings with one another. Our new viral menace has made it difficult to have reasonable patient visits, while we have all learned to use telemedicine as a second best option. On the other hand, telemedicine has offered accessibility and the opportunity to see patients more often and at off-hours. In our experience, first visits are better done in person, so a full physical examination can include a look at the optic discs. For follow up visits, however, incremental changes don't always require an ophthalmoscope.

Unemployment is at a 100 year high in the US. Many of our patients have lost health insurance when their parent has lost a job. Aside from the sudden inability to afford visits or medication, sudden joblessness may lead to depression, anxiety, and food insecurity.

Finally, a focus on race inequality may highlight barriers that were not discussed previously. Health care providers, like all others, must come to grip with their own biases and consider whether their unconscious attitudes may intrude into patient care. Since this is a subject which is no longer a taboo for discussion, we must figure out how to bring this subject into our conversations at the bedside and in clinic.

Further readings

Kelly M, Strelzik J, Langdon R, DiSabella M. Pediatric headache: an overview. *Curr Opin Pediatr.* 2018;30(6):748–754.

Qutby W, Patniyot I, Gelfand A. Telemedicine in pediatric headache: a prospective study. *Neurology.* 2018;90:e1702–e1705.

O'Brien HL, Sk S. Comorbid psychologic conditions in pediatrics headache. *Semin Pediatr Neurol.* 2016;23(1):68–70.

Why does my head hurt?

II

Why does my head hurt? You're not the only one: Epidemiology ☆

2

Rebecca Barmherzig, MD

Epidemiology: For families

So, you have a headache.

The bad news is: *you have a headache.*

The good news is: you are not alone, and there are many things that can be done to help.

Headaches are very common, and affect children and teenagers of all ages, from across the world. Approximately half of school-aged children and 8 out of 10 teenagers have reported a bad headache at some point in their life.[1, 2] In the United States, about 1 out of 6 children report severe or frequent headaches within the past year.[3] Parents often seek medical care to find out the cause of the headaches, or because headaches are affecting their child's life.

Headache history is a key part to helping your clinician make a diagnosis. Your clinician will try to understand all the details of the headache problem, and how it affects your life. We classify headaches based on their characteristics into two general categories, secondary headaches and primary headaches. In secondary headache disorders, the headache can be thought of as a clue to the underlying problem. In primary headache, the headache *is* the underlying problem.

Secondary headaches are caused by another underlying problem, such as a head injury or a viral infection. After asking questions and examining you, your clinician will determine whether there are any "red flags" for a serious condition. It is very rare for a serious condition, like a brain tumor, to present with only headache. This occurs in less than 1% of children. Usually there are other symptoms or exam abnormalities.[4]

Primary headaches are the most common category of headache in children and teens. Primary headaches are not due to another underlying medical problem. Up to three-quarters of children and teens with primary headaches will have a family

---

☆Editor's note: There is much that we know and much that we don't know about how headaches affect children and adolescents. Even if you think you don't know anyone else with bad headaches, you probably do. Migraine is common and disabling, yet patients often cope silently, with invisible pain. Hopefully knowing this will enable you to speak up for yourself, and in turn break down the stigma associated with headache diseases.

Pediatric Headache. https://doi.org/10.1016/B978-0-323-83005-8.00020-3

history of headache. In other words, there is a genetic link to headaches. Whether a headache problem occurs, and how severe it is, can also be influenced by things in the child's environment.[5–7]

The most common primary headache disorder in children and teens is *tension-type headache*. This affects at least 1 in 4 children in their lifetime. Tension-type headaches are often felt all over the head, and are mild to moderate in severity. The headache pain is usually the only symptom, without problems like nausea.

The most common primary headache disorder in children and teens seeking medical attention is *migraine*.[7–9] Migraine is more than "just a headache". The 2017 Global Burden of Diseases Study ranked migraine as the second leading cause of disability worldwide.[10] Studies in children and teens have found that migraine affects children's quality of life as much as diabetes, arthritis, and cancer.[11] Migraine has been described as an invisible illness. Children and teens experiencing a migraine may appear otherwise normal to family, friends, and teachers. Although a migraine might seem invisible, behind the scenes there are important changes happening within the brain. You will read more about this in the chapter on Pathophysiology.

Migraine affects up to 5% of children and approximately 10% of teenagers.[12] Before puberty, it is equally common in boys and girls. After puberty, more girls are affected.[6, 12] Less than a third of children and teens will experience aura symptoms, which are additional neurological symptoms. Most commonly, these are visual symptoms or sensory symptoms affecting one side of the face or body. These symptoms typically evolve over a few minutes, and then resolve completely. They may come before or during the pain of the migraine. Rarely, aura can involve motor weakness.[13–16] This condition, called hemiplegic migraine, can run in families and accounts for only 0.01% of migraine cases in children and adolescents.[17] Chronic migraine, where headache occurs more than half the days in a month, affects between 0.8% and 1.8% of children and adolescents.[18] It is more common in girls and in the later teenage years. Teens with chronic migraine are more likely to report severe headache-related disability and impact on quality of life.[19–22]

In summary, headaches are very common. More children will experience a headache in their lifetime than not. However, all headaches are different, and certainly not all headaches are created equal. Severe or frequent attacks can have a significant impact on day-to-day functioning, school, activities, and mood. *Just because you can't see it, doesn't mean that it is not there.* Molecular studies and functional brain imaging studies have proven that there are many complex changes happening in the brain during a migraine—stay tuned.

Epidemiology: For primary care and specialists

Headache is one of the most common conditions evaluated by healthcare providers. It is prevalent, disabling, underdiagnosed, and undertreated. The estimated mean prevalence of headache in children and adolescents varies between studies and is estimated to be up to 58.4%. Headache is more common in girls than boys, and the prevalence of headache increases from preschool age to adolescence.[6]

Headaches are associated with substantial direct healthcare costs and resource utilization, as well as indirect costs from reduced educational and occupational productivity and quality of life. Migraine alone has an enormous impact on global economics; in 2003 migraine cost the United States $19.6 billion annually and the European Union €27 billion annually.[23, 24] The impact of pediatric headache is especially important to consider during the formative years of childhood and adolescence, where headaches can lead to absence from school, decreased performance, and missed extracurricular activities.[22, 25] The psychosocial and economic burden of headache lends urgency towards better understanding, accurately identifying, and promptly and effectively treating these disorders.

Epidemiological studies are central to understanding the burden, scope, and distribution of headache disorders in children. The lack of standardized case definitions and the heterogeneity in study methodology are among the challenges which contribute to the variability in estimates of prevalence and incidence in the literature.

As noted earlier, headache disorders are classified as primary or secondary. An additional challenge in categorizing pediatric headache using the *International Classification of Headache Disorders, 3rd Edition (ICHD-3)* is that headache disorders in childhood differ from their adult manifestations. Furthermore, the character of pediatric headache disorders can change over time. This may relate to developmental and maturational changes in the brain, such as myelination and synaptic development and reorganization. The two most common primary headache disorders in children are *tension-type headache* and *migraine*, and the distinction clinically between these disorders is far less clear in children than in adults.[26, 27]

Migraine

The literature on pediatric migraine is the most robust among the primary headache disorders in children and adolescents. In girls, the incidence of migraine with aura peaks between 12 and 13 years of age, and the incidence of migraine without aura peaks between 14 and 17 years of age. In boys, the incidence of migraine with aura peaks around 5 years of age, and for migraine without aura between 10 and 11 years of age.[14]

Migraine affects both girls and boys equally at a young age, but more girls than boys in adolescents and young adults. The prevalence of migraine increases with age, from about 7.0% in girls and 4.7% of boys by age 15, up to 9.7% of girls and 6.0% of boys by age 20.[6] The burden of migraine lays not only in the number of children and adolescents it affects, but also in the extent to which they are affected. During a migraine, 60.8% of adolescents report experiencing severe impairment. Evaluating severity and disability surveys, 16.8% of adolescents with migraine report scores in the range of moderate-to-severe disability.

Chronic primary headaches in children and adolescents are particularly challenging to study from an epidemiological perspective, as they can be difficult to diagnostically categorize. There are no criteria specified for children and adolescents for chronic migraine. Since symptoms in children and adolescents can be different than adults, children with chronic headache may not meet the ICHD-3 criteria for a specific headache subtype. The prevalence of chronic migraine in adolescents (ages 12–17) is between 0.8% and 1.8%, with a female preponderance and a peak in the later teenage years. The majority of adolescents surveyed with chronic migraine indicated severe headache-related disability and impact on quality of life. Notwithstanding the degree of impairment, more than half of chronic migraine patients reported they had not seen a healthcare professional for their headaches in the past year.[18, 22]

Migraine is a complex genetic disorder, influenced by both environmental and genetic factors. Most familial migraine results from polygenic changes. Research in genome-wide association studies have revealed many different variants involving genes with roles in both neuronal and vascular pathways. More work is needed to evaluate gene expression and epigenetic factors to better understand how the genetic architecture relates to migraine pathophysiology.[28–30]

A positive family history of migraine is the most impactful risk factor for migraine, conferring a two-fold to three-fold increased risk of developing migraine as compared to people without a family history of migraine. The actual risk may be even higher, as studies have shown that migraine assessed by family member report largely underestimates migraine in relatives. Children and adolescents with a family history of migraine tend to have an earlier onset of headache symptoms and a greater severity than those without a family history.[31–33]

Twin studies and population studies have estimated that half of the variance in migraine prevalence may be attributed to genetic factors. This suggests that environmental risk factors still play an important role.[5, 33–35] In an adult population, migraine has a higher prevalence in the lower income and educational strata.[36] Two hypotheses for this association have been considered. Firstly, in the social causation hypothesis, it is thought that factors relating to lower income such as poor diet, stress, and barriers to accessing healthcare may increase disease prevalence. Conversely, in the social selection hypothesis, those with migraine may be more likely to have a lower income status due to disease-related dysfunction and the downstream effect this has on educational and occupational performance and outcomes.[37, 38]

In adolescents, the same observation holds true only when there is not a parental diagnosis of migraine. With a parental diagnosis of migraine, household income does not have a significant effect on migraine prevalence. This is a curious observation and may suggest that in those with a family history of migraine the biologic predisposition predominates and income strata does not have as strong of a modifying effect.[22]

Several studies have shown a correlation between adverse childhood experiences (ACEs) and headaches. This has been established as a risk factor for early onset and chronicity of headaches in adolescents, and this relationship is independent of a diagnosis of an anxiety disorder or depression.[39–42]

In terms of healthcare utilization in children and adolescent headache, there is often a delay to seeking medical care, and an even greater delay to seeking specialist headache care. A recent study showed that less than 5% of children with migraine who qualified for the use of a preventive medication were started on one while awaiting a neurology referral, and none had been started on a triptan by their primary care physician.[43] Further study evaluating prescribed medications in children with migraine in the United States suggested that more than half were under the care of pediatricians; and less than a quarter were being treated by a neurologist.[44] These findings further emphasize the need for ongoing education among patients, families, and healthcare providers, as inadequate treatment of pediatric migraine is associated with disease progression and chronification.

Tension-type headache

Tension-type headache is the most common primary headache disorder in children and adolescents. There is a wide range in the reported prevalence, from 5% to 25%.[8, 9, 45] The mean age of onset is 7 years old and attack duration is variable, with an average duration of 2 h. Headaches often begin in the afternoon at school. In children, tension-type headache has been postulated to be related to many different risk factors, including psychosocial stressors, musculoskeletal pathology, oro-mandibular dysfunction, or anxiety or depression.[27]

Trigeminal autonomic cephalalgias

Trigeminal autonomic cephalalgias (TACs) are subdivided into: paroxysmal hemicrania, cluster headache; short-lasting unilateral neuralgiform headache attacks with conjunctival injection and tearing (SUNCT); short-lasting unilateral neuralgiform headache attacks with cranial autonomic symptoms (SUNA); and hemicrania continua. These syndromes rarely begin in childhood, and if present, would warrant further workup to exclude for secondary causes. Cluster headache begins in adolescents in a minority of patients (0.03%–0.1%) and has a male predominance of 2.5:1.[46]

Other primary headache disorders

Primary stabbing headache has a prevalence of 3%–5% in children and is associated with a higher incidence of co-morbid migraine or tension-type headache.[47] Other primary headache disorders—such as primary cough headache, primary exercise headache, primary headache associated with sexual activity, and primary thunderclap headache—should be diagnosed in children and adolescents only after appropriate exclusion of a secondary etiology.[27]

New daily persistent headache

New daily persistent headache (NDPH) has a prevalence in the general population of 0.03%–0.1% and is higher in children and adolescents.[48] Among children and adolescents with chronic daily headache, the prevalence of NDPH is 21%–28%.[19, 49] Most children will report a precipitating event such as a febrile illness or minor head injury.

Secondary headache

Secondary headaches in children include headaches attributed to: injury to the head and neck; cranial or cervical vascular disorders; non-vascular intracranial disorders; substance use or withdrawal; infection; disorders of homeostasis; disorders of the head and neck; and psychiatric disorders. The most common cause of secondary headache in children is viral illness. Less than 2.5% of children who undergo neuroimaging to exclude a secondary intracranial cause for headache, are found to have any actionable abnormalities.[50–52] As per the Childhood Brain Tumor Consortium, less than 1% of children with brain tumors present with headache alone, in the absence of other symptoms or signs.[4]

Understanding the classification of headache disorders and evaluating the epidemiological patterns can help identify those groups at highest risk. Evaluating the genetic, environmental, and sociodemographic factors contributing to different types of headache disorders can further provide clues towards better understanding the disease mechanisms and determining the optimal treatment strategies.

References

1. Bille BS. Migraine in school children. *Acta Paediatr Suppl.* 1962;136:1–151.
2. Sillanpää M, Piekkala P. Prevalence of migraine and other headaches in early puberty. *Scand J Prim Health Care.* 1984;2(1):27–32.
3. Lateef TM, Merikangas KR, He J, et al. Headache in a national sample of American children: prevalence and comorbidity. *J Child Neurol.* 2009;24(5):536–543.
4. The Childhood Brain Tumor Consortium. The epidemiology of headache among children with brain tumor. Headache in children with brain tumors. The childhood brain tumor consortium. *J Neurooncol.* 1991;10(1):31–46.
5. Stewart WF, Bigal ME, Kolodner K, Dowson A, Liberman JN, Lipton RB. Familial risk of migraine: variation by proband age at onset and headache severity. *Neurology.* 2006;66:344–388.
6. Abu-Arafeh I, Razak S, Sivaraman B, Graham C. Prevalence of headache and migraine in children and adolescents: a systematic review of population- based studies. *Dev Med Child Neurol.* 2010;52(12):1088–1097.
7. Kienbacher CH, Wöber CH, Zesch HE, et al. Clinical features, classification and prognosis of migraine and tension-type headache in children and adolescents: a long-term follow-up study. *Cephalalgia.* 2006;26:820–830.

8. Laurell K, Larsson B, Eeg-Olofsson O. Prevalence of headache in Swedish schoolchildren, with a focus on tension-type headache. *Cephalalgia*. 2004;24(5):380–388.

9. Wöber-Bingöl C. Epidemiology of migraine and headache in children and adolescents. *Curr Pain Headache Rep*. 2013;17(6):1–11.

10. GBD 2016 Disease and Injury Incidence and Prevalence Collaborators. Global, regional, and national incidence, prevalence, and years lived with disability for 328 diseases and injuries for 195 countries, 1990–2016: a systematic analysis for the Global Burden of Disease Study 2016. *Lancet*. 2017;390(10100):1211–1259.

11. Powers SW, Patton SR, Hommel KA, Hershey AD. Quality of life in childhood migraines: clinical impact and comparison to other chronic illnesses. *Pediatrics*. 2003;112(1 Pt1):e1–e5.

12. Victor TW, Hu X, Campbell JC, Buse DC, Lipton RB. Migraine prevalence by age and sex in the United States: a life-span study. *Cephalalgia*. 2010;30(9):1065–1072.

13. Mavromichalis I, Anagnostopoulos D, Metaxas N, Papanastassiou E. Prevalence of migraine in schoolchildren and some clinical comparisons between migraine with and without aura. *Headache*. 1999;39(10):728–736.

14. Stewart WF, Linet MS, Celentano DD, Van Natta M, Ziegler D. Age and sex-specific rates of migraine with and without visual aura. *Am J Epidemiol*. 1991;134(10):1111–1120.

15. Balestri M, Papetti L, Maiorani D, et al. Features of aura in paediatric migraine diagnosed using the ICHD 3 beta criteria. *Cephalalgia*. 2018;38(11):1742–1747.

16. Noseda R, Burstein R. Migraine pathophysiology: anatomy of the trigeminovascular pathway and associated neurological symptoms, CSD, sensitization and modulation of pain. *Pain*. 2013;154:S44–S53.

17. Lykke Thomsen L, Kirchmann Eriksen M, Faerch Romer S, et al. An epidemiological survey of hemiplegic migraine. *Cephalalgia*. 2002;22(5):361–375.

18. Lipton RB, Manack A, Ricci JA, Chee E, Turkel CC, Winner P. Prevalence and burden of chronic migraine in adolescents: results of the chronic daily headache in adolescents' study (C-dAS). *Headache*. 2011;51:693–706.

19. Bigal ME, Lipton RB, Tepper SJ, Rapoport AM, Sheftell FD. Primary chronic daily headache and its subtypes in adolescents and adults. *Neurology*. 2004;63:843–847.

20. Fuh JL, Wang SJ, Lu SR, Liao YC, Chen SP, Yang CY. Headache disability among adolescents: a student population-based study. *Headache*. 2010;50:210–218.

21. Hershey AD, Powers SW, Vockell AL, LeCates S, Kabbouche MA, Maynard MK. PedMIDAS: development of a questionnaire to assess disability of migraines in children. *Neurology*. 2001;57:2034–2039.

22. Bigal ME, Lipton RB, Winner P, et al. Migraine in adolescents—association with socioeconomic status and family history. *Neurology*. 2007;69:16–25.

23. Andlin-Sobocki P, Jonsson B, Wittchen HU, Olesen J. Cost of disorders of the brain in Europe. *Eur J Neurol*. 2003;12:1–27.

24. Stewart WF, Ricci JA, Chee E, Morganstein D, Lipton R. Lost productive time and cost due to common pain conditions in the US workforce. *JAMA*. 2003;290:2443–2454.

25. Arruda MA, Bigal ME. Migraine and migraine subtypes in preadolescent children: association with school performance. *Neurology*. 2012;79(18):1881–1888.

26. Headache Classification Committee of the International Headache Society (IHS). The International Classification of Headache Disorders, 3rd edition. *Cephalalgia*. 2018;38:1–211.

27. Özge A, Faedda N, Abu-Arafeh I, et al. Experts' opinion about the primary headache diagnostic criteria of the ICHD-3 beta in children and adolescents. *J Headache Pain*. 2017; 18(1):109.

28. Sutherland H, Albury CL, Griffiths LR. Advances in genetics of migraine. *J Headache Pain*. 2019;20(1):72.

29. Ferrari MD, Klever RR, Terwindt GM, Ayata C, van den Maagdenberg AM. Migraine pathophysiology: lessons from mouse models and human genetics. *Lancet Neurol*. 2015;14(1):65–80.

30. Dodick DW. A phase-by-phase review of migraine pathophysiology. *Headache*. 2018;58 (Suppl 1):4–16.

31. Lateef TM, Cui L, Nakamura E, Dozier J, Merikangas K. Accuracy of family history reports of migraine in a community-based family study of migraine. *Headache*. 2015;55(3):407–412.

32. Ottman R, Hong S, Lipton RB. Validity of family history data on severe headache and migraine. *Neurology*. 1993;43(10):1954–1960.

33. Stewart WF, Staffa J, Lipton RB, Ottman R. Familial risk of migraine: a population-based study. *Ann Neurol*. 1997;41:166–172.

34. Mulder EJ, Van Baal C, Gaist D, et al. Genetic and environmental influences on migraine: a twin study across six countries. *Twin Res*. 2003;6(5):422–431.

35. Ulrich V, Gervil M, Fenger K, Olesen J, Russell MB. The prevalence and characteristics of migraine in twins from the general population. *Headache*. 1999;39:173–180.

36. Lipton RB, Bigal ME, Diamond M, Freitag F, Reed ML, Stewart WF. AMPP advisory group. Migraine prevalence, disease burden, and the need for preventive therapy. *Neurology*. 2007;68(5):343–349.

37. Wadsworth ME, Achenbach TM. Explaining the link between low socioeconomic status and psychopathology: testing two mechanisms of the social causation hypothesis. *J Consult Clin Psychol*. 2005;73:1146–1153.

38. Eaton WW, Muntaner C, Bovasso G, Smith C. Socioeconomic status and depressive syndrome: the role of inter- and intra-generational mobility, government assistance, and work environment. *J Health Soc Behav*. 2001;42:277–294.

39. Tietjen GE, Peterlin BL. Childhood abuse and migraine epidemiology, sex differences, and potential mechanisms. *Headache*. 2011;51:869–879.

40. Anda R, Tietjen G, Schulman E, Felitti V, Croft J. Adverse childhood experiences and frequent headaches in adults. *Headache*. 2010;50:1473–1481.

41. Juang KD, Wang SJ, Fuh JL, Lu SR, Chen YS. Association between adolescent chronic daily headache and childhood adversity: a community-based study. *Cephalalgia*. 2004;24:54–59.

42. Fuh JL, Wang SJ, Juang KD, Lu SR, Liao YC, Chen SP. Relationship between childhood physical maltreatment and migraine in adolescents. *Headache*. 2010;50:761–768.

43. Gutta R, Valentini K, Kaur G, Farooqi A, Sivaswamy L. Management of childhood migraine by headache specialist vs non-headache specialists. *Headache*. 2019;1–10.

44. Lai LL, Koh L, Ho JA, Ting A, Obi A. Off-label prescribing for children with migraines in U.S. ambulatory care settings. *J Manag Care Spec Pharm*. 2017;23:382–387.

45. Zwart JA, Dyb G, Holmen TL, Stovner LJ, Sand T. The prevalence of migraine and tension-type headaches among adolescents in Norway. The Nord-Trondelag Health Study (Head-HUNT-Youth), a large population-based epidemiological study. *Cephalalgia*. 2004;24:373–379.

46. Arruda MA, Bonamico L, Stella C. Cluster headache in children and adolescents: ten years of follow-up in three pediatric cases. *Cephalalgia*. 2011;31:1409–1414.

47. Hagler S, Ballaban-Gil K, Robbins MS. Primary stabbing headache in adults and pediatrics: a review. *Curr Pain Headache Rep*. 2014;18(10):450–453.

48. Yamani N, Olesen J. New daily persistent headache: a systematic review on an enigmatic disorder. *J Headache Pain.* 2019;20(1):80.

49. Mack KJ. What incites new daily persistent headache in children? *Pediatr Neurol.* 2004;31(2):122–125.

50. Lewis DW, Qureshi F. Acute headache in children and adolescents presenting to the emergency department. *Headache.* 2000;40(3):200–203.

51. Conicella E, Raucci U, Vanacore N, et al. The child with headache in a pediatric emergency department. *Headache.* 2008;48(7):1005–1011.

52. Alexiou GA, Argyropoulou MI. Neuroimaging in childhood headache: a systematic review. *Pediatr Radiol.* 2013;43(7):777–784.

Pathophysiology of migraine ☆

Carlyn Patterson Gentile, MD, PhD and Ana Recober, MD

For patients and families

The migraine cycle

When people think of migraine, they usually first think of headache or head pain. But migraine is much more than a headache. Migraines come with many other symptoms, not just head pain. Migraines can be split up into different phases, which occur in a predictable cycle. We will describe the brain and nervous system changes that happen at each stage of this cycle:

(1) The *inter-ictal period* is the period between migraines.
(2) The *premonitory period* is a period of increased symptoms that can start hours to days before a headache starts.
(3) *Migraine aura* (occurring in one out of four people with migraine[1]) is a warning that a headache is coming. The most common symptom is a change in vision that starts right before the headache and lasts less than an hour. Other senses can be affected.
(4) *Headache* is the period of head pain that can come along with other symptoms like nausea, and light and sound sensitivity.
(5) The *postdromal period* is the aftermath of the headache. It occurs after the head pain goes away, but the person does not feel like they are back to normal.

In between attacks (interictal). Even when a child is not having migraine headache, they can be extra sensitive to their environment. Lights seem brighter and sounds seem louder and can be uncomfortable. Brain activity in areas that control our senses (e.g., sight, sound, touch) is different and can be increased in people with migraine. Pain and discomfort can be more easily triggered.

The day before (premonitory). Children may behave differently from usual before they get a headache. Several hours to days prior to the headache, they may be more

---

☆Editor's note: Migraine is a complicated disease involving electrochemical changes in the brain. Advancing our understanding of the pathophysiology has enabled us to develop targeted treatments, and from studies of those treatments we have then learned more about pathophysiology. From continued efforts to understand what goes wrong we will learn how to change the trajectory of migraine.

Pediatric Headache. https://doi.org/10.1016/B978-0-323-83005-8.00021-5

sensitive to light and sound, more tired, more irritable, complain of neck pain, and have difficulty concentrating. Frequent yawning and increased urination can also be signs that a migraine headache is coming. These changes have been linked to changes in brain activity.

Migraine aura. One in four people with migraine will experience a warning right before the start of the migraine headache. Migraine aura can take many forms, the most common being changes in vision. Children may experience flashing lights, sparkles, or partial visual loss. Strange smells, tingling or numbness on one side of the body, or one-sided weakness are other types of aura. Auras are caused by a wave of increased activity of brain cells in one part of the brain followed by a period when the brain cells are quiet, most often in the back of the brain that is responsible for vision.

The headache phase. Headache pain can be broken down into two parts. During the first part, i.e., at the start of the throbbing head pain, chemicals are released at the nerve endings of the face and scalp causing nerve irritation. The overactive nerves relay information to the brain that leads to the second part. During the second part, the brain itself becomes more sensitive. Pain pathways within the brain are more active. During this second part, the scalp can become sensitive to the touch. Medications used to stop headache work best before the scalp becomes sensitive, which is why it is important to take medications to treat a migraine headache early.

Aftermath of the headache (postdrome). After the headache goes away, most children will feel tired and have difficulty concentrating. They may even crave certain foods or be very thirsty. These changes can last up to a day, but currently it is unclear what changes in the brain cause this recovery period.

Chronic migraine

Chronic migraine occurs when headache attacks happen very often (at least 15 days a month with 8 of those days being migraine headache). Pain can even be constant with times when the headache becomes more severe. Increased sensitivity of the brain seems to be present all the time in chronic migraine. It appears that the more time a person's brain is in the midst of a migraine, the more likely they are to have a migraine. Having a good rescue therapy to stop a migraine in its tracks, may be important to keep migraines from becoming more frequent.

The effect of puberty and sex hormones

Before puberty, boys and girls get migraine at a similar rate, but after puberty girls get migraine at a higher rate than boys. This may be because of the different effects that sex hormones have on migraine. After puberty, girls can be more likely to have a headache right before or right after their monthly periods. Estrogen and progesterone might both promote migraine headaches, while testosterone may be protective. Migraine related to menstruation is not due to abnormal hormonal levels, but because of the brain's sensitivity to normal hormonal changes. You can read more about this in a chapter related to hormones and headaches.

For general practitioners

It is important to recognize migraine as a complex neurologic disorder of which its hallmark feature, headache, is only one of the many symptoms. For many years, the dominant theory was that migraines resulted from vasodilation of blood vessels. However, it has been demonstrated that vasodilation is not necessary nor sufficient in migraine.[2–5] This revelation has led to a shift from the early vascular hypothesis to the current neurovascular hypothesis of migraine. Migraine is now considered a pathologic brain state involving extensive changes in neurologic function and connectivity.[6]

Migraine cycle

Inter-ictal phase. Between migraines, there is heightened sensitivity to stimuli, including photophobia and phonophobia.[7,8] There is also evidence of increased responses in multiple cortical areas during this phase.[9–16] Both sensory hypersensitivity and greater susceptibility to a migraine may be a consequence of a combination of factors including abnormal interactions between the thalamus (the main sensory relay station of the brain) and the cortex,[17–21] altered connectivity of cortical structures as well as brainstem dysfunction,[17,22–25] and a mismatch between metabolic supply and demand.[26,27]

Premonitory phase. Almost 70% of children with migraine report premonitory symptoms hours to days before the onset of a migraine headache.[28] Premonitory symptoms include fatigue, poor concentration, emotional liability, nausea, yawning, neck discomfort or stiffness, and increased sensory hyper-sensitivity—especially photophobia.[29–31] The nature of these symptoms indicates that migraine is fundamentally a disorder of the central nervous system, which is supported by neurophysiologic changes during the premonitory phase of a migraine.[25,32–35] These symptoms suggest that the beginning of a migraine may start hours to days before the headache and the migraine aura.

Aura. Migraine aura is present in one quarter of individuals.[1] Visual auras are the most common but other aura types include sensory, motor, language, and rarely brainstem symtpoms.[36] The pathogenesis of migraine aura has been attributed to cortical spreading depression (CSD), which consists of a wave of intense cortical neuronal activity followed by a more prolonged period of neuronal activity suppression.[37] CSD may lead to activation of trigeminal nociceptors resulting in head pain.[38] However, migraine often occurs in the absence of aura, premonitory symptoms precede the aura, and migraine aura can occur without headache, arguing that CSD is more likely part of the broader neurologic dysfunction that occurs in migraine.[32]

Headache phase. The headache is typically throbbing and moderate or severe in intensity. This pain is associated with peripheral sensitization of trigeminovascular system caused by release of proinflammatory neuropeptides such as calcitonin gene-related peptide (CGRP) and others, that results in neurogenic inflammation and vasodilation.[39–42] Peripheral stimulation of the trigeminal afferents leads to central sensitization of the brainstem.[43–46] Central sensitization results in cutaneous allodynia and sustained headache.[47,48] Once the central sensitization step is reached, triptans are no longer nearly as effective at treating the attack because they act on peripheral sensitization mechanisms.[49] This is why it is important to advise patients to take the triptan as soon as the headache starts.

Postdrome. Over 80% of children and adolescents report a recovery period lasting up to a day following the headache phase. Most common postdromic symptoms included thirst, tiredness, visual disturbances, food cravings, paresthesias, and ocular pain.[50]

Chronic migraine

Chronic migraine is defined as 15 or more headache days per month for 3 months with at least 8 of those days being migraine headaches.[51] Chronic migraine is characterized by enduring central sensitization and alteration of pain processing pathways.[52–57] Decreased pain thresholds in individuals with chronic compared to episodic migraine support this assertion.[58] Importantly, repeated stimulation of circuitry involved in migraines seems to make the system more vulnerable to persistent central sensitization.[59] High burden of episodic migraine including high headache frequency and ineffective abortive therapy in episodic migraine have been associated with progression to chronic migraine,[60,61] though the causation has not been established. Still, it is likely helpful to have effective treatments for episodic migraine, given the possibility that it may help prevent the transition to chronic migraine.

Sex differences

The prevalence of migraine is similar between boys and girls until puberty, when the prevalence increases for females to a higher degree than for males.[62] Sex differences are important for prognosis as boys are also more likely to have remission of their migraine headaches.[63] Epidemiologic sex difference has led to research in the influence of sex hormones in migraine. There is evidence that estrogen, and estrogen withdrawal in particular, leads to increased susceptibility to a migraine.[64–67] There is also preliminary evidence that testosterone confers a protective influence through anti-inflammatory, and anti-nociceptive properties.[68–70]

For specialists

Over the past 40 years, there have been significant advances of our understanding of migraine pathophysiology. The once dominant vascular hypothesis has been replaced by the neurovascular hypothesis. This shift occurred because there is building evidence of neurologic dysfunction in migraine. Further, vasodilation is not necessary nor sufficient to produce a migraine.[2–5] Currently, migraine is viewed as a cyclical disorder of sensory hyper-sensitivity and brainstem dysfunction manifested as recurrent episodes of headache and other non-pain symptoms.[71] The following section will address the underlying pathophysiology of each phase of the migraine cycle in support of this assertion.

Migraine cycle

Inter-ictal phase. Neurologic dysfunction is evident in between migraines. Sensory hypersensitivity[7,8] and reduced pain thresholds[72] are evident inter-ictally. Hyper-responsivity and lack of habituation of the sensory cortices has been shown by multiple neurophysiologic and neuroimaging modalities,[9–16] which may offer a neural correlate to these symptoms. Hyper-responsivity may result from altered thalamo-cortical connectivity. Abnormal low frequency oscillations localized to the medial dorsal nucleus of the thalamus[17] and increased coherence between low-frequency oscillations of the thalamus and high-frequency oscillations of the visual cortex[18] have been noted inter-ictally. Increased resonance between the thalamus and cortex has been linked to thalamic cells displaying low-threshold calcium spike bursts.[18] These findings are representative of altered network connectivity generally playing a role inter-ictally in migraine. Altered network connectivity has been described in multiple cortical and subcortical brain regions during the inter-ictal period including cerebral cortex,[22–24] brainstem,[25] amygdala,[22] and thalamus[17]. While the consequences of this altered connectivity have not been fully elucidated, it suggests that migraine involves dysfunction in multiple areas. This is consistent with the broad range of symptoms reported in migraine including sensory hypersensitivity, autonomic symptoms, and cognitive dysfunction.[32]

An imbalance between metabolic supply and demand may also contribute. Magnetic resonance spectroscopy (MRS) demonstrates decreased *N*-Acetylaspartate levels indicating abnormal energy metabolism and potential mitochondrial dysfunction.[26] Further, MRS shows abnormalities in glutamate and y-aminobutyric acid (GABA) indicating altered excitability.[26] Increased metabolic demand coupled with impaired metabolic function may help create conditions to precipitate a migraine.[27]

Premonitory phase. Premonitory symptoms, occurring hours to days before the headache phase, are reported in almost 70% of children with migraine.[28] The most common symptoms include fatigue, poor concentration, emotional liability, nausea, yawning, stiff neck and neck discomfort, and increased sensory hyper-sensitivity—especially photophobia.[29–31] The nature of these symptoms indicate that migraine is fundamentally a disorder of the central nervous system. This assertion is supported by the finding that the brain shows increased responses in association with premonitory symptoms measured using neuroimaging and neurophysiologic techniques. Increased hypothalamic activity has been observed[25,33] and may underlie many of these symptoms including polyuria, change in appetite, and mood changes.[32] Increased activity of the brainstem has been observed in the premonitory phase[25] and is associated with nausea.[34] Premonitory photophobia has been associated with increased activity measured in the occipital cortex.[35] Cervical nerve afferents converge with trigeminal nerve afferents in the brainstem and cervical spinal cord, which may explain the occurrence of premonitory neck pain.[73] These findings suggest that the beginning of a migraine may start well before the headache phase and even the migraine aura.

Aura. Migraine aura is present in one quarter of individuals.[1] Visual auras are the most common but other aura types include sensory, motor, language, and brainstem symptoms and can vary within individuals.[36] The pathogenesis of migraine aura has been attributed to cortical spreading depression (CSD). CSD is a common pathologic cortical phenomenon that is also seen following a brain insult including stroke and traumatic brain injury.[74] CSD consists of a wave of intense cortical neuronal activity followed by a more prolonged period of neuronal activity suppression.[37] The initial depolarization of CSD can be triggered by glutamate, and most effectively by activation of the N-methyl-D-aspartate (NMDA) glutamate receptor subtype. The depolarization is associated with dramatic ion shifts. Potassium and hydrogen ions move out of the cells, and sodium, calcium, and chloride ions move into the cell along with water leading to a decrease in the volume of the extracellular space.[37] This wave moves across the cortex at a velocity of 2–4 mm/min. It does not respect vascular territories and is not accompanied by tissue ischemia. It occurs in a linear pattern that is spatially confined to a sulcus or gyrus.[75]

CSD, the proposed pathophysiologic correlate of migraine aura, may lead to activation of trigeminal nociceptors that trigger head pain.[76] It has been proposed that CSD serves as the instigator for activation of the trigeminovascular system based on animal studies. However, this point remains a topic of debate.[77,78] Arguments against this hypothesis are that migraine often occurs in the absence of aura, premonitory symptoms precede migraine aura, and migraine aura can occur without the associated headache. An alternative proposal is that CSD is one component of the much broader neurologic dysfunction that occurs during migraine.[32]

Headache phase. Over the past 40 years, the importance of the trigeminovascular system in migraine pain initiation and continuation has been further elucidated.[79] Head pain starts with peripheral sensitization of trigeminal nerve. Collateral axons from the trigeminal ganglia and dural afferents release proinflammatory neuropeptides such as calcitonin gene-related peptide (CGRP), pituitary adenylate-cyclase activating peptide (PACAP), substance P, and neurokinin A leading to neurogenic inflammation and vasodilation.[39–42] While vasodilation results from release of proinflammatory neuropeptides, it is not necessary nor sufficient to trigger a migraine.[2] This is demonstrated by the findings that vasoactive intestinal peptide causes vasodilation, but does not induce migraine,[3] while sildenafil[4] and nitric oxide[5]-induced migraines are not associated with vasodilation.

Peripheral stimulation of the trigeminal afferents leads to central sensitization as evidenced by neuronal hyper-excitability of the trigeminal nucleus caudalis (TNC) in the brain stem.[43–46] Neuropeptides that are potentially involved include CGRP,[80] glutamate via action on NMDA receptors,[81] and calcium activity.[82] When central sensitization occurs, it leads to cutaneous allodynia and sustained attack.[47,48]

Postdrome. Over 80% of children and adolescents experience a postdromal period that lasts approximately a day following resolution of the headache. Most common postdromal symptoms included thirst, tiredness, visual disturbances, food craving paresthesias, and ocular pain.[50] Little is known about the underlying pathophysiology of the migraine postdrome, but is an important area of future study[83] as it could help to understand the process that leads to resolution of a migraine.

Therapies developed for migraine

The different stages of pain development during a migraine are crucial to understand, from a treatment perspective. This section reviews therapies specifically developed to treat migraine.

Triptans. Triptans are serotonin 5-HT 1B and 5-HT 1D receptor agonists[84] that act on peripheral terminals of meningeal afferents. Therefore, they target peripheral sensitization. Consequently, they are less effective when the migraine progresses to central sensitization. In adults, triptans are 93% effective at stopping a migraine when taken prior to the onset of cutaneous allodynia. This efficacy drops to 15% after the onset of cutaneous allodynia, which is a surrogate marker for central sensitization.[49] Triptans have the potential to inhibit the TNC centrally, but they are likely too large to cross the blood brain barrier.[85] Interestingly, in a rat model, triptans were able to block both peripheral and central sensitization when taken early, but failed to do so once there is evidence of central sensitization.[86] This finding underscores the importance of why taking abortive medications at the start of headache pain is critical; the headache must be stopped before the central sensitization stage is reached.

CGRP antibodies and CGRP antagonists. CGRP acts at multiple levels of the trigeminovascular system. It is important for pain transmission peripherally at the trigeminal ganglion, and also centrally at the TNC.[87] Advances in our understanding on the important role CGRP mechanisms play in migraine pathophysiology has led to the development of two classes of therapeutics that target this system: CGRP antibodies and CGRP antagonists. CGRP antibodies were the first preventive therapy developed specifically for migraine.[88] CGRP antibodies likely act primarily by blocking peripheral CGRP pathways because they are large molecules that cannot cross the blood brain barrier. Relatively low concentrations of CGRP antibodies have been measured centrally in rats, though a central mechanism cannot be excluded.[89] CGRP antagonists have shown efficacy in acute migraine management.[90] There is some evidence that CGRP antagonists may act centrally, though this remains a topic of debate because the antagonists have limited blood-brain barrier permeability.[90]

Chronic migraine

Chronic migraine is defined as 15 or more headache days per month for 3 months with at least 8 of those days being migraine headaches.[51] Pathophysiologic changes in chronic migraine include hyper-excitability, altered metabolism, and persistent central sensitization.[52] Maladaptive changes in neuro-excitability and metabolism of sensory and pain processing pathways are seen in chronic migraine.[53–56] Supportive of persistent central sensitization, pain thresholds are decreased[58] and cutaneous allodynia is more common and severe in individuals with chronic migraine compared with episodic migraine.[91] Further, rats subjected to repeated high intensity stimulation of trigeminal nociceptors develop persistent hyper-excitability in the TNC consistent with central sensitization.[59] This finding indicates that repeated stimulation of the TNC (for instance by multiple migraines) can give rise to a state of persistent central sensitization. This is consistent with the observation that high headache frequency and ineffective abortive therapy in episodic migraine are both risk factors for conversion to chronic migraine.[60,61]

Sex differences

Sex differences, due at least in part to the different effects of male and female sex hormones,[68] play an important role in migraine.[68] The prevalence of migraine is similar in boys and girls until puberty, after that the prevalence increases for both sexes, but with greater rise for females. For many women, the risk of having a migraine is higher between 2 days prior and 3 days after the onset of menstruation.[64] This is attributed to estrogen withdrawal.[65,66] There is more direct evidence that both estrogen and progesterone act on migraine pathophysiology as it increases susceptibility to CSD in mouse models.[67,92] Testosterone, on the other hand, decreases susceptibility to CSD in mouse models[69] and may confer a protective effect in migraine.[68] Furthermore, testosterone has been shown to have anti-inflammatory, and anti-nociceptive properties in other disease states.[70] Additionally, sex hormone differences can lead to differences in brain activity including alterations in pain and sensory processing.[93] It is clear that sex hormones play an important role in migraine, but further research in their role in the pathophysiology of migraine is needed.

References

1. Rasmussen BK, Olesen J. Migraine with aura and migraine without aura: an epidemiological study. *Cephalalgia*. 1992. https://doi.org/10.1046/j.1468-2982.1992.1204221.x.
2. Brennan KC, Charles A. An update on the blood vessel in migraine. *Curr Opin Neurol*. 2010. https://doi.org/10.1097/WCO.0b013e32833821c1.
3. Rahmann A, Wienecke T, Hansen JM, Fahrenkrug J, Olesen J, Ashina M. Vasoactive intestinal peptide causes marked cephalic vasodilation, but does not induce migraine. *Cephalalgia*. 2008. https://doi.org/10.1111/j.1468-2982.2007.01497.x.

4. Kruuse C, Thomsen LL, Birk S, Olesen J. Migraine can be induced by sildenafil without changes in middle cerebral artery diameter. *Brain*. 2003. https://doi.org/10.1093/brain/awg009.

5. Schoonman GG, Van Der Grond J, Kortmann C, Van Der Geest RJ, Terwindt GM, Ferrari MD. Migraine headache is not associated with cerebral or meningeal vasodilatation—a 3T magnetic resonance angiography study. *Brain*. 2008. https://doi.org/10.1093/brain/awn094.

6. Charles A. Migraine: a brain state. *Curr Opin Neurol*. 2013. https://doi.org/10.1097/WCO.0b013e32836085f4.

7. Mulleners WM, Aurora SK, Chronicle EP, Stewart R, Gopal S, Koehler PJ. Self-reported photophobic symptoms in migraineurs and controls are reliable and predict diagnostic category accurately. *Headache*. 2001. https://doi.org/10.1046/j.1526-4610.2001.111006031.x.

8. Ashkenazi A, Mushtaq A, Yang I, Oshinsky ML. Ictal and interictal phonophobia in migraine—a quantitative controlled study. *Cephalalgia*. 2009. https://doi.org/10.1111/j.1468-2982.2008.01834.x.

9. Aurora SK, Barrodale P, Chronicle EP, Mulleners WM. Cortical inhibition is reduced in chronic and episodic migraine and demonstrates a spectrum of illness. *Headache*. 2005. https://doi.org/10.1111/j.1526-4610.2005.05108.x.

10. Aurora SK, Ahmad BK, Welch KMA, Bhardhwaj P, Ramadan NM. Transcranial magnetic stimulation confirms hyperexcitability of occipital cortex in migraine. *Neurology*. 1998. https://doi.org/10.1212/WNL.50.4.1111.

11. Datta R, Aguirre GK, Hu S, Detre JA, Cucchiara B. Interictal cortical hyperresponsiveness in migraine is directly related to the presence of aura. *Cephalalgia*. 2013;33(6):365–374. https://doi.org/10.1177/0333102412474503.

12. Boulloche N, Denuelle M, Payoux P, Fabre N, Trotter Y, Géraud G. Photophobia in migraine: an interictal PET study of cortical hyperexcitability and its modulation by pain. *J Neurol Neurosurg Psychiatry*. 2010. https://doi.org/10.1136/jnnp.2009.190223.

13. Coppola G, Pierelli F, Schoenen J. Is the cerebral cortex hyperexcitable or hyperresponsive in migraine? *Cephalalgia*. 2007. https://doi.org/10.1111/j.1468-2982.2007.01500.x.

14. Coppola G, Pierelli F, Schoenen J. Habituation and migraine. *Neurobiol Learn Mem*. 2009. https://doi.org/10.1016/j.nlm.2008.07.006.

15. Áfra J, Cecchini AP, De Pasqua V, Albert A, Schoenen J. Visual evoked potentials during long periods of pattern-reversal stimulation in migraine. *Brain*. 1998. https://doi.org/10.1093/brain/121.2.233.

16. Aurora SK, Wilkinson F. The brain is hyperexcitable in migraine. *Cephalalgia*. 2007. https://doi.org/10.1111/j.1468-2982.2007.01502.x.

17. Hodkinson DJ, Wilcox SL, Veggeberg R, et al. Increased amplitude of thalamocortical low-frequency oscillations in patients with migraine. *J Neurosci*. 2016. https://doi.org/10.1523/jneurosci.1038-16.2016.

18. Llinas RR, Ribary U, Jeanmonod D, Kronberg E, Mitra PP. Thalamocortical dysrhythmia: a neurological and neuropsychiatric syndrome characterized by magnetoencephalography. *Proc Natl Acad Sci*. 1999. https://doi.org/10.1073/pnas.96.26.15222.

19. De Tommaso M, Ambrosini A, Brighina F, et al. Altered processing of sensory stimuli in patients with migraine. *Nat Rev Neurol*. 2014. https://doi.org/10.1038/nrneurol.2014.14.

20. Angelini L, De Tommaso M, Guido M, et al. Steady-state visual evoked potentials and phase synchronization in migraine patients. *Phys Rev Lett*. 2004. https://doi.org/10.1103/PhysRevLett.93.038103.

21. Coppola G, Ambrosini A, Di Clemente L, et al. Interictal abnormalities of gamma band activity in visual evoked responses in migraine: an indication of thalamocortical dysrhythmia? *Cephalalgia*. 2007. https://doi.org/10.1111/j.1468-2982.2007.01466.x.

22. Chong CD, Gaw N, Fu Y, Li J, Wu T, Schwedt TJ. Migraine classification using magnetic resonance imaging resting-state functional connectivity data. *Cephalalgia.* 2017. https://doi.org/10.1177/0333102416652091.

23. Tedeschi G, Russo A, Conte F, et al. Increased interictal visual network connectivity in patients with migraine with aura. *Cephalalgia.* 2016. https://doi.org/10.1177/0333102415584360.

24. Niddam DM, Lai KL, Fuh JL, Chuang CYN, Chen WT, Wang SJ. Reduced functional connectivity between salience and visual networks in migraine with aura. *Cephalalgia.* 2016. https://doi.org/10.1177/0333102415583144.

25. Schulte LH, May A. The migraine generator revisited: continuous scanning of the migraine cycle over 30 days and three spontaneous attacks. *Brain.* 2016. https://doi.org/10.1093/brain/aww097.

26. Younis S, Hougaard A, Vestergaard MB, Larsson HBW, Ashina M. Migraine and magnetic resonance spectroscopy. *Curr Opin Neurol.* 2017. https://doi.org/10.1097/wco.0000000000000436.

27. Sparaco M, Feleppa M, Lipton RB, Rapoport AM, Bigal ME. Mitochondrial dysfunction and migraine: evidence and hypotheses. *Cephalalgia.* 2006. https://doi.org/10.1111/j.1468-2982.2005.01059.x.

28. Cuvellier JC, Mars A, Vallée L. The prevalence of premonitory symptoms in paediatric migraine: a questionnaire study in 103 children and adolescents. *Cephalalgia.* 2009. https://doi.org/10.1111/j.1468-2982.2009.01854.x.

29. Giffin NJ, Ruggiero L, Lipton RB, et al. Premonitory symptoms in migraine: an electronic diary study. *Neurology.* 2003. https://doi.org/10.1212/01.WNL.0000052998.58526.A9.

30. Quintela E, Castillo J, Muñoz P, Pascual J. Premonitory and resolution symptoms in migraine: a prospective study in 100 unselected patients. *Cephalalgia.* 2006. https://doi.org/10.1111/j.1468-2982.2006.01157.x.

31. Schoonman GG, Evers DJ, Terwindt GM, Van Dijk JG, Ferrari MD. The prevalence of premonitory symptoms in migraine: a questionnaire study in 461 patients. *Cephalalgia.* 2006. https://doi.org/10.1111/j.1468-2982.2006.01195.x.

32. Charles A. The pathophysiology of migraine: implications for clinical management. *Lancet Neurol.* 2018. https://doi.org/10.1016/S1474-4422(17)30435-0.

33. Maniyar FH, Sprenger T, Monteith T, Schankin C, Goadsby PJ. Brain activations in the premonitory phase of nitroglycerin-triggered migraine attacks. *Brain.* 2014. https://doi.org/10.1093/brain/awt320.

34. Maniyar FH, Sprenger T, Schankin C, Goadsby PJ. The origin of nausea in migraine—a PET study. *J Headache Pain.* 2014. https://doi.org/10.1186/1129-2377-15-84.

35. Maniyar FH, Sprenger T, Schankin C, Goadsby PJ. Photic hypersensitivity in the premonitory phase of migraine—a positron emission tomography study. *Eur J Neurol.* 2014. https://doi.org/10.1111/ene.12451.

36. Hansen JM, Goadsby PJ, Charles AC. Variability of clinical features in attacks of migraine with aura. *Cephalalgia.* 2016. https://doi.org/10.1177/0333102415584601.

37. Lauritzen M. Pathophysiology of the migraine aura: the spreading depression theory. *Brain.* 1994. https://doi.org/10.1093/brain/117.1.199.

38. Close LN, Eftekhari S, Wang M, Charles AC, Russo AF. Cortical spreading depression as a site of origin for migraine: role of CGRP. *Cephalalgia.* 2019. https://doi.org/10.1177/0333102418774299.

39. Strassman AM, Raymond SA, Burstein R. Sensitization of meningeal sensory neurons and the origin of headaches. *Nature.* 1996. https://doi.org/10.1038/384560a0.

40. Vaughn AH, Gold MS. Ionic mechanisms underlying inflammatory mediator-induced sensitization of dural afferents. *J Neurosci*. 2010. https://doi.org/10.1523/JNEUROSCI.6053-09.2010.

41. Meßlinger K, Hanesch U, Baumgärtel M, Trost B, Schmidt RF. Innervation of the dura mater encephali of cat and rat: ultrastructure and calcitonin gene-related peptide-like and substance P-like immunoreactivity. *Anat Embryol*. 1993. https://doi.org/10.1007/BF00188214.

42. Dux M, Sántha P, Jancsó G. Capsaicin-sensitive neurogenic sensory vasodilatation in the dura mater of the rat. *J Physiol*. 2003. https://doi.org/10.1113/jphysiol.2003.050633.

43. Hu JW, Sessle BJ, Raboisson P, Dallel R, Woda A. Stimulation of craniofacial muscle afferents induces prolonged facilitatory effects in trigeminal nociceptive brain-stem neurones. *Pain*. 1992. https://doi.org/10.1016/0304-3959(92)90131-T.

44. Burstein R, Yamamura H, Malick A, Strassman AM. Chemical stimulation of the intracranial dura induces enhanced responses to facial stimulation in brain stem trigeminal neurons. *J Neurophysiol*. 1998. https://doi.org/10.1152/jn.1998.79.2.964.

45. Schepelmann K, Ebersberger A, Pawlak M, Oppmann M, Messlinger K. Response properties of trigeminal brain stem neurons with input from dura mater encephali in the rat. *Neuroscience*. 1999. https://doi.org/10.1016/S0306-4522(98)00423-0.

46. Kaube H, Katsarava Z, Przywara S, Drepper J, Ellrich J, Diener HC. Acute migraine headache: possible ensitization of neurons in the spinal trigeminal nucleus? *Neurology*. 2002. https://doi.org/10.1212/WNL.58.8.1234.

47. Edelmayer RM, Vanderah TW, Majuta L, et al. Medullary pain facilitating neurons mediate allodynia in headache-related pain. *Ann Neurol*. 2009. https://doi.org/10.1002/ana.21537.

48. Burstein R. The development of cutaneous allodynia during a migraine attack clinical evidence for the sequential recruitment of spinal and supraspinal nociceptive neurons in migraine. *Brain*. 2000. https://doi.org/10.1093/brain/123.8.1703.

49. Burstein R, Collins B, Jakubowski M. Defeating migraine pain with triptans: a race against the development of cutaneous allodynia. *Ann Neurol*. 2004. https://doi.org/10.1002/ana.10786.

50. Mamouri O, Cuvellier JC, Duhamel A, Vallée L, Nguyen The Tich S. Postdrome symptoms in pediatric migraine: a questionnaire retrospective study by phone in 100 patients. *Cephalalgia*. 2018. https://doi.org/10.1177/0333102417721132.

51. International Headache Society. The international classification of headache disorders, 3rd edition. *Cephalalgia*. 2018;38:1–211. https://doi.org/10.1177/0333102417738202.

52. Mathew NT. Pathophysiology of chronic migraine and mode of action of preventive medications. *Headache*. 2011. https://doi.org/10.1111/j.1526-4610.2011.01955.x.

53. Valfrè W, Rainero I, Bergui M, Pinessi L. Voxel-based morphometry reveals gray matter abnormalities in migraine. *Headache*. 2008. https://doi.org/10.1111/j.1526-4610.2007.00723.x.

54. Fumal A, Laureys S, Di Clemente L, et al. Orbitofrontal cortex involvement in chronic analgesic-overuse headache evolving from episodic migraine. *Brain*. 2006. https://doi.org/10.1093/brain/awh691.

55. Aurora SK, Barrodale PM, Tipton RL, Khodavirdi A. Brainstem dysfunction in chronic migraine as evidenced by neurophysiological and positron emission tomography studies. *Headache*. 2007. https://doi.org/10.1111/j.1526-4610.2007.00853.x.

56. Chen WT, Wang SJ, Fuh JL, Lin CP, Ko YC, Lin YY. Persistent ictal-like visual cortical excitability in chronic migraine. *Pain*. 2011. https://doi.org/10.1016/j.pain.2010.08.047.

57. Schoenen J. Is chronic migraine a never-ending migraine attack? *Pain.* 2011. https://doi.org/10.1016/j.pain.2010.12.002.

58. Kitaj MB, Klink M. Pain thresholds in daily transformed migraine versus episodic migraine headache patients. *Headache.* 2005. https://doi.org/10.1111/j.1526-4610.2005.05179.x.

59. Boyer N, Dallel R, Artola A, Monconduit L. General trigeminospinal central sensitization and impaired descending pain inhibitory controls contribute to migraine progression. *Pain.* 2014. https://doi.org/10.1016/j.pain.2014.03.001.

60. Cho SJ, Chu MK. Risk factors of chronic daily headache or chronic migraine. *Curr Pain Headache Rep.* 2015. https://doi.org/10.1007/s11916-014-0465-9.

61. Bigal ME, Lipton RB. Modifiable risk factors for migraine progression. *Headache.* 2006. https://doi.org/10.1111/j.1526-4610.2006.00577.x.

62. Victor T, Hu X, Campbell J, Buse D, Lipton R. Migraine prevalence by age and sex in the United States: a life-span study. *Cephalalgia.* 2010. https://doi.org/10.1177/0333102409355601.

63. Bille B. A 40-year follow-up of school children with migraine. *Cephalalgia.* 1997. https://doi.org/10.1046/j.1468-2982.1997.1704488.x.

64. MacGregor EA, Hackshaw A. Prevalence of migraine on each day of the natural menstrual cycle. *Neurology.* 2004. https://doi.org/10.1212/01.WNL.0000133134.68143.2E.

65. MacGregor EA. Contraception and headache. *Headache.* 2013. https://doi.org/10.1111/head.12035.

66. Pavlović JM, Allshouse AA, Santoro NF, et al. Sex hormones in women with and without migraine: evidence of migraine-specific hormone profiles. *Neurology.* 2016. https://doi.org/10.1212/WNL.0000000000002798.

67. Eikermann-Haerter K, Dileköz E, Kudo C, et al. Genetic and hormonal factors modulate spreading depression and transient hemiparesis in mouse models of familial hemiplegic migraine type 1. *J Clin Invest.* 2009. https://doi.org/10.1172/JCI36059.

68. Vetvik KG, MacGregor EA. Sex differences in the epidemiology, clinical features, and pathophysiology of migraine. *Lancet Neurol.* 2017. https://doi.org/10.1016/S1474-4422(16)30293-9.

69. Eikermann-Haerter K, Baum MJ, Ferrari MD, Van Den Maagdenberg AMJM, Moskowitz MA, Ayata C. Androgenic suppression of spreading depression in familial hemiplegic migraine type 1 mutant mice. *Ann Neurol.* 2009. https://doi.org/10.1002/ana.21779.

70. Sorge RE, Totsch SK. Sex differences in pain. *J Neurosci Res.* 2017. https://doi.org/10.1002/jnr.23841.

71. Goadsby PJ, Holland PR, Martins-Oliveira M, Hoffmann J, Schankin C, Akerman S. Pathophysiology of migraine: a disorder of sensory processing. *Physiol Rev.* 2017. https://doi.org/10.1152/physrev.00034.2015.

72. Weissman-Fogel I, Sprecher E, Granovsky Y, Yarnitsky D. Repeated noxious stimulation of the skin enhances cutaneous pain perception of migraine patients in-between attacks: clinical evidence for continuous sub-threshold increase in membrane excitability of central trigeminovascular neurons. *Pain.* 2003. https://doi.org/10.1016/S0304-3959(03)00159-3.

73. Goadsby PJ, Knight YE, Hoskin KL. Stimulation of the greater occipital nerve increases metabolic activity in the trigeminal nucleus caudalis and cervical dorsal horn of the cat. *Pain.* 1997. https://doi.org/10.1016/S0304-3959(97)00074-2.

74. Lauritzen M, Dreier JP, Fabricius M, Hartings JA, Graf R, Strong AJ. Clinical relevance of cortical spreading depression in neurological disorders: migraine, malignant stroke, subarachnoid and intracranial hemorrhage, and traumatic brain injury. *J Cereb Blood Flow Metab.* 2011. https://doi.org/10.1038/jcbfm.2010.191.

75. Dahlem MA, Hadjikhani N. Migraine aura: retracting particle-like waves in weakly susceptible cortex. *PLoS One*. 2009. https://doi.org/10.1371/journal.pone.0005007.

76. Moskowitz MA. The neurobiology of vascular head pain. *Ann Neurol*. 1984. https://doi.org/10.1002/ana.410160202.

77. Charles A. Does cortical spreading depression initiate a migraine attack? Maybe not⋯. *Headache*. 2010. https://doi.org/10.1111/j.1526-4610.2010.01646.x.

78. Ayata C. Cortical spreading depression triggers migraine attack: pro. *Headache*. 2010. https://doi.org/10.1111/j.1526-4610.2010.01647.x.

79. Ashina M, Hansen JM, Do TP, Melo-Carrillo A, Burstein R, Moskowitz MA. Migraine and the trigeminovascular system—40 years and counting. *Lancet Neurol*. 2019. https://doi.org/10.1016/S1474-4422(19)30185-1.

80. Jenkins DW, Langmead CJ, Parsons AA, Strijbos PJ. Regulation of calcitonin gene-related peptide release from rat trigeminal nucleus caudalis slices in vitro. *Neurosci Lett*. 2004. https://doi.org/10.1016/j.neulet.2004.05.067.

81. Mitsikostas DD, Sanchez Del Rio M, Waeber C, Moskowitz MA, Cutrer FM. The NMDA receptor antagonist MK-801 reduces capsaicin-induced c-fos expression within rat trigeminal nucleus caudalis. *Pain*. 1998. https://doi.org/10.1016/S0304-3959(98)00051-7.

82. Knight YE, Bartsch T, Kaube H, Goadsby PJ. P/Q-type calcium-channel blockade in the periaqueductal gray facilitates trigeminal nociception: a functional genetic link for migraine? *J Neurosci*. 2002;22:RC213.

83. Bose P, Karsan N, Goadsby PJ. The migraine postdrome. *Continuum (Minneap Minn)*. 2018. https://doi.org/10.1212/CON.0000000000000626.

84. Ong JJY, de Felice M. Migraine treatment: current acute medications and their potential mechanisms of action. *Neurotherapeutics*. 2017. https://doi.org/10.1007/s13311-017-0592-1.

85. Ahn AH, Basbaum AI. Where do triptans act in the treatment of migraine? *Pain*. 2005. https://doi.org/10.1016/j.pain.2005.03.008.

86. Burstein R, Jakubowski M. Analgesic triptan action in an animal model of intracranial pain: a race against the development of central sensitization. *Ann Neurol*. 2004. https://doi.org/10.1002/ana.10785.

87. Edvinsson L. The CGRP pathway in migraine as a viable target for therapies. *Headache*. 2018. https://doi.org/10.1111/head.13305.

88. Edvinsson L. CGRP antibodies as prophylaxis in migraine. *Cell*. 2018. https://doi.org/10.1016/j.cell.2018.11.049.

89. Johnson KW, Morin SM, Wroblewski VJ, Johnson MP. Peripheral and central nervous system distribution of the CGRP neutralizing antibody [125I] galcanezumab in male rats. *Cephalalgia*. 2019. https://doi.org/10.1177/0333102419844711.

90. Holland PR, Goadsby PJ. Targeted CGRP small molecule antagonists for acute migraine therapy. *Neurotherapeutics*. 2018. https://doi.org/10.1007/s13311-018-0617-4.

91. Bigal ME, Ashina S, Burstein R, et al. Prevalence and characteristics of allodynia in headache sufferers: a population study. *Neurology*. 2008. https://doi.org/10.1212/01.wnl.0000310645.31020.b1.

92. Sachs M, Pape HC, Speckmann EJ, Gorji A. The effect of estrogen and progesterone on spreading depression in rat neocortical tissues. *Neurobiol Dis*. 2007. https://doi.org/10.1016/j.nbd.2006.08.013.

93. Faria V, Erpelding N, LeBel A, et al. The migraine brain in transition: girls vs boys. *Pain*. 2015. https://doi.org/10.1097/j.pain.0000000000000292.

Genetics of migraine ☆

4

Andrew D. Hershey, MD, PhD

When asking a family about headaches, many times they can identify multiple family members that intermittently have headaches. Oftentimes, the families view this as normal and have the perception that everybody has headaches. It is only when it becomes a *problem* that the families think that there may be a problem. This recognition that headaches "run in the family" is an early observation by families that headaches may have an inheritable or genetic pattern which can begin the discussion that headaches are a symptom of a disease. The understanding and discussion with a family that, what they are having is a disease with headaches being one of the symptoms, can be one of the first steps to improved treatment and outcome. Although several headache types, including the risk of developing a secondary headache, may have a genetic basis, this chapter will focus on migraine and its genetic component.

For migraine there is a balance between genetic components that are not changeable (i.e., genetic defects or polymorphisms) and genetic modifications (i.e., epigenetics and expression alterations). The modifiable genetic factors can be influenced by both external and internal environmental factors, thus serving as a point of intervention. The impact on fixed and modifiable genetic factors is likely explanation for the variation within families. For recurrent headaches in children and adolescents, the presence of a strong family history of headaches is often observed and has been suggested as a part of the criteria for the diagnosis of migraine.[1]

Understanding the genetic basis of headaches whether primary such as migraine or secondary with genetic risk factors, not only may be useful for the diagnosis but also advances the understanding of the pathophysiology of headaches. This is clearest for migraine where there have been up to 38 different polymorphisms related to migraine identified on large population studies, as well as specific genes identified for the rare migraine sub-types of hemiplegic migraine. The recognition of all these different genetic pathways involved with migraine suggests that migraine is really a

---

☆Editor's note: Dr. Hershey's contribution to our book is based upon the notion that headaches are not "just in your head." He offers advice to our readers as to how to use our understanding of migraine to help patients and families avoid the blame game. He also offers hope that one's fate is not sealed by rotten genes, but that we can overcome or at least minimize the effect of genetic predispositions.

Pediatric Headache. https://doi.org/10.1016/B978-0-323-83005-8.00017-3

polygenic disorder where the phenotypic features seen during the headache are a common end representation of these pathways.

A thorough review of the genetic basis of migraine is beyond the scope of this chapter but having a basic understanding of the foundation of these studies will help in guiding the approaches taken for diagnosis, treatment, and patient education. This extends from the observation of familial basis as observed in population studies to the molecular biology of the identified genes and the pathways involved.

Population studies. One of the central tenets of populations studies is to address whether a given disease occurs more often within a family than odds of it occurring independently. For common diseases like migraine, this high prevalence rate increases the chance occurrence within a family and thus increases the familial associations.

In order to address some of these issues, a study of 4000 individuals from the Danish Central Persons Registry with migraine with aura were compared to an equal number with migraine without aura as the probands.[2] When the results were analyzed, it was found that for migraines without aura, there was a 1.9-fold increased familial risk of having migraine without aura whereas unrelated spouses had a 1.5-fold increased risk, suggesting both genetic and environmental contributions for migraine without aura. The genetic influence was even greater for migraine with aura, with first-degree relatives having a fourfold increased risk of migraine with aura in contrast to no increase in spouses. Additionally, there appeared to be a generational effect seen where the greatest risk for having migraine without aura was seen in the children of probands—3.43-fold increase.[3]

Population Twin Studies. Twin studies are one way to address the question of genetic vs environmental contribution. Twins that are monozygotic (i.e., identical genetic make-up) can be compared to dizygotic twins (i.e., share approximately half their genes), while also adding in the contribution of shared vs independent environmental factors. One such study was based on the New Danish Twin Register of 2026 monozygotic twins and 3334 same-sex dizygotic.[4, 5] When proband comparison was performed, than the pairwise concordance rate was much higher for monozygotic twins (28%) compared with same-sex dizygotic twins (18%). While this study clearly identified a genetic factor in migraine, the lack of complete agreement (i.e., 100% comparison) identified the gap in this approach.

To address this, a population-based twin study of children, aged 8 to 9 years old, found that, of those children reporting a history of headaches, 79% of them were classified as migraine or tension type headaches.[6] Looking at the proband wise concordance, it was highest for monozygotic girls and boys at 0.52 and 0.51, followed by same-sex dizygotic boys and girls at 0.22 and 0.27, while for opposite-sex dizygotic children it was 0.15. This clearly demonstrated the genetic contribution for headaches and in particular, migraine.

Environmental influences. As none of these analyses revealed a 100% concordance, this suggested that there are additional non-genetic factors. To answer this question, researcher tested models of genetic and environmental contributions to explain concordance rates in monozygotic and dizygotic.[7] The best fit was found for a genetics contribution of 61%, while the environment contributed 39%—independent if shared or nonshared.

What do these population and twin studies mean for people affected by headache disorders? The most straight-forward explanation is that migraine is a genetic disease, but there are factors that can be modified to affect the impact of the disease and thus change the expression and outcome. What we can tell the patient is that we can't change your genes, but we can change how the genes are impacting your life.

Molecular Genetics. With the understanding of migraine as a genetic disease, the search for the actual genes continues to advance as we understand more about this polygenic disease.

Familial Hemiplegic Migraine. One of the first migraine disorders to begin to answer this question was familial hemiplegic migraine (FHM). This is a very rare, unique disorder where the patient develops clear one-sided weakness before or during the attack. Currently, the International Classification of Headaches (ICHD-3)[8] classifies this as a type of migraine with aura. In this regard, one must be clear to differentiate a sensory aura in which the patient is numb, thus not getting feedback for movement, from those that are truly weak. In this regard, the identification of the particular genetic mutation may be helpful in confirming the diagnosis, although when the familial nature has been identified, this is rarely needed.

Currently, there are 4 gene mutations identified for FHM – the calcium voltage-gated channel subunit alpha1 A (CACNA1A), the ATPase NA+/K+ transporting subunit alpha 2 (ATP1A2), the sodium voltage-gated channel alpha subunit 1 (SCN1A), and the proline rich transmembrane protein 2 (PRRT2). The first 3 of these are now classified with the corresponding 5th digit in the ICHD-3 as FHM type 1 (ICHD-3 1.2.3.1.1), FHM type 2 (ICHD-3 1.2.3.1.2) and FHM type 3 (ICHD-3 1.2.3.1.4), while the 4th falls into the FHM, other loci (ICHD-3 1.2.3.1.4). It is notable that the first 3 are all ion channels, thus suggesting the neurophysiologic disturbance as the etiology of the FHM. There are now several laboratories that can test for these mutations to provide identification and genetic counseling to the family. An updated review of this information can be found at the dedicated NIH website (https:/ghr.nlm.nih.gov/condition/familial-hemiplegic-migraine).

Migraine. The identification of gene association with migraine has grown significantly, and although most of these are associations and still need to prove direct cause and effect, they are enlightening as to possible etiologies. One of the largest approaches was an international consortium that complied the results of 375,000 individuals and identified 38 unique loci that increased the susceptibility of migraine.[9] This was a large collaborative undertaking and one of the largest advances in understanding the genetics of migraine. These genes can be roughly grouped into four categories: neurological genes, vascular genes, hormonal genes, and inflammatory genes.[10] This observation aligns well with previous hypothesized pathophysiology of migraine, while also demonstrating the widely different pathways that may be involved.

When multiple genes contribute to a single, identified disease we use the term polygenic, and can determine a polygenic risk score.[11] Applying this approach, an analysis can be performed that shows the impact of this risk. Applying such an analysis clearly demonstrated that FHM had the greatest risk score with an odds ratio of 1.96 (1.86–2.07), followed by migraine with typical aura-odds ratio 1.85 (1.79–1.91) and migraine without aura-odds ratio of 1.57 (1.51–1.63).[12] The risk score was highest in children and younger adolescents compared to late adolescents and adults, implying that the genetic contribution is clear for children and adolescents, while diminishing as people get older.

What does this identification of genes mean for patients? It confirms that migraine is a genetic disorder, and that multiple genes are likely to contribute to the headache characteristics and risk factors for progression as well as treatment. Thus, although migraine is a disease, it is a disease that is influenced by multiple different genes whose individual contributions and phenotype, make each persons' headache a little different.

Beyond genetics. As we begin to understand the wide variety of genes involved in migraine, the next step is to determine the impact of these genes and their expression. These areas of research continue to advance our understanding of the biological markers or fingerprints of an individual patient. This approach is exclusively in the research arena and includes genomic expression of mRNA, metabolomics, proteomics, and epigenetics. Through these areas of research, a further understanding of the pathophysiology should help with improved treatment and outcomes.

General practitioners

How can a general practitioner use this information? Having a basic understanding that recurrent headaches, especially migraine, runs in families, efforts to pursue this history can help solidify the diagnosis as well as comfort the patient by relating to other family members. Oftentimes, this is made difficult by several misperceptions that the family may have. This includes anchoring of the onset to a specific life event (i.e., a life stressor or mild head injury), a perception that the headaches of migraine are always severe and disabling when in fact moderate headaches also count, the perception that "doesn't everyone get headaches," or blaming the recurrent headaches on an external factor (i.e., sinus headaches). Beginning to recognize the pattern of recurrent headaches in families helps remove some of these barriers and help progress the concept of migraine as a genetic disease expressed as intermittent headaches of variable frequency.

Specialists

How can this information help a Headache Medicine specialist? Understanding the complexity of migraine as a polygenic disease with multiple genetic pathways involved can support the need for a broad number of treatment approaches needed to improve the outcomes of patients with migraine. This, not only, may include variable acute and preventive medication, but also use of biobehavioral and health habits to influence the pathways as well as potentially alter genomic expression and epigenetic changes. This understanding allows us to work with patients to explain that we may need to continually monitor and modify treatments to find their own unique combination of treatments to improve their headaches. Future treatments based upon genetic profiles are in their infancy, but may play a strong role as our testing gets more specific.

Families

What does this mean for patients and families? Knowing that the most significant risk factor of having headaches in a patient with migraine is genetic helps explain that migraine is a disease and not something that is a fault of the patient. The fact that the impact of these genes can be modified opens up possibilities for improvement, both on the individual and societal level. Having this understanding of migraine as a disease should also help remove some of the stigma that may exist for migraine.

Conclusions

Primary headaches, especially migraine, clearly have a genetic contribution that may be modifiable. The variety of genes identified can be clustered in groups of pathways. This understanding should serve as a strong foundation for the discovery of new treatments of all types and improve outcome. ICHD-3 has begun to recognize this future contribution, holding the 5th digit of the diagnostic coding for this genetic identification. It can be expected that this will continue to grow, as new unique genetic factors are identified. Additionally, as identification of these genes and screening methods and markers are identified, a broad spectrum screening of the genotype in co-association with phenotypic differences may help further identify the pathophysiological processes underlying migraine and chronic migraine. This identification of additional biomarkers should also assist with a more detailed diagnostic analysis of migraine with the variety of the genetic contribution of migraines elucidated.

References

1. Prensky AL, Sommer D. Diagnosis and treatment of migraine in children. *Neurology*. 1979;29:506–510.
2. Russell MB, Iselius L, Olesen J. Migraine without aura and migraine with aura are inherited disorders. *Cephalalgia*. 1996;16:305–309.
3. Russell MB. Genetic epidemiology of migraine and cluster headache. *Cephalalgia*. 1997;17:683–701.
4. Ulrich V, Gervil M, Kyvik KO, Olesen J, Russell MB. Evidence of a genetic factor in migraine with aura: a population-based Danish twin study. *Ann Neurol*. 1999;45 (2):242–246.

5. Gervil M, Ulrich V, Kyvik KO, Olesen J, Russell MB. Migraine without aura: a population-based twin study. *Ann Neurol.* 1999;46(4):606–611.
6. Svensson DA, Larsson B, Bille B, Lichtenstein P. Genetic and environmental influences on recurrent headaches in eight to nine-year-old twins. *Cephalalgia.* 1999;19 (10):866–872.
7. Gervil M, Ulrich V, Kaprio J, Olesen J, Russell MB. The relative role of genetic and environmental factors in migraine without aura. *Neurology.* 1999;53(5):995–999.
8. Headache Classification Committee of the International Headache Society (IHS) The International Classification of Headache Disorders, 3rd edition. *Cephalalgia.* 2018;38 (1):1–211.
9. Gormley P, Anttila V, Winsvold BS, et al. Meta-analysis of 375,000 individuals identifies 38 susceptibility loci for migraine. *Nat Genet.* 2016;48(8):856–866.
10. Persico AM, Verdecchia M, Pinzone V, Guidetti V. Migraine genetics: current findings and future lines of research. *Neurogenetics.* 2015;16(2):77–95.
11. Chalmer MA, Esserlind AL, Olesen J, Hansen TF. Polygenic risk score: use in migraine research. *J Headache Pain.* 2018;19(1):29.
12. Gormley P, Kurki MI, Hiekkala ME, et al. Common variant burden contributes to the familial aggregation of migraine in 1,589 families. *Neuron.* 2018;98(4):743–753.e4.

How did it get so bad?

III

The "episodic syndromes": I.e., what migraine looks like before it "looks like" migraine [☆]

5

Amy A. Gelfand, MD

Introduction

Migraine is much more than a headache. Migraine is actually a disorder of amplified or distorted sensory processing—where lights seem too bright and sounds too loud, where movement worsens the pain and there may be the illusory perception of movement (i.e., vertigo) and nausea/vomiting. There can also be symptoms—such as "brain fog," fatigue, and irritability - in the hours or days preceding and/or following the headache phase. Collectively, these non-headache symptoms and phases of migraine can contribute to migraine-related disability. These symptoms can be more debilitating than the headache itself, at least for some individuals. Some attacks may not even include headache as a symptom. Yet in the public perception, and even in the medical field, migraine continues to be perceived of as predominantly, "just a headache." This narrow recognition of only one slice of migraine can act as a disservice to patients. The problem is even greater for those who have an "episodic syndrome that may be associated with migraine," as these disorders are now referred to in the International Classification of Headache Disorders, 3rd edition (ICHD-3).[1] In this chapter, we will review these episodic syndromes with the view that they *are migraine*—they are just what migraine sometimes looks likes in the young, developing brain. These syndromes can be thought of as early life expressions of the genes that later in life express themselves as "typical" migraine. Saying these disorders *are migraine* does not imply that headache is present during the episodes. Migraine is so, so much more than just a headache. Some of these disorders can occur in adolescents and adults, or start in childhood and persist into adulthood. They are more commonly seen in children and will be presented from "youngest" to "oldest."

☆Editor's note: In these conditions, a baby or older child will present with a set of recurrent symptoms and then may eventually have migraine when older. Sadly, diagnosis is often delayed because we are not smart enough to think about these entities. This causes undue distress for families as their child has recurrent bouts of pain and disability. Making the diagnosis earlier provides a great source of comfort and makes the provider a superhero!

Pediatric Headache. https://doi.org/10.1016/B978-0-323-83005-8.00012-4

Infant colic

All babies cry. Some babies cry more than others. When a healthy and well-fed infant cries excessively, it is referred to as "colic."[2] Approximately, 5%–19% of infants have colic.[3] Crying follows a developmental pattern. Infants generally cry little during the first couple weeks of life. Crying increases around 2 weeks of life, peaks around 5 to 6 weeks of life, then tapers down by 3 months of age.[4, 5] Infant crying also follows a circadian pattern, with more crying in the late afternoon or evening hours.[4] Infant colic may be an amplified version of this normal crying pattern; the infants cry more, and often inconsolably. Inconsolable crying is associated with caregiver frustration and, tragically, shaken baby syndrome—a form of child abuse.[5] For decades infant colic was thought to be due to abdominal pain—either gas or something related to feeding- but those theories don't necessarily fit. All that is clear is that the baby is in distress. It is impossible to know whether from pain or from something else.

A link between migraine and infant colic has been noted now in a number of studies. Children with migraine are more likely to have been colicky as infants.[6–8] Children with tension-type headache are not.[8] In a prospective, population-based cohort study, infant colic was associated with a more than $2\times$ increase in likelihood of migraine without aura by age 18.[9] Mothers with migraine are more likely to have babies with colic, though fathers with migraine are not.[3, 10]

What might explain this link between migraine and infant colic? Remember that migraine is a disorder of amplified or distorted sensory processing, and migraine has a strong genetic link.[11–13] Perhaps babies who inherit migraine genes experience the world differently than those who do not. The new stimuli they encounter in the world may be perceived in an amplified way in their brains. After a long day of amplified stimulation, the infants may express feeling overwhelmed through prolonged crying. If this is the case, then decreasing stimulation around the infant may be helpful. There is some evidence that advising parents to turn down the lights and avoid noisy toys may help with colicky crying.[14] Around the age of 3 months, the infant's brain starts to produce melatonin in a circadian pattern[15] and they can begin to consolidate nighttime sleep. Sleeping for longer stretches may help colicky infants recover from stimulation during the day, leading to less crying around this age. Clearly there is much more to be understood about infant crying in general. However, excessive, fussy crying may be how migraine (read as "excessive sensitivity to stimuli," not headache) looks in the young infant brain.

Key points for families

- Crying may be your baby's way of saying they need a break, particularly if there is a family history of migraine in Mom. Consider limiting the number of people in the room, turning down the lights, avoiding loud sounds, etc. If you find yourself getting overwhelmed, lay the baby down on their back in the crib and leave the room.

Key points for the primary care provider

- If a child you saw for colic as an infant returns later in childhood complaining of headaches with photophobia, phonophobia, and/or nausea/vomiting, think migraine.
- When seeing a colicky baby, ask if there is a maternal history of migraine. If so, consider recommending decreasing stimulation levels, rather than perhaps a change in maternal diet or infant formula.

Key points for the headache specialist

- Asking about a history of infant colic can be informative diagnostically.
- Counsel pregnant women with migraine that they are more likely to have a colicky infant but reassure them that infant colic is time-limited and will pass.

Benign paroxysmal torticollis (BPT)

This disorder typically starts during the first 6 months of infancy and resolves by pre-school age.[16, 17] It is characterized by recurrent episodes of head-tilt (i.e., torticollis), accompanied by irritability, fussing, pallor, and/or nausea/vomiting.[1] Episodes may last for hours to days. The other symptoms may resolve while the head-tilt continues for a longer time. Once the child is old enough to crawl or walk, ataxia (wobbly walking) during episodes may become apparent as well. Attacks usually come at regular intervals. For example, a child may experience an attack every 6 weeks. However, the episodes tend to space further apart as the child ages.

Many children with BPT will have a family history of migraine. Children with BPT may be more likely to develop migraine than other children. This is especially true in children with BPT who have features of migraine—sensitivity to light, sound, or movement—during their attacks.[18] (This may be how migraine looks in the young, developing brain). In some cases, a gene associated with familial hemiplegic migraine (CACNA1A) has been seen in infants with BPT.[19–22]

As BPT is rare, there is limited information about how to treat it. Given the young age of the children, many families may not be interested in a daily preventive medication. Diagnosing BPT and explaining what to expect over time is often adequate. When nausea/vomiting is severe, acute treatment with an anti-nausea medicine may be reasonable.

While called "benign," children with BPT may experience developmental delay.[22, 23] Most often seen is gross motor delay, but delays in other areas have also been reported.[16] It is possible that spending several days a month experiencing a head-tilt makes it harder to progress in gross motor development, rather than delay being indicative of an underlying problem per se. Notably, once the episodes resolve, many of the children do catch up developmentally. There can be an impact on the family as well. As BPT is rare, many pediatricians are not familiar with it and there is commonly a delay in diagnosis. In one study, only 2.4% of pediatricians were aware of BPT.[24] The diagnostic delay and associated testing can be stressful and anxiety-provoking for parents. Parents may also worry about triggering an attack, or about delays in their child's development or their ability to engage in "normal" childhood activities. In one study, Infant Toddler Quality of Life scale scores helped to quantify the impact of BPT on infants and their families.[18] Some children with BPT may go on to develop benign paroxysmal vertigo.[23]

Key points for families

- Talk to your child's pediatrician if you think your child has BPT. Because this is rare, bringing information about it to your child's doctor may help them to make an accurate diagnosis.
- If your child has nausea/vomiting during attacks, ask your child's pediatrician if an anti-nausea medication would be appropriate.

Key points for the primary care provider

- BPT is a disorder characterized by recurrent attacks of head-tilt (torticollis), associated with pallor, irritability, ataxia, and/or nausea/vomiting in an infant or young child. It is important to recognize, in order to avoid diagnostic delay and associated distress for the family.
- Screen children with BPT for developmental delay and refer to services as appropriate.

Key points for the headache specialist

- Ask about a history of BPT, particularly in patients presenting with familial hemiplegic migraine. Consider testing for the CACNA1A mutation.

Benign paroxysmal vertigo (BPV)

While most migrainous phenomena lasts for hours to days, BPV attacks most commonly last for just a few minutes. BPV occurs predominantly in preschool aged children[25] and is one of the more common causes of vertigo in young children.[26, 27] In BPV, attacks of vertigo come "out of the blue"; the child may suddenly appear scared or fall down to the ground. There may be accompanying nystagmus, and epilepsy is on the differential. Attacks usually last for less than 5 min, though they can go for longer. Typically, children outgrow BPT after a few years,[25] but like the other disorders, it can persist.[28] There is often a family history of migraine and children with BPV are more likely to grow up to have migraine.[25, 28]

As attacks are so brief, acute and preventive treatments are not usually needed. If the attacks are occurring multiple times a day, migraine preventive treatment could be considered. In this instance however, often video telemetry would be needed first to rule out epilepsy.

Key points for families

- Ask your child's doctor if you think your child may have BPV.
- Your child's BPV attacks may be frightening to watch. Fortunately, they are generally brief and usually children outgrow them after a couple of years.

Key points for the primary care provider

- Asking about a family history of migraine may help to diagnose BPV.
- Referral to neurology is indicated if the child is having frequent attacks, or there is nystagmus or alteration of consciousness with attacks as epilepsy may need to be ruled out.

Key points for the headache specialist

- If a migraine preventive is indicated, melatonin gummies or propranolol liquid could be considered. Propranolol has been studied for treatment of infantile hemangioma,[29] so safety and dosing in this young age group has been established.

Abdominal migraine

Abdominal migraine involves repeated attacks of abdominal pain. The abdominal pain tends to be all over the belly or periumbilical (i.e., around the "belly button"). The pain feels dull or "just sore."[1] Other symptoms include nausea, vomiting, feeling unwell, looking pale, and/or not wanting to eat.[1] Migrainous symptoms, such as sensitivity to light or sound, may be present.[30] School-aged children are most often affected,[30, 31] though abdominal migraine can also occur in adults.[32] There is often a family history of migraine. Those with abdominal migraine are more likely to go on to develop migraine (i.e., the headache form) once they grow older.[30, 33, 34] The author has also seen children who describe typical visual migraine aura preceding attacks of abdominal migraine.

Even though children localize the pain to their abdomens, it is not clear that anything pathological is occurring in that area. It may be that thalamic processing develops over time, and what is perceived as "abdominal" pain in the young brain will later be perceived as "head" pain in the older brain. While ICHD-3 specifies that if headache is present during attacks, the diagnosis to consider is migraine rather than abdominal migraine,[1] this author has found it hard to draw a distinct line where children cross from one diagnosis to another. It is not unusual to see a child who at age 7 describes attacks of abdominal pain, then by age 10, attacks include both abdominal and head pain, and then by age 12 or 13, attacks are described as headache and the abdomen is no longer mentioned. Calcitonin gene-related peptide (CGRP) is expressed in the gastrointestinal tract, and is involved in migraine pathophysiology.[35] It is possible that CGRP expression patterns evolve over the course of childhood development. For example, in a guinea pig animal model, mesenteric peptidergic nerve plexus density was highest at birth and decreased to half the density by age 2 years.[36] It is also possible that the developmental changes are all occurring in the brain, and how the brain processes, perceives, and localizes signals within the body.

While there has been little research in treating abdominal migraine, a small study demonstrated that pizotifen was superior to placebo for migraine prevention.[37] In the United States, cyproheptadine would probably be the most analogous medication. In our pediatric headache program at the University of California San Francisco, we have successfully treated children with "status abdominal migrainosus" with intravenous dihydroergotamine. However, if we view abdominal migraine as migraine—just a phenotypic variant along the age spectrum—then it follows that anything used to treat migraine could also reasonably be used to treat abdominal migraine.

Key points for families

- Abdominal migraine is best thought of as a form of migraine.
- Abdominal migraine may be treated using treatments used for migraine.

Key points for the primary care provider

- Abdominal migraine symptoms do not necessarily indicate that anything pathologic is occurring in the gastrointestinal tract.

Key points for the headache specialist

- Abdominal migraine may evolve into migraine over the course of several years.
- Consider using migraine treatments for treatment of abdominal migraine.

Cyclical vomiting syndrome (CVS)

Cyclical vomiting syndrome is characterized by repeated episodes of intense nausea and vomiting, often with abdominal pain. Patients tend to wake up out of sleep at a particular time of night with symptoms. For example, a typical history would be, "Every 8 weeks she wakes up between 2:00 and 4:00 am with vomiting, and it lasts for 24 h." The vomiting can be severe. Patients may need to go to the emergency department for rehydration. CVS is most common in school-age children, but teens and adults can be affected.

It is important to ensure that the child is normal in between episodes, and not experiencing developmental regression or delay or seizures. Recurrent vomiting episodes with any of these other red flags would suggest a possible inborn error of metabolism or one of the developmental occipital lobe epilepsies such as Gastaut-type epilepsy or Panayiotopoulos syndrome.[38, 39] Gastrointestinal pathology is also on the differential.

In an adolescent patient presenting with symptoms concerning for CVS, it is essential to ask about cannabis use. This can be done as part of a HEADSS assessment with the adolescent alone. Cannabinoid hyperemesis syndrome (CHS) can mimic CVS and cause episodes of intense nausea/vomiting.[40–43] It most commonly occurs in those who use cannabis daily or near daily, and who have been doing so for months to years, but can occur even with less frequent or shorter duration use.[40, 41] Patients may engage in hot water bathing behavior during episodes, though this is not specific to CHS and can be seen in those with CVS as well. Prolonged use of cannabinoids can lead to downregulation of central cannabinoid receptors (CB1 receptor).[41, 43] Under normal circumstances, endogenous endocannabinoids would be released and bind the CB1 receptors to help prevent nausea when the body is under stress. Downregulation of these receptors inhibits this system. Unfortunately, cannabis is stored in fat tissues, so even once intake has ceased, it can still take weeks to months for stores to empty and receptor patterns to return to normal levels. Thus, symptoms do not necessarily improve with just a few weeks of abstaining from cannabis, which can lead adolescents to conclude that their cannabis use was not the problem. To determine definitively whether cannabis use is contributing to symptoms, several months' abstention may be needed.[43] It is possible that individuals with CVS have a naturally down-regulated CB1 receptor system, and certain genotypes of this receptor are associated with CVS risk.[43, 44] Cannabis use may mimic "primary CVS" by provoking the same phenotype.[41]

Treatment of cyclic vomiting syndrome can be challenging. For one thing, vomiting can be so profuse and rapid in onset that oral routes of administration are often simply untenable. Nasal sprays, intramuscular or subcutaneous injections, and rectal suppository routes may be preferable (though teens generally do not favor the latter). If there is a gap between onset of symptoms and vomiting, oral administration of a rapidly dissolving antiemetic may facilitate administration of oral NSAIDs or triptans. If the patient needs IV fluid rehydration, acute medications can also be given intravenously. For prevention, a trial in children found comparable effectiveness of amitriptyline and cyproheptadine.[45] A second trial comparing amitriptyline to topiramate favored amitriptyline.[46] The neurokinin-1 receptor antagonist, aprepitant, may help both acutely or as a preventive taken twice weekly.[47]

Key points for families

- To avoid emergency department visits plan ahead-of-time with your doctor. Make sure you know what to use as first-line treatment, and what to use for back-up treatment.
- Have an honest conversation with your teenager about cannabis use. Make sure your teenager understands that using cannabis may trigger episodes of vomiting.

Key points for the primary care provider

- Care coordination among multiple specialists may be needed to get to a clear diagnosis of CVS.
- Your long-term relationship with your adolescent patients may make them trust you enough to disclose cannabis use, and you may be best at motivating them to give cannabis cessation a trial of adequate duration.

Key points for headache specialists

- Differential diagnosis for CVS includes inborn errors of metabolism, gastrointestinal pathology, and cannabinoid hyperemesis syndrome.
- Preventive treatment considerations include: amitriptyline, cyproheptadine, and aprepitant.
- Acute treatment may need to be through a non-oral route.

Conclusions

Migraine is a disorder of amplified or distorted sensory perception.[35] The disorders currently referred to in ICHD-3 as "episodic syndromes that may be associated with migraine[1]," namely: benign paroxysmal torticollis, benign paroxysmal vertigo, abdominal migraine, cyclic vomiting syndrome, and infant colic (appendix section), can best be thought of as developmentally phenotypically distinct manifestations of migraine. Formal studies are needed to guide treatment of each sub form. In the meantime, a useful starting point would be to think of them as migraine and to manage them as such.

References

1. Headache Classification Committee of the International Headache Society (IHS) The International Classification of Headache Disorders, 3rd edition. *Cephalalgia*. 2018;38 (1):1–211.
2. Wessel MA, Cobb JC, Jackson EB, Harris Jr GS, Detwiler AC. Paroxysmal fussing in infancy, sometimes called colic. *Pediatrics*. 1954;14(5):421–435.
3. Gelfand AA, Thomas KC, Goadsby PJ. Before the headache: infant colic as an early life expression of migraine. *Neurology*. 2012;79(13):1392–1396.
4. Brazelton TB. Crying in infancy. *Pediatrics*. 1962;29:579–588.
5. Barr RG, Trent RB, Cross J. Age-related incidence curve of hospitalized Shaken Baby Syndrome cases: convergent evidence for crying as a trigger to shaking. *Child Abuse Negl*. 2006;30(1):7–16.
6. Jan MM, Al-Buhairi AR. Is infantile colic a migraine-related phenomenon? *Clin Pediatr (Phila)*. 2001;40(5):295–297.
7. Bruni O, Fabrizi P, Ottaviano S, Cortesi F, Giannotti F, Guidetti V. Prevalence of sleep disorders in childhood and adolescence with headache: a case-control study. *Cephalalgia*. 1997;17(4):492–498.

8. Romanello S, Spiri D, Marcuzzi E, et al. Association between childhood migraine and history of infantile colic. *JAMA*. 2013;309(15):1607–1612.

9. Sillanpaa M, Saarinen M. Infantile colic associated with childhood migraine: a prospective cohort study. *Cephalalgia*. 2015;35:1246–1251.

10. Gelfand AA, Buse DC, Cabana MD, Grimes B, Goadsby PJ, Allen IE. The association between parental migraine and infant colic: a cross-sectional, web-based, US Survey Study. *Headache*. 2019;59(7):988–1001.

11. Gervil M, Ulrich V, Kaprio J, Olesen J, Russell MB. The relative role of genetic and environmental factors in migraine without aura. *Neurology*. 1999;53(5):995–999.

12. Ulrich V, Gervil M, Kyvik KO, Olesen J, Russell MB. Evidence of a genetic factor in migraine with aura: a population-based Danish twin study. *Ann Neurol*. 1999;45 (2):242–246.

13. Russell MB. Is migraine a genetic illness? The various forms of migraine share a common genetic cause. *Neurol Sci*. 2008;29(Suppl 1):S52–S54.

14. McKenzie S. Troublesome crying in infants: effect of advice to reduce stimulation. *Arch Dis Child*. 1991;66(12):1416–1420.

15. Kennaway DJ, Goble FC, Stamp GE. Factors influencing the development of melatonin rhythmicity in humans. *J Clin Endocrinol Metab*. 1996;81(4):1525–1532.

16. Rosman NP, Douglass LM, Sharif UM, Paolini J. The neurology of benign paroxysmal torticollis of infancy: report of 10 new cases and review of the literature. *J Child Neurol*. 2009;24(2):155–160.

17. Drigo P, Carli G, Laverda AM. Benign paroxysmal torticollis of infancy. *Brain Dev*. 2000;22(3):169–172.

18. Greene KA, Lu V, Luciano MS, et al. Benign paroxysmal torticollis: phenotype, natural history, and quality of life. *Pediatr Res*. 2021. https://doi.org/10.1038/s41390-020-01309-1.

19. Giffin NJ, Benton S, Goadsby PJ. Benign paroxysmal torticollis of infancy: four new cases and linkage to CACNA1A mutation. *Dev Med Child Neurol*. 2002;44(7):490–493.

20. Vila-Pueyo M, Gene GG, Flotats-Bastardes M, et al. A loss-of-function CACNA1A mutation causing benign paroxysmal torticollis of infancy. *Eur J Paediatr Neurol*. 2014;18:430–433.

21. Roubertie A, Echenne B, Leydet J, et al. Benign paroxysmal tonic upgaze, benign paroxysmal torticollis, episodic ataxia and CACNA1A mutation in a family. *J Neurol*. 2008;255 (10):1600–1602.

22. Humbertclaude V, Krams B, Nogue E, et al. Benign paroxysmal torticollis, benign paroxysmal vertigo, and benign tonic upward gaze are not benign disorders. *Dev Med Child Neurol*. 2018;60(12):1256–1263.

23. Brodsky J, Kaur K, Shoshany T, Lipson S, Zhou G. Benign paroxysmal migraine variants of infancy and childhood: transitions and clinical features. *Eur J Paediatr Neurol*. 2018;22 (4):667–673.

24. Hadjipanayis A, Efstathiou E, Neubauer D. Benign paroxysmal torticollis of infancy: an underdiagnosed condition. *J Paediatr Child Health*. 2015;51:674–678.

25. Batuecas-Caletrio A, Martin-Sanchez V, Cordero-Civantos C, et al. Is benign paroxysmal vertigo of childhood a migraine precursor? *Eur J Paediatr Neurol*. 2013;17(4):397–400.

26. Davitt M, Delvecchio MT, Aronoff SC. The differential diagnosis of Vertigo in children: a systematic review of 2726 cases. *Pediatr Emerg Care*. 2020;36(8):368–371. https://doi.org/10.1097/PEC.0000000000001281.

27. Lee JD, Kim CH, Hong SM, et al. Prevalence of vestibular and balance disorders in children and adolescents according to age: a multi-center study. *Int J Pediatr Otorhinolaryngol*. 2017;94:36–39.

28. Krams B, Echenne B, Leydet J, Rivier F, Roubertie A. Benign paroxysmal vertigo of childhood: long-term outcome. *Cephalalgia*. 2011;31(4):439–443.

29. Leaute-Labreze C, Hoeger P, Mazereeuw-Hautier J, et al. A randomized, controlled trial of oral propranolol in infantile hemangioma. *N Engl J Med*. 2015;372(8):735–746.

30. Abu-Arafeh I, Russell G. Prevalence and clinical features of abdominal migraine compared with those of migraine headache. *Arch Dis Child*. 1995;72(5):413–417.

31. Mortimer MJ, Kay J, Jaron A. Clinical epidemiology of childhood abdominal migraine in an urban general practice. *Dev Med Child Neurol*. 1993;35(3):243–248.

32. Roberts JE, deShazo RD. Abdominal migraine, another cause of abdominal pain in adults. *Am J Med*. 2012;125(11):1135–1139.

33. Dignan F, Abu-Arafeh I, Russell G. The prognosis of childhood abdominal migraine. *Arch Dis Child*. 2001;84(5):415–418.

34. Symon DN, Russell G, Abu-Arafeh I, Dignan F. Abdominal migraine. *Cephalalgia*. 2003;23(3):242 [author reply 242].

35. Goadsby PJ, Holland PR, Martins-Oliveira M, Hoffmann J, Schankin C, Akerman S. Pathophysiology of migraine: a disorder of sensory processing. *Physiol Rev*. 2017;97(2):553–622.

36. Russell FA, King R, Smillie SJ, Kodji X, Brain SD. Calcitonin gene-related peptide: physiology and pathophysiology. *Physiol Rev*. 2014;94(4):1099–1142.

37. Symon DN, Russell G. Double blind placebo controlled trial of pizotifen syrup in the treatment of abdominal migraine. *Arch Dis Child*. 1995;72(1):48–50.

38. Gelfand AA, Gallagher RC. Cyclic vomiting syndrome versus inborn errors of metabolism: a review with clinical recommendations. *Headache*. 2016;56(1):215–221.

39. Fitzgerald M, Crushell E, Hickey C. Cyclic vomiting syndrome masking a fatal metabolic disease. *Eur J Pediatr*. 2013;172(5):707–710.

40. Simonetto DA, Oxentenko AS, Herman ML, Szostek JH. Cannabinoid hyperemesis: a case series of 98 patients. *Mayo Clin Proc*. 2012;87(2):114–119.

41. Venkatesan T, Levinthal DJ, Li BUK, et al. Role of chronic cannabis use: cyclic vomiting syndrome vs cannabinoid hyperemesis syndrome. *Neurogastroenterol Motil*. 2019;31 (Suppl 2):e13606.

42. Wallace EA, Andrews SE, Garmany CL, Jelley MJ. Cannabinoid hyperemesis syndrome: literature review and proposed diagnosis and treatment algorithm. *South Med J*. 2011;104 (9):659–664.

43. Hasler WL, Levinthal DJ, Tarbell SE, et al. Cyclic vomiting syndrome: pathophysiology, comorbidities, and future research directions. *Neurogastroenterol Motil*. 2019;31(Suppl 2):e13607.

44. Wasilewski A, Lewandowska U, Mosinska P, et al. Cannabinoid receptor type 1 and mu-opioid receptor polymorphisms are associated with cyclic vomiting syndrome. *Am J Gastroenterol*. 2017;112(6):933–939.

45. Badihian N, Saneian H, Badihian S, Yaghini O. Prophylactic therapy of cyclic vomiting syndrome in children: comparison of amitriptyline and cyproheptadine: a randomized clinical trial. *Am J Gastroenterol*. 2018;113(1):135–140.

46. Bagherian Z, Yaghini O, Saneian H, Badihian S. Comparison of the efficacy of amitriptyline and topiramate in prophylaxis of cyclic vomiting syndrome. *Iran J Child Neurol.* 2019;13(1):37–44.
47. Cristofori F, Thapar N, Saliakellis E, et al. Efficacy of the neurokinin-1 receptor antagonist aprepitant in children with cyclical vomiting syndrome. *Aliment Pharmacol Ther.* 2014;40(3):309–317.

Effect of hormones

Ann Pakalnis, MD and Kevin Weber, MD

Effect of hormones: What a headache specialist needs to know

Migraine has long been thought to be more common in boys prior to age 12, and in girls and women after that.[1] Other studies have not shown a difference between boys and girls prior to puberty, or even that girls still have a higher prevalence of migraine than boys prior to puberty.[2] Regardless, prevalence of migraine in women rises sharply at puberty. The increase at puberty is thought to be due to the influence of female sex hormones on migraine. Estrogen is thought to be excitatory, progesterone inhibitory. Cyclic fluctuations in these hormones can contribute to migraine.[3] Estrogen reduces the threshold for cortical spreading depression, the putative mechanism for migraine with aura, whereas testosterone increases the threshold for cortical spreading depression.[4]

That estrogen is excitatory and reduces the threshold for cortical spreading depression is fascinating, since many women have pure menstrual migraine or menstrually-related migraine. The International Classification of Headache Disorders Edition Three (ICHD-3), defines both pure menstrual migraine and menstrually-related migraine in its appendix. Pure menstrual migraine is defined as migraine attacks occurring on day − 2 to + 3 of the menstrual cycle in two out of three cycles, and at no other time during the menstrual cycle. Menstrually-related migraine's definition is similar, with the additional allowance of having migraine attacks outside of menses.[5] Prior to menses, estrogen *decreases*. These declining levels of estrogen correlate with increasing migraine attack frequency.[6] Therefore, it is thought that estrogen *withdrawal* could play a role in pure menstrual migraine and menstrually-related migraine. Accordingly, 70% women using combined oral

---

☆Editor's note: Adult headache clinics are frequented mostly by women. Pediatric practitioners see lots of young boys and girls with headache, but a larger portion of the teenage patients are girls. This comprehensive chapter reviews the literature regarding the connection of hormones to migraine. It helps us unravel the association between migraine with aura and stroke risk and debunks some myths about oral contraceptives in patients with migraine. We learn about how migraine may change during the gender reassignment process. Toward the end, the authors offer advice on how to speak with families about these issues in a gentle but informative way.

Pediatric Headache. https://doi.org/10.1016/B978-0-323-83005-8.00029-X

contraceptives (COCs) reported headaches during the hormone-free "placebo" period at menses in one study.[7]

COCs have long been studied in relationship to migraine. A recent systematic review by the European Headache Federation (EHF) and the European Society of Contraception and Reproductive Health (ESCRH) found that there is low quality evidence for any hormonal interventions in migraine. Desogestrel 75 µg/day was shown to improve migraine in women with both migraine with and without aura, but not necessarily related to menstruation. Studies were limited to women taking this medication for gynecologic (medical or for contraception) reasons and not specifically for migraine. In some women desogestrel actually worsened migraine, and has been found to have an unfavorable side effect profile (bleeding). Extended COC use without placebo hormone-free intervals has been studied in the observational setting and may improve migraine outcomes in women. Only one study looked at strictly migraine patients and only one (a different study) study looked at comparison between traditional 21 day on and 7 day off COC and extended COC use without hormone-free interval. All studies, again, evaluated patients using COCs for gynecologic reasons, not strictly for migraine. Finally, estradiol gel has limited evidence for benefit in menstrual migraine, however the challenge of dosing and timing remains elusive. This was recommended for women with stable, predictable menstrual cycles and brings the risk of withdrawal headache (delayed headache) after the estrogen gel period stops.[5]

The EHF and ESCRH pointed out in the above systematic review and recommendations statement that COCs were not recommended in patients with migraine with aura. There has been concern for long and many studies about the increased risk of stroke in migraine with aura patients taking COCs. A recent systematic review[8] found limited evidence to support that fear. While there was a relative increase stroke risk demonstrated in migraine with aura patients taking COCs, there was not sufficient data to evaluate if this was a (estrogen) dose-dependent relationship. Interestingly, newer studies did not show as strong of a relationship between stroke risk and COC use in migraine patients as the older studies did. Estrogen dosing now tends to be lower than it was in the past.[9] This is a significant opportunity for further study in this area, as many women with migraine with aura could benefit from COCs for gynecologic reasons, and either they or their physicians (or both) are hesitant to prescribe these medications based on concern for stroke risk. It is important to remember that absolute stroke risk remains low even in migraine with aura patients taking COCs, and as always, a risk/benefit discussion between patient and provider is warranted in case of gynecological need for COCs in these patients.

Hormone fluctuation may also play a role in men. A recent study showed a decrease in testosterone levels and relative increase in estrogen levels in men with migraine compared to controls.[10] Another study showed low levels of testosterone in men with chronic migraine,[11] defined by the ICHD-3 as headaches more than 15 days per month, with at least 8 of those days being migraine.[8] Future research will show if supplementing testosterone can be used as a treatment for migraine in men. Limited previous research has shown a role for supplemental testosterone in both men and women with another primary headache, cluster headache.[12]

With an increasing number of transgender adolescents and young adults taking supplemental hormones for gender reassignment, addressing migraine in this population is important. A Dutch survey of male to female transgender individuals on supplemental estrogen after gender reassignment surgery showed a prevalence of 25%, which is similar to that of women in the general population.[13] Another Italian study showed an increase in headaches in male to female transgender patients on supplemental estrogen, as well as a decrease in female to male patients on supplemental testosterone.[14] Further study in this area may focus on treatment options for transgender individuals on supplemental hormones, as well as, if there is any increased stroke risk with supplemental estrogen in this population.

Non-hormonal treatments are commonly used to treat menstrual migraine. A small double-blind, placebo-controlled study of menstrual migraine patients found that a group given 360 mg of magnesium pyrrolidone carboxylic acid supplemented daily for 2 months had reduced headache days vs. placebo,[15] Naproxen 550 mg twice daily from day −7 to day +6 of the menstrual cycle showed reduction of headache days, as well as migraine intensity and duration in menstrual migraine patients.[16] Triptans have also been extensively studied in menstrual migraine. There were two positive trials for frovatriptan 2.5 mg once or twice daily from day −2 to day +4,[17,18] There was one positive trial for naratriptan 1 mg twice daily for five days starting day −2 to day +3.[19] Finally, there was one positive trial for zolmitriptan 2.5 mg twice daily or three times daily from day-2 to day +5.[20] Frovatriptan, naratriptan, and zolmitriptan are three of the longest-acting triptans, so it makes sense why they would be used as prophylaxis in this setting.

A headache specialist should be prepared to ask and receive questions about pure menstrual migraine and menstrually-related migraine management, stroke risk in patients with migraine with aura taking COCs, and hormonal supplementation and migraine. In the years to come, expect further research on these topics as there is a paucity of data, particularly regarding COC estrogen dose and stroke risk and hormonal treatment of menstrual migraine.

The relationship between migraine and hormones: Information to help children and families

Migraine is very common in children and teenagers with about 1 in 10 children and slightly more teenagers suffering from recurrent migraine attacks.[21] Migraine attacks are severe headaches usually occurring in families that often times start to first occur in girls around time of menarche. Monthly hormonal changes are thought to be associated sometimes with onset of migraine especially during the menstrual period.[22] If hormonal changes are affecting headaches, it is important for girls and their families to keep headache diaries to track their monthly headaches and how it relates to their menstrual cycle. Some research has suggested that teen girls with menstrually related migraine had a monthly pattern to their headaches even before their first period.[23] In particular, changes in the hormone estrogen are thought to be most likely to be associated with migraine. This relationship tends to persist going forward into adult years, with migraine about three times more common in adult women than men.[24]

Keeping diaries or journals of headaches is important to keep track of hormonal effects. Good lifestyle practices are important to follow in general, and getting enough exercise and good nutrition and maintaining healthy weight are the first line in management of these headaches. Studies suggest that being significantly overweight can worsen migraine frequency and severity, losing weight can lessen the number of headaches.[25]

When migraine attacks appear to be significantly hormone related, various options for treatment exists in addition to the frequently prescribed medications to take at the onset of a migraine or prevent headaches. Combination oral contraceptives or birth control pills are often prescribed in teenage girls for many reasons, besides for birth control. They can be used to treat acne and also irregular/heavy menstrual periods.[26] Research studies in adult women have shown that combination oral contraceptives containing the hormones estrogen and progesterone can sometimes improve migraine headache frequency, however, sometimes, they can worsen migraine in some. When taking birth control pills with estrogen, most of the migraine attacks tend to happen during the placebo or pill-free week after taking 21 days of active hormone pills. This is probably related to estrogen levels dropping at that time. Omitting the pill free week and going ahead to the next 3 weeks of active hormone present pills can block some of these hormonally related migraine attacks.[27]

In girls with migraine with aura, accompanied by visual changes or numbness in their extremities before the headache, combination oral contraceptives are contraindicated and should be used with caution. There may be some increased risk of stroke in these girls using this combination contraceptive therapy with estrogen and progesterone, although there may be mitigating factors. Other lifestyle issues or medical problems such as cigarette smoking or high blood pressure can increase risk of stroke in teen girls with migraine who are taking this type of birth control pill. Combination oral contraceptives can be used safely in most teen girls with migraine without aura. In some teenagers aura symptoms can start when first using combination birth control pills due to the higher estrogen levels. It is important to discuss with your health care provider, if migraine attacks change their pattern.[28] It is known that pregnancy carries a much higher risk of stroke complications than taking birth control pills. Other alternative forms of contraception should be discussed if increased stroke risk is present, such as migraine with aura, cigarette smoking, high blood pressure or other genetic factors that may be present.

References

1. Abu-Arefeh I, Russell G. Prevalence of headache and migraine in schoolchildren. *BMJ.* 1994;309(6957):765–769. https://doi.org/10.1136/bmj.309.6957.765.
2. Abu-Arafeh I, Razak S, Sivaraman B, Graham C. Prevalence of headache and migraine in children and adolescents: a systematic review of population-based studies. *Dev Med Child Neurol.* 2010;52:1088–1097. https://doi.org/10.1111/j.1469-8749.2010.03793.x.
3. Borsook D, Erpelding N, Lebel A, et al. Sex and the migraine brain. *Neurobiol Dis.* 2014;68:200–214. https://doi.org/10.1016/j.nbd.2014.03.008.
4. Eikermann-Haerter K, Baum MJ, Ferrari MD, van den Maagdenberg AM, Moskowitz MA, Ayata C. Androgenic suppression of spreading depression in familial hemiplegic migraine type 1 mutant mice. *Ann Neurol.* 2009;66(4):564–568. https://doi.org/10.1002/ana.21779.
5. Sacco S, Merki-Feld GS, Ægidius KL, et al. Effect of exogenous estrogens and progestogens on the course of migraine during reproductive age: a consensus statement by the European Headache Federation (EHF) and the European Society of Contraception and Reproductive Health (ESCRH). *J Headache Pain.* 2018;19(1):76. Published 2018 Aug 31. https://doi.org/10.1186/s10194-018-0896-5.
6. MacGregor EA, et al. Incidence of migraine relative to menstrual cycle phases of rising and falling estrogen. *Neurology.* 2006;67(12):2154–2158. Web. 06 Oct. 2019.
7. Sulak PJ, Scow RD, Preece C, Riggs MW, Kuehl TJ. Hormone withdrawal symptoms in oral contracep-tive users. *Obstet Gynecol.* 2000;95:261–266.
8. Headache Classification Committee of the International Headache Society (IHS). The international classification of headache disorders, 3rd edition. *Cephalalgia.* 2018;38:1–211.
9. Sheikh HU, Pavlovic J, Loder E, Burch R. Risk of stroke associated with use of estrogen containing contraceptives in women with migraine: a systematic review. *Headache.* 2018;58:5–21. https://doi.org/10.1111/head.13229.
10. van Oosterhout WPJ, Schoonman GG, van Zwet EW, et al. Female sex hormones in men with migraine. *Neurology.* 2018;91:e374–e381. https://doi.org/10.1212/WNL.0000000000005855.
11. Shields LBE, Seifert T, Shelton BJ, Plato BM. Testosterone levels in men with chronic migraine. *Neurol Int.* 2019;11(2):8079. Published 2019 Jun 19. https://doi.org/10.4081/ni.2019.8079.
12. Stillman MJ. Testosterone replacement therapy for treatment refractory cluster headache. *Headache.* 2006;46:925–933. https://doi.org/10.1111/j.1526-4610.2006.00436.x.
13. Pringsheim T, Gooren L. Migraine prevalence in male to female transsexuals on hormone therapy. *Neurology.* 2004;63(3):593–594.
14. Aloisi AM, Bachiocco V, Costantino A, et al. Cross-sex hormone administration changes pain in transsexual women and men. *Pain.* 2007;132(Suppl 1):S60–S67.
15. Facchinetti F, Sances G, Borella P, Genazzani AR, Nappi G. Magnesium prophylaxis of menstrual migraine: effects on intracellular magnesium. *Headache.* 1991;31:298–301. https://doi.org/10.1111/j.1526-4610.1991.hed3105298.x.
16. Sances G, Martignoni E, Fioroni L, Blandini F, Facchinetti F, Nappi G. Naproxen sodium in menstrual migraine prophylaxis: a double-blind placebo controlled study. *Headache.* 1990;30:705–709. https://doi.org/10.1111/j.1526-4610.1990.hed3011705.x.
17. Silberstein SD, Elkind AH, Schreiber C, Keywood C. A randomized trial of frovatriptan for the intermittent prevention of menstrual migraine. *Neurology.* 2004;63:261.

18. Short-term frovatriptan for the prevention of difficult-to-treat menstrual migraine attacks. *Cephalalgia*. 2009;29:1133.

19. Newman L, Mannix LK, Landy S, et al. Naratriptan as short-term prophylaxis of menstrually associated migraine: a randomized, double-blind, placebo-controlled study. *Headache*. 2001;41:248.

20. Oral zolmitriptan in the short-term prevention of menstrual migraine: a randomized, placebo-controlled study. *CNS Drugs*. 2008;22:877. Abu-Arefeh I, Russell G. prevalence of headache and migraine in schoolchildren. BMJ. 1994:309:765–769.

21. Gunner KB. smith HD: practice guideline and management of migraine headaches in children and adolescents. *J Pediatr Health Care*. 2007;21:327–332.

22. Le Kesche L, Manal LA, Grangoholt MT, et al. Relationship of pain and symptoms to pubertal development in adolescents. *Pain*. 2005;118:201–209.

23. Crawford MJ, Lehman L, Slater S, et al. Menstrual migraine in adolescents. *Headache*. 2009;49:341–347.

24. Bigal M, Liberman JN, Lipton RB. Age-dependent prevalence and clinical features of migraine. *Neurology*. 2006;67:246–251.

25. Hershey AD, Powers SW, Nelson TD, et al. Obesity in the pediatric headache population: a multicenter study. *Headache*. 2009;49:170–177.

26. Burkman RT, Collins JA, Shulman LP, et al. current perspectives on oral contraceptive use. *Am J Obstet Gynecol*. 2001;185:504–512.

27. Sulak P, Willis S, Kuehl T, et al. Headaches and oral contraceptives: impact of eliminating the standard 7-day placebo interval. *Headache*. 2007;47:27–37.

28. Allais G, Gabellari IC, Mana O, et al. Migraine and stroke: the role of oral contraceptives. *Neurol Sci*. 2008;29:S12–S14.

Chronic migraine and other types of primary chronic daily headache[☆]

Serena L. Orr, MD, MSc and Reena Rastogi, MD

Section A: What health care professionals need to know about chronic daily headache in children and adolescents

Introduction

Chronic daily headache (CDH) is a non-specific term that refers to any type of headache that occurs for 15 or more days per month. CDH is not a diagnosis. Although epidemiological studies are scarce, chronic headaches appear to be common in the pediatric age group. United Status population-based data suggest that 3.5% of adolescents experience chronic daily headache (CDH),[1] while data from Taiwan have estimated a prevalence of 1.5%.[2] Data on the incidence of CDH are limited, though one population-based study from Taiwan estimated the incidence at 1.13 per 100 person-years.[3]

There are several primary headaches that can lead to a CDH phenotype. The most common primary headaches causing CDH in the pediatric age group are chronic migraine (CM) and chronic tension-type headache (CTTH) (see Table 1 for International Classification of Headache Disorders 3rd Edition diagnostic criteria[4] and Figs. 1 and 2 for prevalence and incidence). Other primary headaches that can cause CDH in children and adolescents, but that are significantly less common, include: new daily persistent headache, hemicrania continua, chronic cluster headache, chronic paroxysmal hemicrania, chronic short lasting unilateral neuralgiform headaches with cranial autonomic symptoms (SUNA) and chronic short lasting unilateral neuralgiform headaches with conjunctival injection and tearing (SUNCT; see the "Other chronic headaches in children and adolescents" section). In this chapter, the main focus will be on describing the epidemiology, risk factors and preventive

---

[☆]Editor's note: The authors help us classify which headaches can cause daily headache and emphasize that chronic headache is not a diagnosis in itself. In some fashion, regardless of the specific underlying headache diagnosis, all young people who are experiencing daily headache share some common needs: finding a way to have as much normality in life as possible, getting parents and schools to understand, and having a medical provider who can empathize with, believe and support them. The authors describe some rare conditions where only one treatment works. We need to recognize those situations to implement proper intervention to avoid unnecessary delay in diagnosis.

Pediatric Headache. https://doi.org/10.1016/B978-0-323-83005-8.00018-5

Table 1 International Classification of Headache Disorders 3rd Edition (ICHD-3). Diagnostic criteria for chronic migraine and chronic tension-type headache[4]

Criterion	Chronic migraine	Chronic tension-type headache
A	Headache (migraine-like or tension-type-like) on ≥15 days per month for >3 months, fulfilling criteria B and C	Headache occurring on ≥15 days per month for >3 months, fulfilling criteria B–D
B	Occurring in a patient who has had at least five attacks fulfilling criteria B–D for migraine without aura and/or criteria B and C for migraine without aura	Lasting hours to days or unremitting
C	On ≥8 days per month for >3 months, fulfilling any of the following: 1. Criteria C and D for migraine without aura 2. Criteria B and C for migraine with aura 3. Believed by the patient to be migraine at onset and relieved by a triptan or ergot derivative	At least two of the following four characteristics: 1. Bilateral location 2. Pressing or tightening (non-pulsating) quality 3. Mild or moderate intensity 4. Not aggravated by routine physical activity such as walking or climbing stairs
D	Not better accounted for by another ICHD-3 diagnosis	Both of the following: 1. No more than one of photophobia, phonophobia or mild nausea 2. Neither moderate or severe nausea or vomiting
E		Not better accounted for by another ICHD-3 diagnosis

strategies pertaining to chronic migraine, considering that it is the most common cause of CDH seen in pediatric headache practice.[5]

Epidemiology of chronic migraine in children and adolescents

While the epidemiology of chronic migraine (CM) in adults has been well characterized using population-based data and data from cohort studies, comparatively very little has been published on the epidemiology of CM in the pediatric age group. The incidence of CM in adolescents in Taiwan has been estimated at 0.66 per 100 person-years using cohort data from Taitung County, with 2.7% of adolescents with episodic migraine converting to CM within 1–2 years.[3] The prevalence of CM in adolescents in the United States was estimated at 1.75% (95% CI=0.62–2.89) using data from the Chronic Daily Headache in Adolescents Study (C-dAS). Notably, only 0.79% (95% CI=0.0–1.7) of these cases had CM without medication overuse,[1] thereby indicating that, at least in the United States, more than half of the pediatric cases of CDH have medication overuse. In a population-based study of children aged 5 to 12 years living in Brazil, 0.6% of the population was diagnosed with CM.[6] Based on available prevalence estimates, CM accounts for between 7% and 21% of the population cases of chronic daily headache[1,2,7] (see Fig. 1). In the only study that has assessed CM incidence in adolescents, 58.7% of incident CDH cases met diagnostic criteria for CM[3] (see Fig. 2). The observed discrepancy between the proportion of prevalent and incident cases of CDH that are accounted for by CM is likely due, in part, to differences in the populations studied and methodological differences in the studies, but may largely reflect the well-described phenomenon of migraine remission over time, either through remission to an episodic phenotype,[8] or through complete remission.[9–13] In the clinical population, the proportion of CM cases is likely higher than the proportion among population-based cases: in one clinical study, CM accounted for the majority of the cases of CDH seen in a tertiary care pediatric headache clinic.[5] Therefore, CM is likely the most common diagnosis made in pediatric cases of CDH that present to tertiary care settings. It is unknown if this is also true in primary care settings.

According to data from the C-dAS study, in the pediatric age group, CM appears to be more prevalent among females and older adolescents.[1] Aura is not common among adolescents with CM, with only 20% reporting that they experience aura.[1] In addition to the prevalence of CM being higher in females as compared to males, this is also true of the incidence of CM[3] (see Fig. 2).

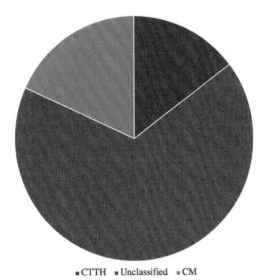

■ CTTH   ■ Unclassified   ■ CM

FIG. 1

ICHD diagnoses among population-based cases of prevalent adolescent CDH. *The estimates displayed in the figure were generated by pooling together data from the two pediatric CDH prevalence studies.[1, 2]

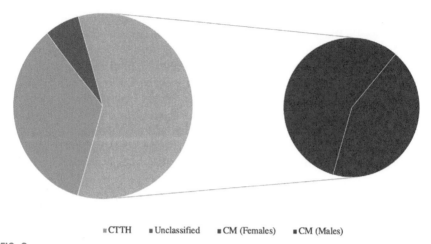

■ CTTH   ■ Unclassified   ■ CM (Females)   ■ CM (Males)

FIG. 2

ICHD diagnoses among population-based cases of incident adolescent CDH. *The estimates displayed in the figure were generated using data from the single study that has assessed incident CDH subtypes in a population-based sample from Taiwan.[3]

Burden of disease associated with chronic migraine in children and adolescents

Given that migraine is the second most prevalent cause of years lived with disability among all diseases across the lifespan,[14] one would expect that children and adolescents with CM are significantly disabled. Indeed, adolescents with CM on average have a severe level of impact on their lives attributed to migraine, and experience significant migraine-related disability.[1,15–18] A majority of adolescents with CDH report that their headaches have a significant impact on their ability to learn in school,[7] and data from a study using objective measures of school performance support the fact that academic performance is inferior in children with CM as compared to their peers.[6] In addition, a small proportion of affected adolescents (though a larger proportion as compared to healthy peers) ultimately drop out of school.[7] In addition to the educational impacts of CM on children and adolescents, these youth also experience significant disability in the home, social and extra-curricular spheres.[1,16]

It is known that the costs associated with CM are significantly higher than the costs associated with episodic migraine in the adult population.[19–24] Unfortunately, data on the costs associated with pediatric CM have not been estimated. Surprisingly, given the degree of disability associated with pediatric CM, population-based studies have illustrated that the majority of these children and adolescents had not visited a health care provider in the past year, and this was true both in American and Taiwanese populations.[1,2,7] This could be due to a multitude of factors, including stigma, inadequate education in the general population around care and treatment options, or due to the fact that CM is more prevalent among adolescents of lower socioeconomic status[6] who may not have adequate access to care. Alternately, given that it has been shown that patients with CM presenting to a tertiary care pediatric headache clinic have less confidence in their treatment plan as compared to patients with episodic migraine, patient expectations may be a barrier to accessing care for a variety of reasons (e.g., lack of knowledge about the breadth of treatment options or disillusionment due to prior unsuccessful attempts at treatment and contact with the healthcare system). In summary, based on the available data, it appears that there is an unmet treatment need reflected by the fact that the majority of children and adolescents with CM are not receiving care and it is unclear why this gap exists.

Risk factors for migraine chronification in children and adolescents

A variety of clinical parameters have been identified as risk factors for progression to chronic migraine in the adult population.[25] The phenomenon of migraine chronification and risk factors that may contribute to this process have been understudied in children and adolescents. Preliminary evidence suggests that depression,[3,7,26] high baseline headache frequency,[3] acute medication overuse,[3,7] obesity,[3] and low socioeconomic status[3] contribute to disease progression to chronic migraine in children and adolescents (see Fig. 3). Of the risk factors studied to date, depression appears

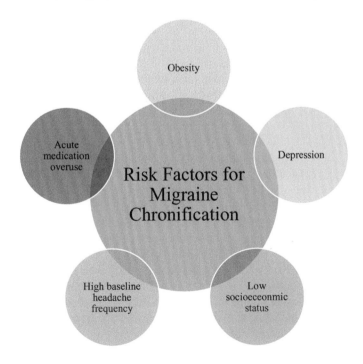

FIG. 3

Risk factors for progression from episodic to chronic migraine in children and adolescents.

to have the most consistent evidence supporting its role in disease progression.[3,7,26] It remains unclear if these risk factors will be validated in other pediatric samples, and why they may contribute to disease progression. Some of the identified risk factors, such as high baseline headache frequency and medication overuse, may be linked with migraine chronification through the phenomenon of central sensitization,[27] which can biologically predispose individuals to increasing attack frequencies. Overall, the small number of studies that have examined risk factors for progression to pediatric CM and methodological limitations in the published literature (e.g., in how outcomes and predictors were ascertained and in the external validity of the results) should compel further research into this important area. It is especially critical for the research community to identify modifiable risk factors for migraine progression, considering that early intervention in pediatric migraine may result in disease modification and a more favorable long-term prognosis.[12,28]

Prevention of migraine chronification in children and adolescents

In some individuals, episodic migraine can worsen in frequency over time until the headaches are occurring 15 days or more per month, often daily or almost daily. This is considered chronification of migraine or transformed migraine (TM).[29] Transformed migraine is considered a complication of migraine and is not a formal diagnosis on its own. By ICHD-3 criteria, this diagnosis is chronic migraine (CM).[4] The incidence of chronic migraine in children has not been well studied. It is not clear if all people with migraine have the ability to progress to chronic migraine or if some individuals are genetically predisposed to this transformation.[30] There are data to suggest a biologic predisposition to chronic migraine in children. In a large study in Brazil, it was found that if a mother had chronic daily headache (CDH), the risk of CDH in the child increased almost 13-fold.[30]

Early intervention prior to migraine chronification is key to preventing migraine-related disability. This is most beneficial while the patient is still in the episodic migraine phase. Unfortunately, studies show that children and adolescents tend to have low healthcare and medication utilization for headaches,[1,2,7] similar to findings seen in adults.[29] Early diagnosis and treatment of migraine without aura is important in order to prevent chronic migraine.[12,28] A study looking at the prognosis of children and adolescents under the care of a healthcare provider showed that the majority of patients who receive care for migraine headache tend to have good outcomes that are likely sustained in the long-term.[26] Preventive treatment can be initiated in patients having frequent attacks or in whom the use of acute medications puts them at risk for medication overuse headache in order to reduce headache frequency and prevent transformation to chronic migraine.[28,29,31] This can be in the form of both pharmacologic and non-pharmacologic treatment, such as lifestyle management, depending on the needs of each individual patient.

In patients who have a high frequency of headaches, it is important to avoid medication overuse.[29,30,32] Medication overuse headache (MOH) is defined by the ICHD-3 as headache occurring 15 or more days per month in a patient with pre-existing primary headache as a result of regular overuse of acute headache medication.[4] MOH is a common cause of migraine chronification[29,30] and it is estimated that over half of the adolescents with chronic migraine in the United States also overuse acute medications.[32] Whether this is the cause, or the effect of the chronic headaches is not well understood. Treatment is to avoid or limit use of symptomatic medications,[32,33] although this does not always lead to improvement in headache frequency.[32] Table 3, below, lists the various acute pain medications according to their limits of use. Addition of a prophylactic medication can also be beneficial as well as consideration of psychological support for medication overuse.[29,33]

It is also essential to address potential co-existing disorders that can lead to chronification in children and adolescents with migraine.[7,29] The most common of these comorbid conditions that are known to be risk factors for migraine chronification in children and adolescents include depression, anxiety, and obesity.[2,7,26] Early identification of these risk factors is important in order to determine the appropriate treatment for the patient and intervene before headaches become chronic.[26,28,29] Children with migraine should be screened for depression and anxiety. Non-pharmacological treatments such as cognitive behavioral therapy or biofeedback should be initiated once these risk factors are identified.[15,31] Patients should be referred to a psychiatrist for pharmacologic treatment of depression or anxiety as deemed necessary. A weight management program including diet and exercise may be beneficial for children and adolescents with obesity.[34] Use of certain medications for migraine prophylaxis that address comorbidities can be advantageous for these patients, for instance, using topiramate for obesity with avoidance of medications such as tricyclic antidepressants, cyproheptadine, or divalproex which promote weight gain.[35]

Other chronic headaches in children and adolescents
Chronic tension-type headache

Chronic tension-type headache (CTTH) is the second most common headache leading to CDH in the pediatric population, after chronic migraine.[1,2] The prevalence of CTTH found in the CDH population for children is highly variable in studies.[36,37] Results of the C-dAS (Chronic Daily Headache in Adolescents Study) found that CTTH frequency was only 2.8% in adolescents with CDH, compared to CM in 20.9% of adolescents with CDH, and the remainder of the CDHs were unclassified.[1] However, in a study of 115 children and adolescents (age 3 to 15 years) with CDH, the frequency of CTTH was overwhelmingly high, with 81% of patients fulfilling criteria for CTTH. Tension-type headaches were the only headache type seen in 63.5% of the patients, while others had mixed tension-type headaches and migraine.[36] It is important to note that in children with tension-type headaches, features of migraine can often be seen, at times making the diagnosis somewhat unclear.[37] The diagnostic criteria of CTTH can be found in Table 1, above. CTTH is defined as a mild to moderate headache that occurs 15 or more days per month and may have bilateral location, a pressing or tightening quality, no more than one of photophobia, phonophobia or mild nausea, and is not aggravated by routine physical activity.[4] Children with CTTH often exhibit significant impairment in daily functioning, with high rates of school absence and low school performance.[38,39] CTTH is likely caused by both internal and external stressors.[39] Chronic diseases and stressful emotional or physical events are known risk factors for the development of CTTH.[36] As with CM, it is important to assess for medication overuse. Treatment is similar to that of CM, with a multimodal and multidisciplinary approach including lifestyle management, psychological (cognitive behavioral therapy, relaxation, biofeedback) interventions, and prophylactic pharmacological treatment.[37–39]

Chronic cluster headache

Cluster headache (CH) falls under the category of trigeminal autonomic cephalalgias (TACs), which all have similar clinical features of unilateral headache with cranial parasympathetic autonomic symptoms seen ipsilateral to the headache. The various TACs are distinguished by the frequency of attacks and also include paroxysmal hemicrania (PH), short-lasting unilateral neuralgiform headaches (SUNCT/SUNA), and hemicrania continua (HC). These will be discussed below. TACs are considered a diagnosis of exclusion, requiring neuroimaging with magnetic resonance imaging (MRI) of the brain, and with particular attention to the pituitary and cavernous sinus region.[40] CH consists of severe unilateral pain in the orbital, supraorbital, or temporal region, lasting 15–180 min, associated with ipsilateral autonomic symptoms, and occurring at a frequency of between one every other day and 8 per day. The ICHD-3 diagnostic criteria of CH is listed in Table 2, below. Chronic CH is characterized by cluster headaches occurring without a remission period, or with a remission period of <3 months, lasting for at least 1 year.[4] CH is rare in the pediatric population. It is estimated that the prevalence of CH in children aged 0–18 years is anywhere from 0.09% to 0.1%[41,42] and it is estimated that 10% to 20% of these children have chronic CH, similar to the prevalence seen in adults.[42] There are numerous case series reporting CH in children as young as 1 year of age, though in most case reports the onset of CH is in the 2nd decade of life.[43] Unlike in adults, in which there is a male predominance, CH in children seems to have a fairly equal male to female ratio.[41,44] The diagnosis is difficult to make, especially in children, as the symptoms are often misdiagnosed as other conditions.[41,43,45] CH is often misdiagnosed as migraine as migraine is much more common in children, and symptoms of photophobia, phonophobia, and nausea may be present with CH.[45] It may also be that autonomic symptoms are less apparent in children, making the diagnosis even more difficult in this population.[42] Treatment of pediatric CH is based on the available data on treatment in the adult population, as there are no randomized controlled trials on CH treatment in children.[44]

Table 2 ICHD-3 diagnostic criteria for trigeminal autonomic cephalalgias (TACs).[4]

Criterion	Cluster headache	Paroxysmal hemicrania	Short-lasting unilateral neuralgiform headache attacks	Hemicrania continua
A	At least 5 attacks fulfilling criteria B–D	At least 20 attacks fulfilling criteria B–E	At least 20 attacks fulfilling criteria B–D	Unilateral headache fulfilling criteria B–D
B	Severe or very severe unilateral orbital, supraorbital and/or temporal pain lasting 15–180 min	Severe unilateral orbital, supraorbital and/or temporal pain lasting 2–30 min	Moderate or severe unilateral head pain, with orbital, supraorbital, temporal and/or other trigeminal distribution, lasting for 1–600 s and occurring as single stabs, series of stabs or in a saw-tooth pattern	Present for >3 months, with exacerbations of moderate or greater intensity
	Either or both of the following: **1.** At least one of the following symptoms or signs, ipsilateral to the headache: – Conjunctival injection and/or lacrimation – Nasal congestion and/or rhinorrhea – Eyelid oedema – Forehead and facial sweating – Miosis and/or ptosis **2.** A sense of restlessness or agitation	Either or both of the following: **1.** At least one of the following symptoms or signs, ipsilateral to the headache: – Conjunctival injection and/or lacrimation – Nasal congestion and/or rhinorrhea – Eyelid oedema – Forehead and facial sweating – Miosis and/or ptosis **2.** A sense of restlessness or agitation	At least one of the following five cranial autonomic symptoms or signs, ipsilateral to the pain: **1.** Conjunctival injection and/or lacrimation **2.** Nasal congestion and/or rhinorrhoea **3.** Eyelid oedema **4.** Forehead and facial sweating **5.** Forehead and facial flushing **6.** Sensation of fullness in the ear **7.** Miosis and/or ptosis	Either or both of the following: **1.** At least one of the following symptoms or signs, ipsilateral to the headache: – Conjunctival injection and/or lacrimation – Nasal congestion and/or rhinorrhea – Eyelid oedema – Forehead and facial sweating – Miosis and/or ptosis **2.** A sense of restlessness or agitation, or aggravation of the pain by movement

Continued

Table 2 ICHD-3 diagnostic criteria for trigeminal autonomic cephalalgias (TACs).[4] —Cont'd

Criterion	Cluster headache	Paroxysmal hemicrania	Short-lasting unilateral neuralgiform headache attacks	Hemicrania continua
D	Occurring with a frequency between one every other day and 8 per day	Occurring with a frequency of >5 per day	Occurring with a frequency of at least one a day	Responds absolutely to therapeutic doses of indomethacin
E	Not better accounted for by another ICHD-3 diagnosis	Prevented absolutely by therapeutic doses of indomethacin	Not better accounted for by another ICHD-3 diagnosis	Not better accounted for by another ICHD-3 diagnosis
F		Not better accounted for by another ICHD-3 diagnosis		

Chronic paroxysmal hemicrania

Paroxysmal hemicrania (PH) is another TAC which is unique in the fact that it is remarkably responsive to treatment with indomethacin.[40,46] For this reason, it is important to correctly identify the diagnosis and to distinguish it from CH.[47] PH is even rarer in children than CH and there is no epidemiologic data available in this population, although the frequency is likely similar to what is seen in adults.[40] Table 2 below lists the diagnostic criteria. PH involves attacks of severe unilateral orbital, supraorbital, or temporal pain, lasting 2–30 min, associated with ipsilateral autonomic symptoms, and occurring >5 times per day. The responsiveness to indomethacin is part of the ICHD-3 diagnostic criteria. The chronic form of PH must occur without a remission period, or with remissions lasting <3 months, for at least 1 year.[4] In adults, about 80% suffer from chronic PH and only 20% have episodic PH. Similarly, in a study of 628 chronic pediatric headache patients, five patients (0.8%) were diagnosed with PH and three patients (0.5%) with probable PH. Of these eight patients, five of them had chronic PH. The age of onset for these patients ranged from 2.5 years to 12.9 years, with the average being 5.9 years.[46]

Chronic SUNCT (short-lasting unilateral neuralgiform headaches with conjunctival injection and tearing) and SUNA (short-lasting unilateral neuralgiform headaches with cranial autonomic symptoms

SUNCT and SUNA are considered subcategories of short-lasting unilateral neuralgiform headaches in the ICHD-3 (see Table 2). These consist of moderate to severe unilateral head pain in the trigeminal distribution, lasting for 1–600 s, occurring as a single stab, series of stabs, or in a saw-tooth pattern, and associated with ipsilateral autonomic symptoms. SUNCT is associated with conjunctival injection and tearing, while SUNA is only associated with one or neither of these symptoms. Chronic SUNCT and SUNA are attacks occurring for more than 1 year without remission, or with a remission period of <3 months, for at least 1 year.[4] SUNCT and SUNA are usually seen in middle aged or older patients, typically between the ages of 40 to 70 years. They are extremely rare in the pediatric population and there is no epidemiologic data available for the pediatric population.[40] There are very few case reports of pediatric SUNCT or SUNA, including secondary cases,[47] and, to our knowledge, there is no reported chronic pediatric SUNCT or SUNA in the literature.

Hemicrania continua

Hemicrania continua (HC) is considered one of the chronic daily headaches (CDH), as by definition it is chronic, and the pain can be continuous. It is a unilateral headache that is present for >3 months and associated with ipsilateral cranial autonomic symptoms. It is also absolutely responsive to indomethacin (see Table 2). There is a remitting subtype, which is not present daily or continuously, but has interruptions for at least 24 h. The unremitting subtype is daily and continuous for at least 1 year, without remission periods of 24 h or more.[4] It is typically not described in children and adolescents,[47,48] though onset is reported from 10 to 58 years of age.[48] The incidence in adults is about 1% of patients with daily headaches and most patients are female. Typical age of onset is 30 to 50 years.[49]

Section B: What patients and their families need to know about chronic daily headache in children and adolescents

Chronic daily headache (CDH) is a term used to describe any type of headache that occurs on at least 15 days per month; it is not a diagnosis. There is likely regional variation in how common it is, with studies reporting that anywhere from 1.5% to 3.5% of youth suffer from CDH.[1,2] There are a variety of causes of CDH.

The most common headaches that cause CDH in children and adolescents are chronic tension-type headache (CTTH) and chronic migraine (CM). CTTH is the cause of CDH in about 15% of cases and CM is the cause in about 18% of cases.[1,2] These numbers are based on studies done in the general population. In children and adolescents who visit headache clinics for their CDH, CM is the most common diagnosis made.[5] Table 1 lists the current diagnostic criteria for CTTH and CM and highlights some of the features of these headaches. Although both are associated with at least 15 headache days per month, these disorders are quite different. Essentially, CTTH is a disorder associated with mild-to-moderate headaches that usually occur on both sides of the head, that feel pressure-like and that aren't associated with other symptoms except for, in some cases, light or sound sensitivity. In contrast, CM is a disorder associated with moderate-severe headaches that can occur on one side or both sides of the head, that can feel pulsating and that are associated with other symptoms: both light and sound sensitivity, or nausea and/or vomiting. Children and adolescents with CM may also experience other symptoms such as an aura, which is like a warning sign that happens before the headache and that involves neurological symptoms like vision changes or tingling in a part of the body. Autonomic symptoms, like runny eyes or nose, red eyes or facial sweating, can occur with CM. There may also be allodynia during the headache, which is an abnormal sensitivity that occurs in the head and/or neck and causes non-painful sensations to feel painful or to worsen the headache.[4] For example, wearing a ponytail or a hat may feel unpleasant or cause the headache to intensify. Females and older adolescents are more likely to suffer from CM than males and younger adolescents and children.[1,3] Aside from CTTH and CM, there are several other headaches that can cause CDH, though they are each individually quite rare in children. These are in the category of trigeminal autonomic cephalalgias (TACs): hemicrania continua, chronic cluster headache, chronic paroxysmal hemicrania, chronic short lasting unilateral neuralgiform headaches with cranial autonomic symptoms (SUNA), and chronic short lasting unilateral neuralgiform headaches with conjunctival injection and tearing (SUNCT). See Table 2 for the definitions of these headache types.[4]

Children and adolescents with CDH experience significant disability. In the case of CM, children and adolescents often have difficulty functioning at school, at home and in their extra-curricular activities due to migraine.[1,6,7,15–18] They report more difficulty learning than their peers,[7] have lower academic performance[6] and might be at higher risk of dropping out of school.[7] Unfortunately, despite the disability associated with CM, it appears that a majority of children and adolescents with this condition are not receiving medical care for it.[1,2,7] Although the reasons for this are unclear, there is a clear need to improve access to care for children and adolescents with CM and other forms of CDH. Without accessing medical care, it can be very challenging to get a diagnosis and appropriate treatment.

Because of how disabling it is, the medical community is trying to understand how to prevent CDH in the first place. In some children, migraine can go from being episodic (less than 15 headache days per month) to chronic (15 or more headache days per month) over time. It can be helpful to start treatment early while the headaches are still episodic, in order to prevent migraine from becoming chronic. Treatment can be as simple as making modifications to lifestyle factors such as getting adequate sleep, regular exercise, drinking enough water, eating right, avoiding caffeine, and managing stress.[31] There are certain vitamins that can be taken daily which are helpful for migraine, though the data are limited in kids. Finally, sometimes a daily medicine which is meant to prevent headaches needs to be started, and can be initiated even if a child is having three or more attacks of migraine per month, depending on how disabling the headaches are.[28,29,31] These treatments can often help prevent the development of chronic migraine and other headaches.

One of the most common reasons for progressing from having episodic headaches to chronic headaches is using too much pain medication to try and stop the pain. This is called acute medication overuse and can lead to medication overuse headache (MOH) in susceptible individuals. MOH is diagnosed in a person who already has headaches but is having 15 or more days per month of headache as a result of overusing acute medicine such as over-the-counter or prescription medicines for pain relief. Children and adolescents with a pre-existing headache disorder (e.g., migraine or tension-type headache) can develop CDH from using any acute pain medication too frequently. The limit of use above which the medication can be associated with worsening headache depends on the type of medication that is being overused. Table 3 lists these acute pain medications according to their limits of use. The treatment for MOH is to stop using the medicine that is causing the headaches to be worse. Sometimes a medicine that is taken daily to prevent headaches is also started to try to reduce the headaches that are occurring. Behavioral interventions can also help to reduce overuse of medicines for headaches.[29,30,32,33]

Aside from overusing acute pain medications, several other factors may increase the risk of progressing from having less frequent headaches to CDH. This has been best studied in CM. Children and adolescents who are obese, of lower socioeconomic status, who have more headaches at baseline and who suffer from depression or anxiety are more likely to experience worsening of migraine over time and to progress from episodic (less than 15 headache days per month) to chronic (more than 15

Table 3 Limits of use for acute pain medications.

Do NOT use on greater than 10 days per month (>2 days/week)	Do NOT use on greater than 15 days per month (>3 days/week)
• Ergotamines (e.g., dihydroergotamine) • Opioids (e.g., morphine, hydromorphone) • Triptans (e.g., sumatriptan, rizatriptan) • Barbiturates (e.g., bultalbital) • Combination drugs (e.g., Tylenol 3, Excedrin) • Multiple drug classes not overused individually	• Acetaminophen • Non-steroidal anti-inflammatory medications (e.g., ibuprofen, naproxen) • Other non-opioid analgesics (e.g., acetylsalicylic acid)

headache days per month) migraine (see Fig. 3).[3,7,26] Depression, in particular, appears to consistently predict progression to CM in the available studies.[3,7,26] It is still unclear if treating the risk factors that can be treated (i.e., obesity, depression, and high baseline headache frequency) can reduce the risk of progressing to CM, although it is important to address these factors. Treatments for depression and anxiety include a type of therapy called cognitive behavioral therapy, which is also a treatment that has been proven in children and adolescents with migraine.[15] A weight management program with diet and exercise can be helpful for obesity. However, some studies suggest that getting a diagnosis of migraine early results in better outcomes.[12,28] Based on this, it is likely that early medical care that includes treatment of these risk factors would play a role in preventing the progression to CM. Therefore, the medical community needs to study these risk factors in more depth and how we may intervene early to prevent CDH in the first place.

References

1. Lipton RB, Manack A, Ricci JA, Chee E, Turkel CC, Winner P. Prevalence and burden of chronic migraine in adolescents: results of the chronic daily headache in adolescents study (C-dAS). *Headache*. 2011;51(5):693–706.
2. Wang SJ, Fuh JL, Lu SR. Chronic daily headache in adolescents: an 8-year follow-up study. *Neurology*. 2006;66:193–197.
3. Lu S-R, Fuh J-L, Wang S-J, et al. Incidence and risk factors of chronic daily headache in young adolescents: a school cohort study. *Pediatrics*. 2013;132(1):e9–16.
4. Headache Classification Committee of the International Headache Society. The International Classification of Headache Disorders, 3rd edition. *Cephalalgia*. 2018;38(1):1–211.
5. Bigal M, Lipton R, Tepper S, Rapoport A, Sheftell F. Primary chronic daily headache and its subtypes in adolescents and adults. *Neurology*. 2004;63:843–847.
6. Arruda MA, Bigal ME. Migraine and migraine subtypes in preadolescent children: association with school performance. *Neurology*. 2012;79(18):1881–1888.

7. Wang S, Fuh J, Lu S, Juang K. Outcomes and predictors of chronic daily headache in adolescents: a 2-year longitudinal study. *Neurology*. 2007;68(8):591–596.
8. Serrano D, Lipton RB, Scher AI, et al. Fluctuations in episodic and chronic migraine status over the course of 1 year: implications for diagnosis, treatment and clinical trial design. *J Headache Pain*. 2017;18(1):1–12.
9. Bille B. A 40-year follow-up of school children with migraine. *Cephalalgia*. 1997;17:488–491.
10. Monastero R, Camarda C, Pipia C, Camarda R. Prognosis of migraine headaches in adolescents: a 10-year follow-up study. *Neurology*. 2006;67(8):1353–1356.
11. Guidetti V, Galli F. Evolution of headache in childhood and adolescence: an 8-year follow-up. *Cephalalgia*. 1998;18(7):449–454.
12. Galinski M, Sidhoum S, Cimerman P, Perrin O, Annequin D, Tourniaire B. Early diagnosis of migraine necessary in children: 10-year follow-up. *Pediatr Neurol*. 2015;53 (4):319–323.
13. Virtanen R, Aromaa M, Rautava P, et al. Changing headache from preschool age to puberty. A controlled study. *Cephalalgia*. 2007;27(4):294–303.
14. James SL, Abate D, Abate KH, et al. Global, regional, and national incidence, prevalence, and years lived with disability for 354 diseases and injuries for 195 countries and territories, 1990-2017: a systematic analysis for the Global Burden of Disease Study 2017. *Lancet*. 2018;392:1789–1858.
15. Powers SW, Kashikar-Zuck SM, Allen JR, et al. Cognitive behavioral therapy plus amitriptyline for chronic migraine in children and adolescents: a randomized clinical trial. *JAMA*. 2013;310(24):2622–2630.
16. Hershey AD, Powers SW, Lecates S, Kabbouche MA, Maynard MK. PedMIDAS: development of a questionnaire to assess disability of migraines in children. *Neurology*. 2001;57:2034–2039.
17. Kacperski J, O'Brien HL, Hershey AD, et al. Headache frequency and level of disability altered by expectations and confidence in treatment plan. In: *Headache*. 2012:896 Conference(var.pagings).
18. Kabbouche M, O'Brien H, Hershey AD. OnabotulinumtoxinA in pediatric chronic daily headache. *Curr Neurol Neurosci Rep*. 2012;12(2):114–117.
19. Stewart WF, Wood GC, Manack A, Varon SF, Buse DC, Lipton RB. Employment and work impact of chronic migraine and episodic migraine. *J Occup Environ Med*. 2010;52(1):8–14.
20. Osumili B, McCrone P, Cousins S, Ridsdale L. The economic cost of patients with migraine headache referred to specialist clinics. *Headache*. 2018;58(2):287–294.
21. Stokes M, Becker WJ, Lipton RB, et al. Cost of health care among patients with chronic and episodic migraine in Canada and the USA: results from the international burden of migraine study (IBMS). *Headache*. 2011;51(7):1058–1077.
22. Munakata J, Hazard E, Serrano D, et al. Economic burden of transformed migraine: results from the American Migraine Prevalence and Prevention (AMPP) Study. *Headache*. 2009;49:498–508.
23. Serrano D, Manack AN, Reed ML, Buse DC, Varon SF, Lipton RB. Cost and predictors of lost productive time in chronic migraine and episodic migraine: results from the American Migraine Prevalence and Prevention (AMPP) Study. *Value Health*. 2013;16(1):31–38.
24. Berra E, Sances G, De Icco R, et al. Cost of chronic and episodic migraine: a pilot study from a tertiary headache centre in northern Italy. *J Headache Pain*. 2015;16(1):1–8.

25. Buse DC, Greisman JD, Baigi K, Lipton RB. Migraine progression: a systematic review. *Headache*. 2019;59:306–338.
26. Orr SL, Turner A, Kabbouche MA, et al. Predictors of short-term prognosis while in pediatric headache care: an observational study. *Headache*. 2019;59(4):543–555.
27. May A, Schulte LH. Chronic migraine: risk factors, mechanisms and treatment. *Nat Rev Neurol*. 2016;12(8):455–464.
28. Charles JA, Peterlin BL, Rapoport AM, Linder SL, Kabbouche MA, Sheftell FD. Favorable outcome of early treatment of new onset child and adolescent migraine-implications for disease modification. *J Headache Pain*. 2009;10(4):227–233.
29. Manzoni GC, Camarda C, Torelli P. Chronification of migraine: what clinical strategies to combat it? *Neurol Sci*. 2013;34(1):57–60.
30. Bigal ME, Lipton RB. Migraine chronification. *Curr Neurol Neurosci Rep*. 2011;11(2):139–148.
31. Rastogi RG, Borrero-Mejias C, Hickman C, Lewis KS, Little R. Management of episodic migraine in children and adolescents: a practical approach. *Curr Neurol Neurosci Rep*. 2018;18(12):103.
32. Gelfand AA, Goadsby PJ. Medication overuse in children and adolescents. *Curr Pain Headache Rep*. 2014;18(7):428.
33. Chiappedi M, Balottin U. Medication overuse headache in children and adolescents. *Curr Pain Headache Rep*. 2014;18(4):404.
34. Pakalnis A, Kring D. Chronic daily headache, medication overuse, and obesity in children and adolescents. *J Child Neurol*. 2012;27(5):577–580.
35. Bigal ME, Lipton RB. Modifiable risk factors for migraine progression. *Headache*. 2006;46(9):1334–1343.
36. Abu-Arafeh I. Chronic tension-type headache in children and adolescents. *Cephalalgia*. 2001;21(8):830–836.
37. Anttila P. Tension-type headache in children and adolescents. *Curr Pain Headache Rep*. 2004;8(6):500–504.
38. Claar RL, Kaczynski KJ, Minster A, McDonald-Nolan L, Level AA. School functioning and chronic tension headaches in adolescents: improvement only after multidisciplinary evaluation. *J Child Neurol*. 2012;28(6):719–724.
39. Przekop P, Przekop A, Haviland M. Multimodal compared to pharmacologic treatments for chronic tension-type headache in adolescents. *J Bodyw Mov Ther*. 2016;20(4):715–721.
40. Mack KJ, Goadsby P. Trigeminal autonomic cephalalgias in children and adolescents: cluster headache and related conditions. *Semin Pediatr Neurol*. 2016;23(1):23–26.
41. Mariani R, Capuano A, Torriero R, et al. Cluster headache in childhood: case series from a pediatric headache center. *J Child Neurol*. 2014;29(1):62–65.
42. Antonaci F, Alfei E, Piazza F, De Cillis I, Balottin U. Therapy-resistant cluster headache in childhood: case report and literature review. *Cephalalgia*. 2010;30(2):233–238.
43. Taga A, Manzoni GC, Russo M, Paglia MV, Torelli P. Childhood-onset cluster headache: observations from a personal case-series and review of the literature. *Headache*. 2018;58(3):443–454.
44. Arruda MA, Bonamico L, Stella C, Bordini CA, Bigal ME. Cluster headache in children and adolescents: ten years of follow-up in three pediatric cases. *Cephalalgia*. 2011;31(13):1409–1414.
45. VanderPluym J. Cluster headache: special considerations for treatment of female patients of reproductive age and pediatric patients. *Curr Neurol Neurosci Rep*. 2016;16(1):5.

46. Blankenburg M, Hechler T, Dubbel G, Wamsler C, Zernikow B. Paroxysmal hemicrania in children—symptoms, diagnostic criteria, therapy and outcome. *Cephalalgia*. 2009;29 (8):873–882.
47. Lambru G, Byrne S. Trigeminal autonomic cephalalgias in children and adolescents. *Neurol Sci*. 2018;39(1):105–106.
48. Moorjani BI, Rothner AD. Indomethacin-responsive headaches and children and adolescents. *Semin Pediatr Neurol*. 2001;8(1):40–45.
49. Burish MJ, Rozen TD. Trigeminal autonomic cephalalgias. *Neurol Clin*. 2019;37(4): 847–869.

Comorbidities in children and adolescents ☆

Jason L. Ziplow, MD and Dawn C. Buse, PhD

Introduction

A comorbidity is defined as "a greater than chance association between two conditions in the same individual."[1] Studying and understanding comorbidities, especially with migraine and other severe headache, can help to provide insight into underlying disease pathophysiology which can then be used to guide treatment formulation and ongoing management. In addition, comorbidities can occasionally have implications that interfere with diagnosis or lead to over diagnosis of a given condition, so knowing this information can help improve diagnostic accuracy. Learning about comorbid diagnoses can also help inform the general knowledge about disease progression and provide more information about a disorder's natural history.

In adults with headache, there are several well-studied comorbidities, which include cardiovascular disorders like stroke,[2–5] psychiatric disorders such as anxiety and depression,[6–8] inflammatory conditions like asthma and allergic rhinitis,[9, 10] neurologic diseases like epilepsy,[11, 12] sleep disorders including restless leg syndrome and insomnia[13, 14] as well as chronic pain conditions such as fibromyalgia.[15] However, trying to apply this data to children and adolescents ignores the physiologic differences that distinguish this population from adults. In doing so, there is the risk of making misleading assumptions that could impact the diagnosis and treatment of this population. Studying the pediatric population independently presents its own challenges, because designing studies for children and adolescents specifically raises certain ethical considerations. Nevertheless, it is important for these studies to be conducted. In the information provided below, we hope to review the most up-to-date and relevant research available on comorbidities for children and adolescents with headache, while acknowledging its limitations (Tables 1 and 2).

☆ Editor's note: Taking care of patients requires getting to know them as people. People with headaches often also have other issues that crop up. Often, as headaches get worse so do other conditions. Comorbidity is defined well in the first paragraph. It implies that two conditions occur in the same patient. No causality is implied. All we know is that these two entities group together. Getting to know your patient with headache means being comfortable acknowledging their comorbidities and forming a plan to address them.

Pediatric Headache. https://doi.org/10.1016/B978-0-323-83005-8.00007-0

Table 1 Summary of the evidence of comorbidities in pediatric headache.

Comorbidity	Summary of evidence	Assessments	Medical and biobehavioral management
Psychological disorders			
Depression/anxiety	Some positive associations with anxiety and depressive symptoms and headache, particularly migraine. However, there is no directionality known about the relationship and little data to support associations with clinically significant generalized anxiety disorder and major depressive disorder[18-20,22]	PAT,[24] SDQ[21] *GAD-7, MINI, PHQ-9, PROMIS, PSC, CDI[19,21,110]	Referral for psychological interventions (e.g., CBT, biofeedback)[21,25] *SSRIs[25]
Alexithymia	Higher levels of alexithymia in patients with headache compared to controls. Compared to migraine and control groups, patients with TTH may test higher on alexithymia testing and had greater difficulty in identifying feelings[26-28]	Toronto Alexithymia Scale[27,28] Symptom Checklist 90-R[27,28] Alexithymia Questionnaire for Children[27,28]	Identification, referral for psychological interventions (e.g., MBT)[29]
Functional disorders	Functional movement disorders are associated with chronic more than episodic migraine.[30] Migraine, but not TTH is associated with functional gastrointestinal disorders.[32] Functional constipation is associated with TTH, but not migraine[31]	Fahn and Williams Criteria[30] Rome III/IV Criteria[31,32] Functional Disability Inventory[34]	Migraine therapy (e.g., patient education, preventive medication, trigger avoidance)[35] Mindfulness-based stress reduction[34]
Obesity	Recurrent headaches associated with being overweight (greater in patients with migraine than TTH). Some associations between elevated BMI and increased	Height, weight, BMI percentile Child Eating Behavior Questionnaire[47] Dutch Eating Behavior	Management of nutrition/dietary behaviors, physical exercise, CBT[38,43]

Condition	Clinical association	Diagnostic considerations	Treatment considerations
	headache frequency/disability. Some associations with intake of high-fat/sugary items and migraine severity[37-42,44,45,47,111]	Questionnaire[47] Food Intake Questionnaire[47]	
Epilepsy	Risk of epilepsy in patients with migraine higher than those with TTH. Increased incidence of both migraine in patients with epilepsy and epilepsy in patients with migraine. However, infrequent cooccurrence of headache and epilepsy[49-54]	Electroencephalogram Magnetic resonance imaging[50,52,54] *Consider genetic testing[50,52,54]	AEDs (e.g., valproate, topiramate), *Ketogenic/modified Atkins diet[50] *Behavioral interventions (e.g., progressive muscle relaxation, focused-attention)[56]
Atopic disorders (allergic conjunctivitis, allergic rhinitis, atopic dermatitis, asthma)	Higher incidence of overall headaches in patients with allergic conjunctivitis (especially migraine without aura). Higher incidence of migraine without aura in patients with allergic rhinitis. Higher cooccurrence of atopic dermatitis in patients with migraine than other headache subtypes. Asthma more common in adolescents with migraine than nonspecific headaches[51,58-64]	Symptomatic diagnosis[62-64] GINA Guidelines[62]	Antiasthmatic/antiallergic therapies (e.g., inhaled or nasal corticosteroids)[62] GINA Guidelines[62]
Neurodevelopmental and neurobehavioral issues *ADHD*	While there are some studies to show an association between ADHD and primary headaches (especially migraine),[65-67] others suggest no association or associations with impaired attention span and hyperactivity/impulsivity only[69,70]	DSM Criteria,[69] MTA-SNAP-IV Scale[69] *CBCL, SDQ[69]	No headache-specific considerations reported

Continued

Table 1 Summary of the evidence of comorbidities in pediatric headache. *Continued*

Comorbidity	Summary of evidence	Assessments	Medical and biobehavioral management
Visual attention	Patients with migraine show more difficulty with selective and alternate attention[72] as well as visual motor integration,[71] which suggests partial disturbance of visual processing. Treatment of migraine can help improve this difference[74]	Trail Making Test A and B,[72] Letter Cancellation Test,[72] Test of Visual Attention (3rd Edition),[72] Visual Evoked Potentials[73]	Prophylactic migraine medications[74] Visuospatial Software Training[71]
Auditory processing	Impairments in temporal processing and selective auditory attention (deficits in auditory processing in a noisy background)[75] seen in children with migraine[76]	GIN, DPT, SSI, NVDT[76]	No headache-specific considerations reported
Nocturnal/sleep disorder			
Narcolepsy	Limited data show that migraine is an independent risk factor for narcolepsy development in children[78]	ICSD-3 Criteria[79] MSLT[79]	Sleep hygiene (regular sleep-wake cycles).[79] Avoidance of medications that could exacerbate headache (e.g., stimulants)[80]
Bruxism	Although some studies have shown and association between episodic migraine/TTH and bruxism, the rates described in the studies are within typical frequency range for the general population.[80-83] However, in children with bruxism, more headaches may be reported[84]	Children's Sleep Habits Questionnaire[85] Polysomnography[82]	Stress management, sleep hygiene, behavioral therapies, biofeedback[84]

RLS	In patients with migraine and TTH there is a higher frequency of RLS, but no significant difference between migraine and TTH[87-89]	Pediatric IRLSSG Criteria[86] ICSD-3 Criteria[79] Serum ferritin level[89]	Sleep hygiene, CBT, distraction techiniques[79,86] Iron supplementation[84]
Celiac disease	Some studies show an association between patients with celiac disease and headache (including migraine, TTH, and chronic headache).[90-96] However, others show no higher prevalence of celiac disease in patients with migraine compared with healthy controls[97,98]	Serum TTG IgA antibodies[97] Total serum IgA[97] Duodenal biopsy[97]	Gluten-free diet[95,99]

*Requires further explanation.

Abbreviations: ADHD, attention deficit-hyperactivity disorder; AEDs, antiepileptic drugs; BMI, body mass index; CBCL, child behavioral checklist; CBT, cognitive behavioral therapy; CDI, child depression inventory; DPT, duration pattern test; DSM, diagnostic and statistical manual of mental disorders; GAD-7, generalized anxiety disorder 7-item scale; GIN, gaps-in-noise; GINA, global initiative for asthma; ICSD-3, international classification of sleep disorders, third edition; IgA, immunoglobulin A; IRLSSG, International Restless Leg Syndrome Study Group; MBT, mentalization-based treatment; MINI, mini international; MSLT, mean sleep latency testing; NVDT, neuropsychiatric interview nonverbal dichotic test; PAT, psychosocial assessment tool 2.0; PHQ-9, patient health questionnaire; PROMIS, patient-reported outcomes measurement information system; PSC, pediatric symptoms checklist; RLS, restless leg syndrome; SDQ, strength and difficulties questionnaire; SSI, synthetic sentence identification test; SSRIs, selective serotonin reuptake inhibitors; TTG, tissue transglutaminase; TTH, tension type headache.

Table 2 Psychometric validation for children and adolescents for selected instruments.

Test name	Test content and diagnostic use(s)	Data for use in children and adolescents
PHQ-9	9-Item questionnaire used to screen for major depressive disorder	Studied best in ages 13–17 years old with good sensitivity (89.5%) and specificity (77.5%)[94]
GAD-7	7-Item questionnaire used to screen for generalized anxiety disorder	Studies in patients 12–17 years old with "acceptable specificity and sensitivity for detecting clinically significant anxiety symptoms"[95]
Fahn and Williams criteria	Set of criteria used to diagnose psychogenic movement disorders	Initially proposed criteria were validated for use in children by Kirsch and Mink[31, 96]
Rome criteria	Set of criteria used to identify functional gastrointestinal disorders	Specific pediatric questionnaires and criteria that have been validated. Rome III Criteria were released in 2006 and revised Rome IV Criteria were released in 2016[97]
Trail making test	2-Part test with 15 targets (in the pediatric version) used to test visual attention, processing speed, and executive functioning[98]	Validated child-specific version and studied in children with acquired and neurodevelopmental disorders from varying causes (e.g., learning disabilities, epilepsy, traumatic brain injury)[98]
Letter cancellation test	Measures visual attention by timing the subject as they mark a letter as it appears in a list of letters[99]	Validated for use in children with establishment of norms in children[100]
Test of visual attention, 3rd edition	Computerized test comprised of 3 different tasks used to evaluate visual attention[101]	Normative data for children and adolescents in the Brazilian version of the test exist[101]
Visual evoked potential	Provides "diagnostic information on the functional integrity of the visual system"[102]	Data to supports its use including algorithms for interpretation in children exist[102, 103]
GIN	Tests auditory temporal resolution by playing segments of noise with silent intervals and asking the subject to identify when they are heard[71]	Initially created for adults, but found to be acceptable to be used in children as young as 7 years old[104]
DPT	Evaluates auditory temporal ordering by playing 3 tones where one is of different duration the subject then has to identify[71, 105]	Has been used repeatedly in children and adolescents as well as adults[105]

Table 2 Psychometric validation for children and adolescents for selected instruments. *Continued*

Test name	Test content and diagnostic use(s)	Data for use in children and adolescents
SSI	Evaluation of auditory processing by requesting the subject point out a picture indicated by a recording[71, 106]	Pediatric version called the pediatric speech intelligibility test for use in children greater than 3 years old[106]
NVDT	Evaluation of auditory processing by providing nonverbal auditory stimuli in a 2-step process including each ear[71]	Used in a Brazilian study to evaluate children who had experienced strokes[107]

Abbreviations: DPT, *duration pattern test*; GAD 7, *generalized anxiety disorder 7-item scale*; GIN, *gaps in noise*; NVDT, *nonverbal dichotic test*; PHQ-9, *patient health questionnaire*; SSI, *synthetic sentence identification test*.

For general providers and headache specialists
Psychological disorders

Anxiety and depression. In the adult headache population, several studies have shown associations with psychological disorders such as anxiety and depression.[6–8, 16, 17] However, while in the pediatric population some associations with the *symptoms* related to anxiety and depression have been shown, studies have not been able to show specific associations with anxiety and depressive *disorders*.[18–22] Criteria for Major Depressive Disorder and Generalized Anxiety Disorder as well as many other related conditions are listed in the Diagnostic and Statistical Manual of Mental Disorders (DSM-5).[23] Common screening tools used in-office to help diagnose patients with anxiety and/or depression include the 7-item Generalized Anxiety Disorder Scale (GAD-7) and 9-Item Patient Health Questionnaire (PHQ-9). These are available for use, free of charge and can be accessed at: www.phqscreeners.com. The issue with these tools, specifically in trying to diagnose patients with headache, is that there is substantial overlap between the symptoms of anxiety and depression assessed during these inventories and the symptoms of headache.[19, 20] For example, the questions in the PHQ-9 that deal with poor appetite or poor concentration and in the GAD-7 that deal with being restless can all be seen independently in patients who have headaches, which may lead to false-positive comorbid diagnoses. As such, some research has looked into better overall assessments to use in patient with tension-type headache (TTH) and migraine, leading to the implementation of the Psychosocial Assessment Tool 2.0 (PAT) by some healthcare providers.[24] Once patients are identified as needing further assessment and treatment based on these screening tools, they should be treated and/or referred for interventions such as Cognitive Behavioral Therapy (CBT) and Biofeedback, which have shown independent efficacy in pediatric headache patients, and/or medication treatment if needed.[21, 25]

Alexithymia. Alexithymia is characterized by a difficulty in emotional regulation and verbalizing emotional expression.[26–28] Associations between children and adolescents with TTH and alexithymia have been shown in several studies.[26–28] These findings are suggestive of some incomplete or immature cognitive and emotional development[26] in this population that could point towards an underlying pathologic neurodevelopmental mechanism. In screening for alexithymia in these patients, the Toronto Alexithymia Scale, Symptom Checklist 90-R, and Alexithymia Questionnaire for Children have been utilized specifically in this population.[27, 28] Should this condition cause impairment in important aspects of social or academic functioning, referral for psychological interventions such as mentalization-based treatment, as well as other general cognitive behavioral, developmental, and educational therapies may be of benefit for management of alexithymia.[29]

Functional disorders. Functional disorders represent a wide array of phenotypes and include such manifestations as movement disorders and gastrointestinal symptoms. Different types of functional disorders are associated with different types of headache. Specifically, functional movement disorders (especially nonepileptic spells, tremor, functional syncopal spells, and gait disorders), have been associated more with people having chronic migraine than those with episodic migraine.[31] Functional gastrointestinal disorders such as functional constipation is associated with TTH[33] whereas other functional gastrointestinal disorders like functional dyspepsia and IBS are associated more with migraine.[32] Identification of functional gastrointestinal disorders can be achieved through use of the Rome IV criteria questionnaires (which require a fee for use)[32, 33] whereas functional movement disorders can be recognized utilizing the Fahn and Williams Criteria.[31, 96] The Functional Disability Inventory can be used in adolescents with chronic pain disorders to assess their physical and functional impairments and help identify the need for additional therapeutic options.[34] Treatment involves mindfulness based stress reduction[34] and avoidance of migraine triggers, and preventive medications if indicated.[35]

Obesity

Several population- and clinic-based studies in children and adolescents, have shown some associations between being overweight/obese and having migraine.[36–43, 46, 108, 109] In addition, an elevated BMI has been shown to be correlated with an increase in both headache frequency and disability from headache.[37] One possible etiology of this, as proposed by a study from Ray et al., is that obesogenic eating behaviors (including the consumption of high fat and sugary items) are correlated with migraine frequency and headache disability.[44] Shared mechanisms of both obesity and migraine include involvement of the hypothalamus including the orexin system, serotonin system, the calcitonin gene-related protein (CGRP), and adipocytokines such as leptin and adiponectin.[39–41, 110] Many of these proposed shared mechanisms deal with satiety and food intake behaviors as well as pain and inflammation.[40, 110] In addition, both migraine and obesity have strong genetic predispositions. Assessment of obesity in these individuals includes more than just measurement of height, weight, and calculation of BMI, but also assessment of eating behaviors, food intake, and activity level.[44] Management of nutrition as well as dietary behaviors and physical exercise has been showed to be beneficial for both treatment of obesity as well as headache.[37, 39, 46, 108] CBT has also been shown to be of value in this population.[46] As diet is often dictated by the family, and parents specifically, it is imperative to involve the parents in this treatment plan. Without parental support and participation, it can be almost impossible to effect change in the child alone. Family therapy, group nutrition, counselling, group exercise plans, and/or physical therapy may benefit the entire family as well as the patient.

Epilepsy

Studies have shown that although headache and epilepsy co-occur infrequently, there is a higher incidence of migraine in children and adolescents with epilepsy and vice versa.[47–52] However, this same pattern does not hold true with TTH.[51] In patients with epilepsy, headaches can be a phenomenon preictally, interictally, or postictally, which can sometimes lead to diagnostic confusion.[48, 49, 52] Also complicating matters, occipital lobe seizures can present similarly to migraine aura.[50, 52] Shared mechanisms have been postulated to include that epileptic discharges lead to activation of the trigeminovascular systems with subsequent migraine development and/or lead to the cortical spreading depression associated with migraine.[49, 52] Evaluation of patients with both epilepsy and migraine requires a thorough history to try and distinguish features of both migraine and epilepsy, an electroencephalogram to provide further data about epileptiform activity, and possible genetic testing. Some genetic polymorphisms have been identified as possible contributing factors in these patients.[48, 49] Imaging, specifically Magnetic Resonance Imaging (MRI), can be useful at identifying possible seizure foci, however its utility in headache evaluation is usually in patients with abnormal neurologic exams or worrisome symptomatology.[48] While acute treatments for migraine and epilepsy differ, prophylactic regimens for both disorders may include antiepileptic medications such as topiramate and valproic acid as well as some limited data to support the ketogenic diet/modified Atkins diet as adjunctive therapy.[48] While there is not specific data in children to suggest whether behavioral therapies might be helpful in epilepsy treatment, there have been studies showing that cognitive behavioral therapy and relaxation therapies using progressive muscle relaxation can be beneficial in headache reduction as well as the management of epilepsy among adults.[111] An adult multicenter randomized control trial has shown that behavioral therapies such as progressive muscle relaxation and control focused-attention activity with extremity movements can significantly reduce seizure frequency.[53] Thus, there could likely be benefit to behavioral therapies for pediatric patients with both migraine and epilepsy, but currently there are not enough data to support this recommendation.

Atopic disorders

Atopic disorders are those disorders that involve genetic predisposition for Immuno-globulin E production after allergen exposure and includes allergic conjunctivitis, allergic rhinitis, atopic dermatitis, and asthma.[112] In patients with migraine headache, associations with higher incidence and co-occurrence of atopic disease exist.[54–60] In patients with allergic conjunctivitis and allergic rhinitis there is a higher incidence of migraine without aura.[59, 60] Atopic dermatitis and asthma also both co-occur more frequently in patients with migraine over other types of headache.[56–58] In addition, patients with persistent asthma were more likely to have a higher number of monthly migraine episodes compared to those with intermittent asthma.[58] The significance of these disorders co-occurring gives insight into the possible role of inflammation mediated by mast cells.[54] Atopic disorders are usually symptomatic,[58–60] yet the Global Initiative for Asthma (GINA) guidelines exist to help both with diagnosis and asthma management. Treatment for atopic disorders usually involves inhaled or nasal corticosteroids, however, there is some data to suggest that this may also decrease risk of migraine in children and adolescents.[58] Because of this, screening for atopic disorders may be helpful for treatment planning in patients with migraine.[56] Conversely, in patients presenting with atopic disorders, screening for migraine may aid overall disease management.[59, 60]

Neurodevelopmental and neurobehavioral issues

Attention deficit hyperactivity disorder (ADHD). Both primary headache subtypes and ADHD are common pediatric diagnoses that can impact a child's learning and social interactions. Research into the possible associations between the two has shown mixed results; some studies have shown that there is some association between ADHD and primary headaches (specifically migraine, although others show specific associations with TTH as well),[61–63, 113] however other studies have shown no association or that some of the primary symptoms of ADHD like hyperactivity/impulsivity and impaired attentiveness (but not formal ADHD diagnosis) are associated with headache.[64, 65, 113] In the studies showing associations between headache and ADHD, increased ADHD risk is associated with increased headache frequency.[63] However, some of the research has been limited by the screening tools such as the Childhood and Behavioral Checklist (CBCL), which asks limited questions on inattentive symptoms, for example.[64] Criteria for ADHD are listed in the Diagnostic and Statistical Manual of Mental Disorders (DSM-5).[23] Other assessment tools used for diagnosis of ADHD include the Multimodal Treatment Study of Children with ADHD-Swanson, Nola, and Pelham IV Scale (MTA-SNAP-IV scale).[64] Targeted treatments towards patients with both ADHD and headache still require further research.

Visual attention. Selective and alternate attention as well as visual motor integration are skills involved with visual processing and attention. Children and adolescents with migraine have shown more difficulty in these tasks than have age-matched peers from the general population, suggestive of at least partial disturbance of visual processing in migraine.[66, 67] This disturbance may, in part, lead to a disturbance in academic performance. An array of assessments in these patients can be performed to assess visual attention and processing including Trail Making Test A and B, the Letter Cancellation Test, Test of Visual Attention (3rd edition), and Visual Evoked Potentials.[66, 69] Interestingly, treatment of migraine with prophylactic medications has been shown to improve children's ability to perform visual attention tasks to a level comparable to their healthy peers.[68] Visual attention-specific treatment may include various neuropsychological therapeutic approaches including specialized Visuospatial Software training.[67]

Auditory processing. Deficits in auditory processing in a noisy background (selective auditory attention) as well as temporal processing impairments are seen specifically in children with migraine although some studies show no difference in performance between children and adolescents with migraine and TTH.[70, 71] Specialized screening tools performed to assess for impairments in auditory processing include the Duration Pattern Test (DPT), Synthetic Sentence Identification Test (SSI), Nonverbal Dichotic Test (NVDT)[71]. Unlike with visual attention, little research exists to suggest specific treatment options to improve auditory processing in patients with migraine/headache although we suggest avoidance of noisy backgrounds, for these patients.

Nocturnal/sleep disorders

Narcolepsy. Narcolepsy is a rare disorder that normally develops by mid-adolescence that involves disruption of the control of the sleep-wake cycle.[114] According to some research, migraine represents an independent risk factor for the development of narcolepsy.[72] Given the relationship between migraine and narcolepsy, the latter is mediated by destruction of orexin-producing neurons in the hypothalamus, some additional light can be shed on the pathogenesis of migraine.[72] Diagnosing narcolepsy can be achieved by using Mean Sleep Latency Testing (MSLT) as well as criteria from the International Classification of Sleep Disorders, Third Edition (ICSD-3).[73] In treating patients with both narcolepsy and headache, some common treatment themes exist including sleep hygiene (such as trying to maintain regular sleep-wake cycles). However, some treatments for narcolepsy include stimulants, which can result in headache independently, so avoiding these medications when possible may be a specific consideration for this population.[74]

Bruxism. Involuntary nocturnal teeth grinding and jaw clenching, also known as bruxism, has been researched in the context of headache in children and adolescents. Some studies have shown that there is an association between episodic migraine as well as TTH and bruxism.[75] However, the rates that have been reported in these studies are within the typical frequency range seen in the general population.[74, 76, 77] On the other hand, one study has shown that children with bruxism may be more likely to report headaches.[78] Assessing for nocturnal bruxism can be achieved through completing the Children's Sleep Habits Questionnaire or by using polysomnography.[76, 79] Once a diagnosis of bruxism has been made, management includes biofeedback, stress management techniques, sleep hygiene, and behavioral therapies which have also shown efficacy in patients with headache.[78]

Restless leg syndrome (RLS). RLS is characterized by an almost uncontrollable urge to move the legs that can also be connected to abnormal or unpleasant sensations such as tingling or "ants crawling" on the skin.[83] While studying this disorder in the context of children and adolescents with headache, it was found that in both migraine and TTH, there is a higher frequency of RLS than in the general population.[74, 80–82] However, no difference was found between people with migraine and those with TTH.[82] Diagnostic criteria have been compiled by the Pediatric International RLS Study Group and can be used along with serum ferritin to aid in diagnosis.[82, 83] In children and adolescents with low serum ferritin, iron supplementation may be helpful whereas sleep hygiene, CBT, and distraction techniques can be useful for all patients with this comorbidity.[78, 83]

Celiac disease

Celiac disease occurs when the body produces antibodies to gluten which subsequently results in damage to the small intestine. In people with headache, the comorbidity of these conditions has been studied and although some studies do show an association between celiac disease and headache,[84–90] while others do not.[91, 92] In those that do, headache subtypes such as migraine, TTH, and chronic headache all seem to share in this association with celiac disease.[84–90] Aside from symptom assessment in these patients, blood testing including serum antibodies to tissue transglutaminase as well a total levels of immunoglobulin A helps with the diagnosis.[91] In addition to this, duodenal biopsies are used to help confirm the diagnosis.[91] Given the mixed research, there are no strict recommendations about screening every headache patient for celiac disease.[92] However, in those that do, studies have shown that initiation of the gluten-free diet leads to both celiac disease symptom reduction as well as improvement in headaches.[89, 93] The concept of gluten being a migraine trigger is popular among people with migraine, in the lay press, and on social media. There is no empirical evidence for or against this belief; however, youth with migraine should be encouraged to eat a healthy, balanced diet, and stay on a regular, routine eating schedule.

How to facilitate successful biobehavioral referrals

Biobehavioral treatments including cognitive behavioral therapy, relaxation training, biofeedback, and healthy lifestyle habits are empirically supported treatments for many of the comorbidities reviewed in this section as well as having good evidence for benefit in migraine and chronic tension type headache management. However, there are challenges inherent in facilitating successful referrals for treatment and/or educating patients and their families about these approaches. Access and openness to treatment are affected by a range of factors that fall into two categories: (1) factors related to broader health care systems, and (2) factors related to the patient. Ernst and colleagues review these challenges as well as provide responses to Frequently Asked Questions and challenges to behavioral therapies, links to websites, apps, and online programs, sample behavioral protocols, and other very useful information on facilitating successful biobehavioral referrals for pediatric migraine management in their open access (free) 2015 manuscript.[115] They explain that with regard to factors related to broader health care systems, health care professional knowledge of biobehavioral interventions, previous patient exposure to biobehavioral interventions, and health care professional-patient communication is central to patient and family acceptance of biobehavioral approaches. They report that persuasive communication, combined with empathic and nonjudgmental listening to the patient and caregivers' concerns, perspectives, and questions also improve openness to multidisciplinary migraine management. They review how the Motivational Interviewing model can be used by healthcare professionals to examine patients' (and caregivers') motivation to change, openness to treatment, and likelihood of referral follow-through.[116] This is a valuable technique to enhancing adherence and motivation to any and all types of treatment as well as reducing frustration and increasing self-efficacy for the healthcare professional. While biobehavioral therapies may or may not be focused on treating a psychological condition, they are often provided by mental health professionals and therefore can be associated with stigma. The manner in which the referring healthcare professional presents the suggested biobehavioral therapy and explains its method of improving migraine, other primary headache and/or any of the comorbidities reviewed may be a deciding factor as to whether a patient and/or his family will consider a biobehavioral treatment. Discussing benefits, any associated risks and costs in a similar manner to that in which medical interventions are discussed is very important. For example, the biobehavioral therapy should be written in the Electronic Health Record and patient summary in the same list as any prescribed pharmacologic therapies.[117] Building rapport with patients and establishing therapeutic relationships based on a collaborative approach to health care and migraine management is important to the referral process, because patients may be more open to suggestions and more likely to follow through with appointments and referrals if they have a greater sense of trust in their health care professionals or medical teams. Open communication using active listening has been established to lead to higher levels of patient-provider trust and rapport. Effective communication techniques include using open-ended questions and the ask-tell-ask technique to confirm understanding and agreement.[118–120] In cases where access is limited by financial, geographic, and time barriers, new technologies including web-based, smart phone-based, and telemedicine-based programs may provide solutions.[115, 121, 122]

For patients and families

There is substantial research in the field of identifying medical and psychological comorbidities in children and adolescents with headache. One of the purposes of knowing the comorbidities associated with different types of primary headaches is to screen and treat patients where appropriate for comorbidities that could ultimately affect disease outcomes, management, and patient quality of life. However, unnecessary screening for disorders that do not have good evidence of being comorbid with headaches can be invasive, time-consuming, and expensive. That being said, knowing how and when to seek care for co-occurring disorders can be difficult, so the section below will help provide some guidance.

The healthcare professional managing migraine and/or headache may initiate screening for comorbidities, although patients and family members can provide helpful context by sharing family history as well as reporting symptoms, which may or may not appear to be related to the migraine or headache. In the case of a comorbidity related to sleep, the patient may be referred to a specialist for a sleep study, and/or a psychological for behavioral sleep management or biofeedback. In the case of obesity, the patient may be referred to an endocrinologist, a dietician, physical therapy, and/or a psychologist. In the case of comorbidity related to psychological, emotional or cognitive factors, the patient may be referred to a psychologist, neuropsychologist and/or psychiatrist, or simply advised to seek therapy (which may include medication therapy, neuropsychological testing, cognitive behavioral therapy (CBT), relaxation training or biofeedback among other treatments). In many cases, these treatments will not only improve the psychological, cognitive or emotional condition, quality of life, and academic engagement, but also have direct effects improving migraine.[123]

As well as treating psychiatric comorbidities such as depression, anxiety, obesity, and insomnia, biobehavioral treatments have proven efficacy in migraine management and are recommended as a component of migraine management for children and adolescents by the American Academy of Neurology.[124] These therapies are often covered by health insurance. If your healthcare professional does not provide a specific referral, providers can often be found through the websites of the following organizations: The Association for Applied Psychophysiology and Biofeedback (www.AAPB.org), the Biofeedback Certification International Alliance (www.bcia.org), the Association for Behavioral and Cognitive Therapies (www.abct.org), the Society of Behavioral Medicine (www.sbm.org), and the American Psychiatric Association (www.psychiatry.org). In addition, people can learn and practice some of the techniques such as relaxation training and mindfulness practices through free or low-cost programs available on the internet or apps.[115, 121, 122]

Disclosures

(1) Jason L. Ziplow, MD has no disclosures.
(2) Dawn C. Buse, PhD, in the past 12 months, has received grant support from NIH/FDA and Amgen. She has received compensation for consulting from Allergan, Amgen, Avanir, Biohaven, Lilly, Promeius, and Teva. She is a co-founder and stockholder in Unison Mind. She is on the editorial board of *Current Pain and Headache Reports*.

References

1. Feinstein AR. The pre-therapeutic classification of co-morbidity in chronic disease. *J Chronic Dis.* 1970;23(7):455–468.
2. Mahmoud AN, Mentias A, Elgendy AY, et al. Migraine and the risk of cardiovascular and cerebrovascular events: a meta-analysis of 16 cohort studies including 1 152 407 subjects. *BMJ Open.* 2018;8(3), e020498.
3. Adelborg K, Szepligeti SK, Holland-Bill L, et al. Migraine and risk of cardiovascular diseases: Danish population based matched cohort study. *BMJ.* 2018;360:k96.
4. Schurks M, Rist PM, Bigal ME, Buring JE, Lipton RB, Kurth T. Migraine and cardiovascular disease: systematic review and meta-analysis. *BMJ.* 2009;339:b3914.
5. Hu X, Zhou Y, Zhao H, Peng C. Migraine and the risk of stroke: an updated meta-analysis of prospective cohort studies. *Neurol Sci.* 2017;38(1):33–40.
6. Buse DC, Silberstein SD, Manack AN, Papapetropoulos S, Lipton RB. Psychiatric comorbidities of episodic and chronic migraine. *J Neurol.* 2013;260(8):1960–1969.
7. Minen MT, Begasse De Dhaem O, Kroon Van Diest A, et al. Migraine and its psychiatric comorbidities. *J Neurol Neurosurg Psychiatry.* 2016;87(7):741–749.
8. Lampl C, Thomas H, Tassorelli C, et al. Headache, depression and anxiety: associations in the Eurolight project. *J Headache Pain.* 2016;17:59.
9. Aamodt AH, Stovner LJ, Langhammer A, Hagen K, Zwart JA. Is headache related to asthma, hay fever, and chronic bronchitis? The Head-HUNT Study. *Headache.* 2007;47(2):204–212.
10. Martin VT, Fanning KM, Serrano D, Buse DC, Reed ML, Lipton RB. Asthma is a risk factor for new onset chronic migraine: results from the American migraine prevalence and prevention study. *Headache.* 2016;56(1):118–131.
11. Nye BL, Thadani VM. Migraine and epilepsy: review of the literature. *Headache.* 2015;55(3):359–380.
12. Keezer MR, Bauer PR, Ferrari MD, Sander JW. The comorbid relationship between migraine and epilepsy: a systematic review and meta-analysis. *Eur J Neurol.* 2015;22 (7):1038–1047.
13. Vgontzas A, Pavlovic JM. Sleep disorders and migraine: review of literature and potential pathophysiology mechanisms. *Headache.* 2018;58(7):1030–1039.
14. Buse DC, Rains JC, Pavlovic JM, et al. Sleep disorders among people with migraine: results from the chronic migraine epidemiology and outcomes (CaMEO) study. *Headache.* 2019;59(1):32–45.
15. Wang KA, Wang JC, Lin CL, Tseng CH. Association between fibromyalgia syndrome and peptic ulcer disease development. *PLoS One.* 2017;12(4), e0175370.
16. Muneer A, Farooq A, Farooq JH, Qurashi MS, Kiani IA, Farooq JS. Frequency of primary headache syndromes in patients with a major depressive disorder. *Cureus.* 2018;10 (6), e2747.
17. Breslau N, Lipton RB, Stewart WF, Schultz LR, Welch KM. Comorbidity of migraine and depression: investigating potential etiology and prognosis. *Neurology.* 2003;60 (8):1308–1312.
18. Blaauw BA, Dyb G, Hagen K, et al. The relationship of anxiety, depression and behavioral problems with recurrent headache in late adolescence - a young-HUNT follow-up study. *J Headache Pain.* 2015;16:10.

19. Gelfand AA. Psychiatric comorbidity and paediatric migraine: examining the evidence. *Curr Opin Neurol*. 2015;28(3):261–264.
20. Powers SW, Gilman DK, Hershey AD. Headache and psychological functioning in children and adolescents. *Headache*. 2006;46(9):1404–1415.
21. O'Brien HL, Slater SK. Comorbid psychological conditions in pediatric headache. *Semin Pediatr Neurol*. 2016;23(1):68–70.
22. Blaauw BA, Dyb G, Hagen K, et al. Anxiety, depression and behavioral problems among adolescents with recurrent headache: the young-HUNT study. *J Headache Pain*. 2014;15:38.
23. Force. APAAPAD-T. *Diagnostic and Statistical Manual of Mental Disorders: DSM-5*. 5th ed. Arlington, VA: American Psychiatric Association; 2013. Washington, D.C.: American Psychiatric Association, ©2013. ©2013.
24. Law EF, Powers SW, Blume H, Palermo TM. Screening family and psychosocial risk in pediatric migraine and tension-type headache: validation of the psychosocial assessment tool (PAT). *Headache*. 2019;59(9):1516–1529.
25. Blume HK, Brockman LN, Breuner CC. Biofeedback therapy for pediatric headache: factors associated with response. *Headache*. 2012;52(9):1377–1386.
26. Natalucci G, Faedda N, Calderoni D, Cerutti R, Verdecchia P, Guidetti V. Headache and alexithymia in children and adolescents: what is the connection? *Front Psychol*. 2018;9:48.
27. Gatta M, Spitaleri C, Balottin U, et al. Alexithymic characteristics in pediatric patients with primary headache: a comparison between migraine and tension-type headache. *J Headache Pain*. 2015;16:98.
28. Cerutti R, Valastro C, Tarantino S, et al. Alexithymia and psychopathological symptoms in adolescent outpatients and mothers suffering from migraines: a case control study. *J Headache Pain*. 2016;17:39.
29. Lof J, Clinton D, Kaldo V, Ryden G. Symptom, alexithymia and self-image outcomes of Mentalisation-based treatment for borderline personality disorder: a naturalistic study. *BMC Psychiatry*. 2018;18(1):185.
30. Qubty W, Gelfand AA. Psychological and behavioral issues in the management of migraine in children and adolescents. *Curr Pain Headache Rep*. 2016;20(12):69.
31. Youssef PE, Mack KJ. Abnormal movements in children with migraine. *J Child Neurol*. 2015;30(3):285–288.
32. Le Gal J, Michel JF, Rinaldi VE, et al. Association between functional gastrointestinal disorders and migraine in children and adolescents: a case-control study. *Lancet Gastroenterol Hepatol*. 2016;1(2):114–121.
33. Inaloo S, Dehghani SM, Hashemi SM, Heydari M, Heydari ST. Comorbidity of headache and functional constipation in children: a cross-sectional survey. *Turk J Gastroenterol*. 2014;25(5):508–511.
34. Ali A, Weiss TR, Dutton A, et al. Mindfulness-based stress reduction for adolescents with functional somatic syndromes: a pilot cohort study. *J Pediatr*. 2017;183:184–190.
35. Bonvanie IJ, Kallesoe KH, Janssens KAM, Schroder A, Rosmalen JGM, Rask CU. Psychological interventions for children with functional somatic symptoms: a systematic review and meta-analysis. *J Pediatr*. 2017;187:272–281 [e217].
36. Robberstad L, Dyb G, Hagen K, Stovner LJ, Holmen TL, Zwart JA. An unfavorable lifestyle and recurrent headaches among adolescents: the HUNT study. *Neurology*. 2010;75(8):712–717.

37. Hershey AD, Powers SW, Nelson TD, et al. Obesity in the pediatric headache population: a multicenter study. *Headache.* 2009;49(2):170–177.
38. Ravid S, Shahar E, Schiff A, Gordon S. Obesity in children with headaches: association with headache type, frequency, and disability. *Headache.* 2013;53(6):954–961.
39. Eidlitz Markus T, Toldo I. Obesity and migraine in childhood. *Curr Pain Headache Rep.* 2018;22(6):42.
40. Peterlin BL, Rapoport AM, Kurth T. Migraine and obesity: epidemiology, mechanisms, and implications. *Headache.* 2010;50(4):631–648.
41. Farello G, Ferrara P, Antenucci A, Basti C, Verrotti A. The link between obesity and migraine in childhood: a systematic review. *Ital J Pediatr.* 2017;43(1):27.
42. Pinhas-Hamiel O, Frumin K, Gabis L, et al. Headaches in overweight children and adolescents referred to a tertiary-care center in Israel. *Obesity (Silver Spring).* 2008;16 (3):659–663.
43. Oakley CB, Scher AI, Recober A, Peterlin BL. Headache and obesity in the pediatric population. *Curr Pain Headache Rep.* 2014;18(5):416.
44. Ray S, Singh SB, Halford JC, Harrold JA, Kumar R. A pilot study of obesogenic eating behaviors in children with migraine. *J Child Neurol.* 2016;31(7):895–898.
45. Chai NC, Scher AI, Moghekar A, Bond DS, Peterlin BL. Obesity and headache: part I—a systematic review of the epidemiology of obesity and headache. *Headache.* 2014;54 (2):219–234.
46. Verrotti A, Agostinelli S, D'Egidio C, et al. Impact of a weight loss program on migraine in obese adolescents. *Eur J Neurol.* 2013;20(2):394–397.
47. Papavasiliou AS, Bregianni M, Nikaina I, Kotsalis C, Paraskevoulakos E, Bazigou H. Pediatric headache and epilepsy comorbidity in the pragmatic clinical setting. *Neuropediatrics.* 2016;47(2):107–111.
48. Oakley CB, Kossoff EH. Migraine and epilepsy in the pediatric population. *Curr Pain Headache Rep.* 2014;18(3):402.
49. Jacobs H, Singhi S, Gladstein J. Medical comorbidities in pediatric headache. *Semin Pediatr Neurol.* 2016;23(1):60–67.
50. Sowell MK, Youssef PE. The comorbidity of migraine and epilepsy in children and adolescents. *Semin Pediatr Neurol.* 2016;23(1):83–91.
51. Toldo I, Perissinotto E, Menegazzo F, et al. Comorbidity between headache and epilepsy in a pediatric headache center. *J Headache Pain.* 2010;11(3):235–240.
52. Rajapakse T, Buchhalter J. The borderland of migraine and epilepsy in children. *Headache.* 2016;56(6):1071–1080.
53. Haut SR, Lipton RB, Cornes S, et al. Behavioral interventions as a treatment for epilepsy: a multicenter randomized controlled trial. *Neurology.* 2018;90(11):e963–e970.
54. Lateef TM, Cui L, Nelson KB, Nakamura EF, Merikangas KR. Physical comorbidity of migraine and other headaches in US adolescents. *J Pediatr.* 2012;161(2):308–313 e301.
55. Lateef TM, Merikangas KR, He J, et al. Headache in a national sample of American children: prevalence and comorbidity. *J Child Neurol.* 2009;24(5):536–543.
56. Ozge A, Oksuz N, Ayta S, et al. Atopic disorders are more common in childhood migraine and correlated headache phenotype. *Pediatr Int.* 2014;56(6):868–872.
57. Shreberk-Hassidim R, Hassidim A, Gronovich Y, Dalal A, Molho-Pessach V, Zlotogorski A. Atopic dermatitis in Israeli adolescents from 1998 to 2013: trends in time and association with migraine. *Pediatr Dermatol.* 2017;34(3):247–252.

58. Aupiais C, Wanin S, Romanello S, et al. Association between migraine and atopic diseases in childhood: a potential protective role of anti-allergic drugs. *Headache*. 2017;57 (4):612–624.

59. Wang IC, Tsai JD, Lin CL, Shen TC, Li TC, Wei CC. Allergic rhinitis and associated risk of migraine among children: a nationwide population-based cohort study. *Int Forum Allergy Rhinol*. 2016;6(3):322–327.

60. Wang IC, Tsai JD, Shen TC, Lin CL, Li TC, Wei CC. Allergic conjunctivitis and the associated risk of migraine among children: a nationwide population-based cohort study. *Ocul Immunol Inflamm*. 2017;25(6):802–810.

61. Kutuk MO, Tufan AE, Guler G, et al. Migraine and associated comorbidities are three times more frequent in children with ADHD and their mothers. *Brain and Development*. 2018;40(10):857–864.

62. Jameson ND, Sheppard BK, Lateef TM, Vande Voort JL, He JP, Merikangas KR. Medical comorbidity of attention-deficit/hyperactivity disorder in US adolescents. *J Child Neurol*. 2016;31(11):1282–1289.

63. Salem H, Vivas D, Cao F, Kazimi IF, Teixeira AL, Zeni CP. ADHD is associated with migraine: a systematic review and meta-analysis. *Eur Child Adolesc Psychiatry*. 2018;27 (3):267–277.

64. Bellini B, Arruda M, Cescut A, et al. Headache and comorbidity in children and adolescents. *J Headache Pain*. 2013;14:79.

65. Parisi P, Verrotti A, Paolino MC, et al. Headache and attention deficit and hyperactivity disorder in children: common condition with complex relation and disabling consequences. *Epilepsy Behav*. 2014;32:72–75.

66. Villa TR, Correa Moutran AR, Sobirai Diaz LA, et al. Visual attention in children with migraine: a controlled comparative study. *Cephalalgia*. 2009;29(6):631–634.

67. Precenzano F, Ruberto M, Parisi L, et al. Visual-spatial training efficacy in children affected by migraine without aura: a multicenter study. *Neuropsychiatr Dis Treat*. 2017;13:253–258.

68. Villa TR, Agessi LM, Moutran AR, Gabbai AA, Carvalho DS. Visual attention in children with migraine: the importance of prophylaxis. *J Child Neurol*. 2016;31(5):569–572.

69. Oelkers-Ax R, Bender S, Just U, et al. Pattern-reversal visual-evoked potentials in children with migraine and other primary headache: evidence for maturation disorder? *Pain*. 2004;108(3):267–275.

70. Ciriaco A, Russo A, Monzani D, et al. A preliminary study on the relationship between central auditory processing and childhood primary headaches in the intercritical phase. *J Headache Pain*. 2013;14:69.

71. Agessi LM, Villa TR, Carvalho DS, Pereira LD. Auditory processing in children with migraine: a controlled study. *Neuropediatrics*. 2017;48(2):123–126.

72. Yang CP, Hsieh ML, Chiang JH, Chang HY, Hsieh VC. Migraine and risk of narcolepsy in children: a nationwide longitudinal study. *PLoS One*. 2017;12(12), e0189231.

73. Hintze JP, Paruthi S. Sleep in the pediatric population. *Sleep Med Clin*. 2016;11(1):91–103.

74. Dosi C, Figura M, Ferri R, Bruni O. Sleep and headache. *Semin Pediatr Neurol*. 2015;22 (2):105–112.

75. Vendrame M, Kaleyias J, Valencia I, Legido A, Kothare SV. Polysomnographic findings in children with headaches. *Pediatr Neurol*. 2008;39(1):6–11.

76. Masuko AH, Villa TR, Pradella-Hallinan M, et al. Prevalence of bruxism in children with episodic migraine–a case-control study with polysomnography. *BMC Res Notes*. 2014;7:298.

77. Peskersoy C, Peker S, Kaya A, Unalp A, Gokay N. Evaluation of the relationship between migraine disorder andoral comorbidities: multicenter randomized clinical trial. *Turk J Med Sci*. 2016;46(3):712–718.

78. Guidetti V, Dosi C, Bruni O. The relationship between sleep and headache in children: implications for treatment. *Cephalalgia*. 2014;34(10):767–776.

79. Miller VA, Palermo TM, Powers SW, Scher MS, Hershey AD. Migraine headaches and sleep disturbances in children. *Headache*. 2003;43(4):362–368.

80. Angriman M, Cortese S, Bruni O. Somatic and neuropsychiatric comorbidities in pediatric restless legs syndrome: a systematic review of the literature. *Sleep Med Rev*. 2017;34:34–45.

81. Seidel S, Bock A, Schlegel W, et al. Increased RLS prevalence in children and adolescents with migraine: a case-control study. *Cephalalgia*. 2012;32(9):693–699.

82. Sevindik MS, Demirci S, Goksan B, et al. Accompanying migrainous features in pediatric migraine patients with restless legs syndrome. *Neurol Sci*. 2017;38(9):1677–1681.

83. Becker PM, Novak M. Diagnosis, comorbidities, and management of restless legs syndrome. *Curr Med Res Opin*. 2014;30(8):1441–1460.

84. Zelnik N, Pacht A, Obeid R, Lerner A. Range of neurologic disorders in patients with celiac disease. *Pediatrics*. 2004;113(6):1672–1676.

85. Roche Herrero MC, Arcas Martinez J, Martinez-Bermejo A, et al. The prevalence of headache in a population of patients with coeliac disease. *Rev Neurol*. 2001;32 (4):301–309.

86. Assa A, Frenkel-Nir Y, Tzur D, Katz LH, Shamir R. Large population study shows that adolescents with celiac disease have an increased risk of multiple autoimmune and non-autoimmune comorbidities. *Acta Paediatr*. 2017;106(6):967–972.

87. Lionetti E, Francavilla R, Maiuri L, et al. Headache in pediatric patients with celiac disease and its prevalence as a diagnostic clue. *J Pediatr Gastroenterol Nutr*. 2009;49 (2):202–207.

88. Zis P, Julian T, Hadjivassiliou M. Headache associated with coeliac disease: a systematic review and meta-analysis. *Nutrients*. 2018;10(10).

89. Diaconu G, Burlea M, Grigore I, Anton DT, Trandafir LM. Celiac disease with neurologic manifestations in children. *Rev Med Chir Soc Med Nat Iasi*. 2013;117(1):88–94.

90. Nenna R, Petrarca L, Verdecchia P, et al. Celiac disease in a large cohort of children and adolescents with recurrent headache: a retrospective study. *Dig Liver Dis*. 2016;48 (5):495–498.

91. Balci O, Yilmaz D, Sezer T, Hizli S. Is celiac disease an etiological factor in children with migraine? *J Child Neurol*. 2016;31(7):929–931.

92. Inaloo S, Dehghani SM, Farzadi F, Haghighat M, Imanieh MH. A comparative study of celiac disease in children with migraine headache and a normal control group. *Turk J Gastroenterol*. 2011;22(1):32–35.

93. Jericho H, Sansotta N, Guandalini S. Extraintestinal manifestations of celiac disease: effectiveness of the gluten-free diet. *J Pediatr Gastroenterol Nutr*. 2017;65(1):75–79.

94. Richardson LP, McCauley E, Grossman DC, et al. Evaluation of the patient health questionnaire-9 item for detecting major depression among adolescents. *Pediatrics*. 2010;126(6):1117–1123.

95. Mossman SA, Luft MJ, Schroeder HK, et al. The generalized anxiety disorder 7-item scale in adolescents with generalized anxiety disorder: signal detection and validation. *Ann Clin Psychiatry*. 2017;29(4):227–234A.

96. Kirsch DB, Mink JW. Psychogenic movement disorders in children. *Pediatr Neurol*. 2004;30(1):1–6.

97. Koppen IJ, Nurko S, Saps M, Di Lorenzo C, Benninga MA. The pediatric Rome IV criteria: what's new? *Expert Rev Gastroenterol Hepatol.* 2017;11(3):193–201.

98. Thaler NS, Allen DN, Hart JS, Boucher JR, McMurray JC, Mayfield J. Neurocognitive correlates of the trail making test for older children in patients with traumatic brain injury. *Arch Clin Neuropsychol.* 2012;27(4):446–452.

99. Uttl B, Pilkenton-Taylor C. Letter cancellation performance across the adult life span. *Clin Neuropsychol.* 2001;15(4):521–530.

100. Pradhan B, Nagendra HR. Normative data for the letter-cancellation task in school children. *Int J Yoga.* 2008;1(2):72–75.

101. Duchesne M, Mattos P. Normalization of a computerized visual attention test (TAVIS). *Arq Neuropsiquiatr.* 1997;55(1):62–69.

102. Kim J, Sung IY, Ko EJ, Jung M. Visual evoked potential in children with developmental disorders: correlation with neurodevelopmental outcomes. *Ann Rehabil Med.* 2018;42 (2):305–312.

103. Renault FNRFGABCC-GF. Flash visual evoked potentials: maturation from birth to 15 years of age. *Invest Ophthalmol Vis Sci.* 2011;52(14).

104. Shinn JB, Chermak GD, Musiek FE. GIN (gaps-in-noise) performance in the pediatric population. *J Am Acad Audiol.* 2009;20(4):229–238.

105. Delecrode CR, Cardoso ACV, Frizzo ACF, Guida HL. Testes tonais de padrão de frequência e duração no Brasil: revisão de literatura. *Revista CEFAC.* 2014;16:283–293.

106. Vellozo FF, Delaméa APL, Garcia MV. Design of a sentence identification test with pictures (TIS-F) based on the pediatric speech intelligibility test. *Revista CEFAC.* 2017;19:773–781.

107. Ortiz KZ, Pereira LD. *Teste não-verbal de escuta direcionada.* São Paulo, Brazil: Lovise; 1997:231.

108. Kossoff EH, Huffman J, Turner Z, Gladstein J. Use of the modified Atkins diet for adolescents with chronic daily headache. *Cephalalgia.* 2010;30(8):1014–1016.

109. Pakalnis A, Kring D. Chronic daily headache, medication overuse, and obesity in children and adolescents. *J Child Neurol.* 2012;27(5):577–580.

110. Chai NC, Bond DS, Moghekar A, Scher AI, Peterlin BL. Obesity and headache: part II–potential mechanism and treatment considerations. *Headache.* 2014;54(3):459–471.

111. Kroon Van Diest AM, Powers SW. Cognitive behavioral therapy for pediatric headache and migraine: why to prescribe and what new research is critical for advancing integrated biobehavioral care. *Headache.* 2019;59(2):289–297.

112. Borish L. Allergic rhinitis: systemic inflammation and implications for management. *J Allergy Clin Immunol.* 2003;112(6):1021–1031.

113. Genizi J, Gordon S, Kerem NC, Srugo I, Shahar E, Ravid S. Primary headaches, attention deficit disorder and learning disabilities in children and adolescents. *J Headache Pain.* 2013;14:54.

114. Okun ML, Lin L, Pelin Z, Hong S, Mignot E. Clinical aspects of narcolepsy-cataplexy across ethnic groups. *Sleep.* 2002;25(1):27–35.

115. Ernst MM, O'Brien HL, Powers SW. Cognitive-behavioral therapy: how medical providers can increase patient and family openness and access to evidence-based multimodal therapy for pediatric migraine. *Headache.* 2015;55(10):1382–1396.

116. Shinitzky HE, Kub J. The art of motivating behavior change: the use of motivational interviewing to promote health. *Public Health Nurs.* 2001;18(3):178–185.

117. Perez-Munoz A, Buse DC, Andrasik F. Behavioral interventions for migraine. *Neurol Clin.* 2019;37(4):789–813.

118. Lipton RB, Hahn SR, Cady RK, et al. In-office discussions of migraine: results from the American migraine communication study. *J Gen Intern Med.* 2008;23(8):1145–1151.
119. Hahn SR, Lipton RB, Sheftell FD, et al. Healthcare provider-patient communication and migraine assessment: results of the American migraine communication study, phase II. *Curr Med Res Opin.* 2008;24(6):1711–1718.
120. Buse DC, Lipton RB. Facilitating communication with patients for improved migraine outcomes. *Curr Pain Headache Rep.* 2008;12(3):230–236.
121. Minen MT, Torous J, Raynowska J, et al. Electronic behavioral interventions for headache: a systematic review. *J Headache Pain.* 2016;17:51.
122. Mosadeghi-Nik M, Askari MS, Fatehi F. Mobile health (mHealth) for headache disorders: a review of the evidence base. *J Telemed Telecare.* 2016;22(8):472–477.
123. Powers SW, Andrasik F. Biobehavioral treatment, disability, and psychological effects of pediatric headache. *Pediatr Ann.* 2005;34(6):461–465.
124. Oskoui M, Pringsheim T, Billinghurst L, et al. Practice guideline update summary: pharmacologic treatment for pediatric migraine prevention: report of the guideline development, dissemination, and implementation Subcommittee of the American Academy of Neurology and the American Headache Society. *Headache.* 2019;59(8):1144–1157.

New daily persistent headache ☆

Rachel Neely, MSHS, PA-C and Frank R. Berenson, MD

New daily persistent headache (NDPH) is an often-refractory headache which presents with sudden onset. The day on which the patient develops the headache is distinct, and the time of onset is clearly remembered by the patient, with the pain becoming continuous and unremitting within 24 h.[1] Though a subset of children and adolescents with NDPH will respond quite nicely to treatment, unfortunately, many continue to experience daily headaches for years to come. Secondary etiologies must be excluded in patients in whom NDPH is suspected, as misdiagnosis can lead to inappropriate treatment and poor outcomes. Once a diagnosis is established, the importance of early intervention cannot be overemphasized. These daily headaches can lead to missed school and extracurricular activities, as well as anxiety, depression, and significant strain upon the family. The onus is often on the primary care provider, who typically has first contact with the child with NDPH, to diagnose appropriately and treat aggressively, or to refer the patient to a headache specialist.

To make an accurate diagnosis, it is critical that the provider recognize an abrupt onset headache which rapidly escalates to a continuous headache within 24 h. A thorough workup must also be performed to exclude secondary causes. NDPH typically occurs in patients without any significant prior headache history, though it can occur in those with preexisting tension-type headache or migraine. In those with prior headache history, there should be no report of an increase in headache days before the onset of daily headaches. If the patient has prior history of tension-type headache or migraine, the presence of medication overuse during, or following the development of their daily headaches excludes NDPH as the primary diagnosis. Acute traumatic headaches, headaches attributed to low cerebrospinal fluid pressure (such as spontaneous intracranial hypotension), and headaches attributed to high cerebrospinal fluid pressure (such as idiopathic intracranial hypertension) are considered secondary headaches and are not classified as NDPH.[1] These conditions will need to be ruled out by appropriate diagnostic evaluation.

☆Editor's note: Headache specialists recognize that NDPH can be challenging to treat. As the authors suggest, treatment options need to be tailored to disability, but the confident reassurance we dispense so easily to those with migraine cannot be doled out so readily to families of a youngster with NDPH. Just giving the condition a name can be helpful. We use what we use for other headache conditions and hope for the best.

Pediatric Headache. https://doi.org/10.1016/B978-0-323-83005-8.00015-X

As defined in the third edition of the International Classification of Headache Disorders (ICHD-3),[a] patients with NDPH have unremitting headaches which occur daily, and last all day for at least 3 months. The patient is classified as having *probable NDPH* when the headaches have been present for less than 3 months, with all other diagnostic features identical to those seen in NDPH.[1]

The quality of pain reported by children with NDPH may be nondescript. The pain is commonly bilateral in location and moderate in intensity, though it can be seen on any aspect of the head and range in intensity from mild to severe. In some, there are overlapping migrainous features. These may include pulsing/throbbing quality, unilateral location, photophobia, phonophobia, nausea and/or vomiting, and worsening by physical activity.[2-5] The slow progression of headache frequency in those with chronic tension-type headache or chronic migraine is sharply contrasted by the rapid onset of NDPH.[6] Careful history-taking alone should differentiate NDPH from chronic tension-type headache, chronic migraine, and rare daily headache conditions such as hemicrania continua.

In our experience, early diagnosis and treatment often decreases functional disability and in some cases prevents it. It is critical that the provider listen attentively to patients and their families while taking the history and take care not to be dismissive of complaints of daily headaches regardless of how "well" the child may appear in front of the provider. This advice applies for all headache patients, regardless of diagnosis. Pain ratings are often difficult to obtain from younger patients using validated scales, and we find using impairment of activities (no impairment equating to mild, some impairment equating to moderate, and complete impairment indicating severe intensity) to be clinically useful measures. Creating a strong therapeutic alliance is instrumental in directing appropriate diagnostic workup and therapeutic management, which can at times be lengthy and taxing on patients as well as their families (Table 1).

Table 1 ICHD-3 criteria for NDPH.

NDPH diagnostic criteria:
A Persistent headache fulfilling criteria B and C
B Distinct and clearly remembered onset, with pain becoming continuous and unremitting within 24 h
C Present for >3 months
D Not better accounted for by another ICHD-3 diagnosis[1]

[a]ICHD-3 is published as the first issue of *Cephalalgia* in 2018. It is a systematic classification system for headache with explicit diagnostic criteria for each condition as agreed upon by the Classification Committee of the International Headache Society and supported by research.

Epidemiology

NDPH has higher prevalence in children and adolescents than in adults. Studies conducted at various tertiary headache centers throughout the United States and abroad have shown NDPH to be present in 13%–35% of children with chronic daily headache (defined as headache for at least 15 days in a period of 1 month, over at least a 3 month period, and with no secondary cause).[4,7–13] In comparison, it is estimated that up to 10.8% of adult patients with chronic daily headache have NDPH.[11] Kung et al. found that NDPH is more prevalent in girls compared to boys (with a female: male ratio of 1.8). In their study, which included patients aged 6–18 years with chronic daily headache, the mean age of onset of NDPH was 14.2 years.[4] The majority of patients with NDPH described in both the pediatric and the adult literature are Caucasian,[2,4,13,14] although this may reflect selection bias as to who gets to a headache clinic.

A retrospective review published by Grengs and Mack in 2016 evaluated the temporal onset of NDPH in school-aged children seen at a tertiary care center. Interestingly, there was a statistically significant increase in headache onset in the months of September and January, months traditionally associated with return to school following a break at the end of the prior semester.[15] The authors postulate that the action of returning to school may trigger the onset of NDPH. We suspect that this correlates with a significant stress trigger.

In adults, mood disorders have been shown to have higher prevalence in NDPH patients compared to healthy subjects. A cross-sectional study conducted in India looked at the prevalence of depression, anxiety, pain somatization, and catastrophizing in NDPH patients. Among these adult NDPH patients, severe anxiety was evident in 65.5%, and severe depression was present in 40%.[16] Though few pediatric studies have explored this association, in our clinical experience, mood disorders appear highly prevalent in pediatric NDPH patients. Baron and Rothner reported straight-A report cards and excessive extracurricular activities as possible risk factors for NDPH chronification.[6] However, this reflects co-morbidity but not causality.

Pathogenesis

Unfortunately, little is known about the pathogenesis of NDPH. There is a paucity of data regarding this condition, especially in the pediatric population. Thus the etiology of these headaches is largely speculative. Some authors have theorized that NDPH results from glial cell activation precipitated by prior viral illness or infection, psychological stress, invasive surgical procedure, mild to moderate head injury, or other provoking events. These events could lead to the continuous production of cytokines, triggering a chronic inflammatory response and the production of pain.[2,3,5,12,14] In an abstract from 2004, the authors found that in 34 children and adolescents with NDPH, 15% (5 patients) developed NDPH following an infection, 15%

(5 patients) had a history of preceding mild to moderate head injury, and 12% (4 patients) had significant psychosocial stressors.[17]

A number of researchers have explored whether an infectious trigger exists for NDPH. Diaz-Mitoma and colleagues hypothesized that activation of latent Epstein-Barr virus (EBV) may play a role in the development of NDPH. In their study, 84% of 32 NDPH patients had evidence of an active EBV infection compared to only 25% of 32 age- and gender- matched controls.[18] In a retrospective chart review by Li and Rozen, EBV antibody titers were positive for past infection in 5 of 7 patients (71%) tested, though there was no evidence of active infection.[3] Others have found no evidence of past or prior EBV infection in their NDPH patients, but have identified evidence of other infections, including herpes simplex virus (HSV) and cytomegalovirus (CMV).[5] Additional proposed infectious triggers include *Salmonella*, adenovirus, toxoplasmosis, herpes zoster virus, and *Escherichia coli* urinary tract infections.[19]

A temporal relationship between NDPH and exposure to pesticides, certain medications (including antibiotics, terbinafine, and progesterone), and massage treatment has also been observed in adults.[14] Rozen and colleagues also suspect that cervical joint hypermobility may play a role. Hypothetically, irritation of the cervical facet and atlanto-axial region, as well as stimulation of the C1-C3 cervical nerve roots in individuals with hypermobility could bring on daily head pain through activation of the trigemino-cervical complex. This may be especially relevant in cases of NDPH following surgical procedures due to extension of the neck with intubation.[14,20,21] Additionally, defective internal jugular venous drainage has been suggested as a potential trigger.[22]

Interestingly, Rozen and Swidan found elevated levels of TNF alpha in the CSF samples of 19 out of 20 NDPH patients from an inpatient headache unit, lending support to the role of pro-inflammatory cytokines in the pathogenesis of NDPH.[23] TNF alpha can activate the production of calcitonin gene-related peptide, a protein that is known to play a major role in the pathogenesis of other headache disorders, including migraine and cluster headache. Though the implications of elevated levels of TNF alpha in the CSF of NDPH patients remain entirely theoretical, these findings may suggest that NDPH is not a consequence of a specific infectious agent, but instead results from a nonspecific inflammatory response to illness, physical or emotional stress, or other significant change in the environment.[7]

Workup

Diagnostic workup should include laboratory studies to exclude metabolic derangements and inflammatory disorders as secondary causes. Blood work should include complete blood count with differential, comprehensive metabolic panel, thyroid studies, and sedimentation rate. In our practice, we additionally check vitamin D and vitamin B12 levels, as well as antinuclear antibodies (ANA) with reflex. Obtaining EBV IgG and IgM titers is reasonable, though the significance of elevated EBV titers when identified is unknown. Some headache specialists advocate for having titers drawn for CMV, human herpesvirus 6, and parvovirus, and others consider testing for West Nile and Lyme disease potentially useful.[7,24] Although there is no targeted treatment for most of these illnesses, identifying a potential causative agent as a trigger can be reassuring for families.[7]

Regarding neuroimaging, we recommend a gadolinium-enhanced MRI of the brain with MRV in all NDPH or probable NDPH patients to exclude spontaneous CSF leak, cerebral venous sinus thrombosis, inflammatory processes, and other potential intracranial pathology that can mimic the presentation of NDPH. In treatment-refractory patients, a lumbar puncture may be necessary to exclude a high-pressure headache without papilledema, low pressure headache, or a CNS inflammatory disorder.[13]

Treatment

We recommend that the provider tailor the treatment approach to the patient's level of functional disability, which is measured by frequency of missed school and social events, and impairment of daily activities. The spectrum of disability observed in the NDPH patient population is quite wide. The patient without disability remains in school without impairment of their day-to-day routine, while other patients are so significantly disabled that they have withdrawn from traditional school programs entirely. The goal of therapy is to allow the patient to return to (or remain in) a state of normal function.

For the patient without disability, we recommend initiating treatment with a course of oral steroids 5–7 days in duration. Though the literature regarding the use of steroids in NDPH is sparse, with only rare findings of patient improvement with cycled intravenous steroids[24,25], in our clinical experience, a relatively short steroid pulse provides significant clinical benefit to a small subset of patients.

Any of the daily medications used for migraine and tension headache may be of potential benefit for the patient with NDPH, including neuromodulators such as topiramate or valproic acid; tricyclic antidepressants such as amitriptyline or nortriptyline; or beta blockers such as propranolol. If there is no clinical improvement within 6–8 weeks on a given daily enteral medication, we recommend transitioning to a medication with a different mechanism of action. If there is partial response, we recommend continuing therapy, titrating further, or adding another agent.

Selection of an oral preventive should be directed by the semiology of the headache (i.e., higher consideration of topiramate if more migrainous in character, versus a tricyclic antidepressant if more tension-type), while also taking the potential side-effect profile of the medication into consideration. Again, though this approach has proven helpful in our clinical experience, there is very limited data to support the selection of one oral medication over another.

We have found nerve blocks to be quite beneficial as well, and these are commonly used by pediatric headache specialists to treat patients with NDPH. In our practice, we use a combination of lidocaine and bupivacaine. Other specialists may use bupivacaine alone or in combination with steroids.[26] We often offer these in conjunction with titration of daily medications. If the response is poor, we then consider cycling intravenous medication in an inpatient setting. For refractory cases, Botox (onabotulinumtoxinA) injections, a prolonged course of steroids, leukotriene inhibitors, or perhaps anticalcitonin gene-related peptide monoclonal antibodies may be of benefit. Biofeedback, relaxation therapy, or acupuncture may also be helpful.

For those with significant disability, we have found that early admission to the hospital for cycled intravenous medication is beneficial. Rather than prolonging school absences and potentially increasing patient deconditioning by waiting weeks for daily enteral meds to show effect, inpatient admission allows for a potentially rapid return to function. We recommend starting with serial intravenous infusions of diphenhydramine, prochlorperazine, and ketorolac, with transition to intravenous dihydroergotamine if poor response within 24–48 h. If these measures are ineffective, we recommend serial infusions of magnesium or valproate sodium. In our practice, typical duration of such inpatient admissions is 3–4 days, with discharge at that point if no response. Preventive enteral medication including neuromodulators, tricyclic antidepressants, and antihypertensives, among others, can be initiated prior to discharge to help prevent headache recurrence. If inpatient therapy fails to bring benefit, we recommend proceeding with nerve blocks, Botox (onabotulinumtoxinA) injections, or a trial of a prolonged course of steroids in the outpatient setting.

Prognosis

Despite aggressive treatment measures, NDPH is often quite treatment-refractory. This can be tremendously frustrating for the patient, the family, as well as the provider. It has been postulated that there may be two types of NDPH: (1) a form which can resolve spontaneously within several months; and (2) a form which is refractory to even the most aggressive forms of treatment. In our clinical practice, the latter form is by far more prevalent. In a small cohort study of 28 children and adolescents with NDPH by Wintrich and Rothner, 20 patients (71%) reported headaches 6 months to 2 years later, and only 8 patients (29%) were headache-free. Despite these high statistics regarding persistent headache, it is encouraging that 79% of these 28 patients had Migraine Disability Assessment (MIDAS) scores that indicated normal function.[27]

NDPH: What families need to know

New daily persistent headache (NDPH) is a headache that develops on a given day and persists all day, every day from that time onward. To you and your child, these headaches may have seemed to come "out of the blue" and just won't go away. Your child will likely recall where they were and what they were doing when the headache first started. For many, headache onset occurs during unremarkable circumstances, such as while sitting at home playing video games, socializing with friends at a birthday party, or concentrating at school during a math test.

Usually, the child who develops NDPH did not complain of frequent or severe headaches before the start of their daily headaches. NDPH is sometimes diagnosed in patients who already have another type of headache, such as migraine headache or tension-type headache, but then develop *new* headaches without any increase or significant change in the prior headache pattern.

Typically, over the counter and oral prescription medications for headache do not provide relief from these daily headaches. For many, even infusions of medication into the vein do not alleviate the pain. In other words, these headaches are often quite resistant to treatment. These headaches and their significant impact on day-to-day function can be alarming to families. For many, the mind often jumps to the worst-case scenario: brain tumor, brain bleed, severe infection, or other life-threatening conditions.

Fortunately, patients with NDPH do not suffer from any of the above. Testing is always ordered to exclude potential medical causes. Your provider may want to obtain a scan of your child's brain (MRI), as well as laboratory (blood sample) studies. In some cases, your provider may even want to have a small amount of spinal fluid drawn (a procedure called a "spinal tap") to check the pressure around the brain and look for markers of inflammation. Some providers will also order special blood tests to look for evidence of recent infection. If any of the tests for infection return positive, it is possible that a virus could have contributed to the development of your child's headache. In patients with NDPH, this testing frequently comes back normal.

We still do not know the exact cause of NDPH. Of the few studies exploring this question, there have been some findings to support that a viral illness could have played a role, at least in some cases. Others suspect that mild head trauma or recent surgery on a part of the body besides the brain (such as having the appendix removed) may trigger these headaches. However, for many patients, no specific trigger is identified.

Your child may be prescribed medications including steroids, antidepressants, antiseizure medications, and blood pressure medications, among others. Other treatments include learning relaxation techniques through biofeedback, or participating in other types of therapy. In some cases, patients are admitted to the hospital for several days to receive cycled intravenous medications. The goal of treatment is not only to reduce or eliminate your child's headaches, but also to allow your child to remain in school, enjoy daily activities, and return to normal function.

Though this type of headache is difficult to treat in most cases, and some patients continue to experience daily headaches despite therapy, many do see good improvement. It is crucial that you be an advocate for your child, and that you establish a partnership with a provider who is experienced in caring for children with NDPH. By creating a solid relationship with your provider and working through the challenges of diagnosis and treatment, one step at a time, it is possible to gain significant improvement and control of your child's headaches so that your child can lead a normal life.

References

1. Headache Classification Committee of the International Headache Society (IHS) the international classification of headache disorders, 3rd edition. *Cephalalgia*. 2018; 38(1):1–211.
2. Robbins MS, Grosberg BM, Napchan U, Crystal SC, Lipton RB. Clinical and prognostic subforms of new daily-persistent headache. *Neurology*. 2010;74(17):1358–1364.
3. Li D, Rozen T. The clinical characteristics of new daily persistent headache. *Cephalalgia*. 2002;22(1):66–69.
4. Kung E, Tepper S, Rapoport A, Sheftell F, Bigal M. New daily persistent headache in the pediatric population. *Cephalalgia*. 2009;29(1):17–22.
5. Meineri P, Torre E, Rota E, Grasso E. New daily persistent headache: clinical and serological characteristics in a retrospective study. *Neurol Sci*. 2004;25(S3).
6. Baron E, Rothner A. New daily persistent headache in children and adolescents. *Curr Neurol Neurosci Rep*. 2010;10(2):127–132.
7. Mack K. New daily persistent headache in children and adults. *Curr Pain Headache Rep*. 2009;13(1):47–51.
8. Gladstein J, Holden E. Chronic daily headache in children and adolescents: a 2-year prospective study. *Headache*. 1996;36(6):349–351.
9. Koenig M, Gladstein J, McCarter R, Hershey A, Wasiewski W. The Pediatric Committee of the Amer. Chronic daily headache in children and adolescents presenting to tertiary headache clinics. *Headache*. 2002;42(6):491–500.
10. Mack K. What incites new daily persistent headache in children? *Pediatr Neurol*. 2004; 31(2):122–125.
11. Bigal M, Lipton R, Tepper S, Rapoport A, Sheftell F. Primary chronic daily headache and its subtypes in adolescents and adults. *Neurology*. 2004;63(5):843–847.
12. Takase Y, Nakano M, Tatsumi C, Matsuyama T. Clinical features, effectiveness of drug-based treatment, and prognosis of new daily persistent headache (NDPH): 30 cases in Japan. *Cephalalgia*. 2004;24(11):955–959.
13. Yamani N, Olesen J. New daily persistent headache: a systematic review on an enigmatic disorder. *J Headache Pain*. 2019;20(1).
14. Rozen TD. Triggering events and new daily persistent headache: age and gender differences and insights on pathogenesis-a clinic-based study. *Headache*. 2015;56(1):164–173.
15. Grengs LR, Mack KJ. New daily persistent headache is most likely to begin at the start of school. *J Child Neurol*. 2016;31(7):864–868.
16. Uniyal R, Paliwal VK, Tripathi A. Psychiatric comorbidity in new daily persistent headache: a cross-sectional study. *Eur J Pain*. 2017;21(6):1031–1038.
17. Abdelsalam HHM, Guo Y, Rothner AD. New daily persistent headache in children and adolescents [abstract]. *Ann Neurol*. 2004;56:S83–S131.
18. Diaz-Mitoma F, Vanast WJ, Tyrrell DL. Increased frequency of Epstein-Barr virus excretion in patients with new daily persistent headaches. *Lancet*. 1987;1(8530):411–415. https:/doi.org/10.1016/s0140-6736(87)90119-x.
19. Santoni JR, Santoni-Williams CJ. Headache and painful lymphadenopathy in extracranial or systemic infection: etiology of new daily persistent headaches. *Intern Med*. 1993; 32(7):530–532.
20. Rozen T, Roth J, Denenberg N. Cervical spine joint hypermobility: a possible predisposing factor for new daily persistent headache. *Cephalalgia*. 2006;26(10):1182–1185.

21. Bartsch T, Goadsby PJ. The trigeminocervical complex and migraine: current concepts and synthesis. *Curr Pain Headache Rep.* 2003;7(5):371–376.
22. Donnet A, Levrier O. A consecutive series of ten cases of new daily persistent headache: Clinical presentation and morphology of the venous system. *Neurology.* 2009;72(Suppl. 3):A419.
23. Rozen T, Swidan SZ. Elevation of CSF tumor necrosis factor α levels in new daily persistent headache and treatment refractory chronic migraine. *Headache.* 2007;47(7):1050–1055.
24. Rozen T. New daily persistent headache: clinical perspective. *Headache.* 2011;51(4):641–649.
25. Rozen T. New daily persistent headache: an update. *Curr Pain Headache Rep.* 2014;18(7):431.
26. Szperka CL, Gelfand AA, Hershey AD. Patterns of use of peripheral nerve blocks and trigger point injections for pediatric headache: results of a survey of the American headache society pediatric and adolescent section. *Headache.* 2016;56(10):1597–1607.
27. Wintrich S, Rothner D. New daily persistent headaches–follow up and outcome in children and adolescents. *Headache.* 2010;50(Suppl. 1):s23.

Posttraumatic headaches in youth ☆

10

Shannon Babineau, MD and Heidi K. Blume, MD

Introduction

Concussion and mild traumatic brain injury (TBI) are very common in pediatrics, and headache is one of the most common and most troubling symptoms following head injury. Persistent posttraumatic headaches (PTH) can also be one of the most challenging headache syndromes to manage. This is a relatively new area of research, and there are few studies to help us determine which treatments are most likely to be effective for a particular child. In this chapter, we will review the current definitions and risk factors for PTH in children and teens. We will discuss PTH in a step-wise manner; (a) a section to help families understand PTH and what they can do to manage these headaches, (b) information that can be used in a primary care setting, and (c) more detailed information that a headache specialist may consider when headaches are disabling and persistent for weeks or months following injury. This chapter will discuss the subacute and chronic phases of PTH. The acute management of concussion and TBI on the sidelines or in the ED, is outside the scope of this book, but the CDC has many resources on this topic on their website, www.cdc.gov/traumaticbraininjury/index.html.

Information about posttraumatic headache for families

- **How does posttraumatic headache happen?** The mechanisms that lead to headache after trauma are complicated and multifactorial. There is still a lot that medical professionals do not understand about concussion, and persisting symptoms like headache. Head trauma can trigger a cascade of problematic events that include an inflammatory response, and changes in how the nerve cells

---

☆Editor's note: The treatment for concussions has undergone radical changes over the years. We used to insist on "brain rest," where we advised patients to essentially do nothing for a prolonged period of time. We took away their screens, friends, and light. We've learned since then that this is unnecessary and can actually lead to prolongation of symptoms. The authors present a data driven and practical approach to management that employs common sense incremental return to activities based upon how each individual youngster heals. They explain head injury in a way that is useful for practitioners and patients alike.

Pediatric Headache. https://doi.org/10.1016/B978-0-323-83005-8.00016-1

function and communicate with each other. These initial changes are irritating to the brain and nerves in the head and neck and frequently lead to the perception of pain in the head, or headache. The brain gets to work healing these changes as soon as they happen. However, it often takes weeks for this to occur, which is why the symptoms of concussion may take weeks to resolve. In a subset of people, the healing process does not shut down the pain signals that were initially triggered by the head injury. We believe that for people with prolonged headache after concussion, nerve cells may communicate differently than before the concussion, and the brain can become rewired so that pain becomes the new "normal." The pain system continues to act as though there is an irritant or ongoing injury even after the irritant (concussion) is resolved and there is no ongoing injury. The brain learns pain, and this can lead to headaches that continue well after the concussion has resolved.

- **Steps to feeling better:** Initially after a concussion it is important to rest and recover. Good initial concussion care does require meeting with your health care provider, taking frequent breaks, pacing during cognitive activity, and avoiding high-risk contact activities. Most kids with concussion will recover back to normal within 1–2 weeks. However, if symptoms continue for several weeks, continued withdrawal from school and physical activity can cause more harm than good. The more we learn about concussion, the more we learn how important return to physical activity can be, in concussion recovery. If you were an athlete before your concussion, it is helpful to start returning to a routine of regular exercise (without risk of head trauma), starting with light activities that don't make your symptoms worse, and slowly increasing your activity over time. If your headaches are significantly worsened by physical activity, you may need to build up slowly and recondition yourself, particularly if you have not been doing much physical activity for a long time. It may be helpful to work together with a trainer or physical therapist who knows about "subthreshold exercise" training as a treatment for concussion. You may need to adjust your activity to accommodate your headaches, including avoiding activities with a lot of bouncing. Often running can trigger or worsen headaches, so activities like stationary bike riding and swimming are easier to start with.

It is also important to take care of your body and avoid activities that are known to worsen headaches. You can read the chapters on healthy habits for migraine management for more detail. In brief: get enough sleep, hydrate, eat well, and take care of your emotional health. Children and teenagers are often sleep deprived. It is important to know how much sleep you need at your age, and to try your best to get it. It is important to stay well hydrated and it is important to eat regularly throughout the day with protein and healthy snacks.

It can be very difficult to adjust to the effects that concussion and headache can have on your life. It's hard because you go from feeling healthy and active, to feeling miserable and experiencing a lot of pain and other symptoms overnight. In addition, concussion cannot be seen by other people. It is easy to identify and care for someone who has a broken leg and needs a cast and crutches. However, there are no outward signs that you are suffering with concussion and posttraumatic headache. You are not alone, but it may feel like it. Posttraumatic headache can make you feel powerless over your body. Talking about how all of this makes you feel and starting to find ways to make yourself feel more powerful and in control of your body and feelings can be very important in recovering and learning to live with the new symptoms. Having someone to help you with this is very important. Consider reaching out to a therapist in your area that can help you with this process.

As you are recovering, it is important to be realistic with your activities. As you learn to adjust to how you feel, you may not be able to take all of the classes you want to take or do all the after school activities you want to do right away. While you learn how to manage your symptoms, you have to give yourself time. You are going to need extra time to take care of yourself because you need time for sleep, exercise, and going to additional doctor's appointments or therapy appointments. If you don't give yourself this time, and instead fill it with honors classes and other clubs, you are not giving your body what it needs and you are likely to prolong your symptoms. You may need to have a period of months or even a school year where you shift your priorities. That doesn't mean you will not be able to return to other activities or classes in the future but taking this time will allow you to recovery more fully and with a greater chance of success. However, it is equally important to continue with some of the things that are important to you, as we know that curling up in a ball on the couch in a dark room and stopping all normal activity will actually make symptoms last longer.

- **How to navigate school**: Returning to school for a full day when you are suffering with headaches can be very difficult. There are many things in the school environment that make headaches worse-it is loud, bright, and you are there for long hours. However, returning to school as normally and regularly as possible, will ultimately help your symptoms improve and get you back to doing the things you need and want to do. There are going to be days that you really don't feel well, and it may be necessary to skip a few hours or the full day. If this occurs with high frequency, though, you will fall behind and get out of your routine, which is worse overall for your headaches. It is helpful to have some tricks, for the time when you don't feel well in school, that can help you feel better and allow you to return to class without having to go home. Sometimes having rest periods built into the day can be helpful. Having some treatments to use at the nurse's office like cool compresses, a dark resting spot, meditation, as well as medication can also be beneficial. You may need adjustments in your schoolwork on days when you don't feel well to help allow the additional rest needed. Overall, it is important to speak with your school about the symptoms you are still having and what types of activities might make them worse. It is helpful to have an agreement with the school about certain accommodations you may need, usually done with a 504 plan. If your school is not familiar with options for management of school work after concussion, the CDC "Heads Up" concussion program has on-line resources everyone can access and use. (www.cdc.gov/headsup/.)

- **Long term prognosis.** While the majority of people recover within 3 months after concussion, there are people who continue to have headaches long after sustaining a concussion. Even these people can ultimately get better, even after a year or more. It is best to plan for the worst and hope for the best. There are many techniques available to help manage headaches that range from different lifestyle measures, alternative therapies, and medication. Speak with your doctor about what is right for you. There is no reason to suffer with headaches for months or years waiting for them to resolve. The longer your brain spends with pain, the more it gets used to it. Intervening with these therapies will not prolong recovery and may in fact speed up the resolution of the headaches; and if it doesn't, and you continue to have headaches, you will learn more quickly about how to cope with them and return to your life where you are in control.

Information for primary care clinicians
What is "posttraumatic headache"?

The CDC defines a TBI as "disruption in the normal function of the brain that can be caused by a bump, blow, or jolt to the head, or penetrating head injury." The formal definition of PTH by the International Classification of Headache Disorders-3 is a headache that develops within 7 days of TBI that is not "better accounted for by another diagnosis."[1] The headache that occurs after a TBI can have many different characteristics, including migrainous (accompanied by photophobia, phonophobia, nausea, vomiting), tension type symptoms, or occipital neuralgia, but PTHs may also be more difficult to characterize than primary headache syndromes.[2, 3] PTH is also often associated with other postconcussion symptoms including mood changes, problems with balance, sleep disturbance, and cognitive changes. These other concussion symptoms may also exacerbate headache frequency and severity, which can complicate the management of PTH.

It can be helpful to attempt to determine if the PTH fits into a "subclass" of headache using ICHD-3 criteria. Almost all the primary headache syndrome phenotypes, migraine, tension, cluster, primary stabbing headaches have been described after head trauma.[4, 5] The majority of PTH in children meet criteria for migraine.[3] In addition, identifying migrainous phenotype in a patient can aid in prognostication. Patients with migrainous PTH often have more symptoms from the concussion, including lower cognitive scores and poorer balance on testing, and thus greater disability.[6, 7] Interestingly, cervicogenic headache is more common in PTH patients, seen in up to 20%, than in the general pediatric headache population,[3] which is not surprising given the likelihood of neck trauma or whiplash associated with mild TBI.

Most children who sustain a concussion will recover to baseline within a few weeks without significant sequelae,[8-10] and this information is vital for the child and their family to understand.[11] However, some will develop symptoms that can persist for weeks or months, which can cause significant disability, loss of school time and loss of participation in sports and other extracurricular activities.

Red flags: Most children with concussion do not need neuroimaging or other tests. There are well established guidelines regarding when neuroimaging should be considered immediately following TBI, this includes those with some combination of the following risk factors:

- Age younger than 2 years
- Vomiting
- Loss of consciousness
- Severe mechanism of injury
- Severe or worsening headache
- Amnesia
- Nonfrontal scalp hematoma
- Glasgow Coma Scale score less than 15
- Clinical suspicion for skull fracture[12]

In addition, providers may consider neuroimaging, with MRI or CT scan, or other testing, if the child has increasing headaches, new neurological symptoms, new severe headache greater than a week after injury, or symptoms of another disorder that could be causing headaches.

Pathophysiology of PTH

There is little that we understand definitively about the pathophysiology of PTH. Given the high proportion of patients with a migrainous phenotype to their PTH, as well as the efficacy of several medications used typically in migraine, it is likely that the trigeminovascular system is involved in the generation of PTH. The effect of a traumatic injury on the brain may be like the effect of cortical spreading depression (one of the mechanisms of migraine activation) on the brain. Both entities lead to ionic changes, excessive neurotransmitter/neuropeptide release, inflammatory cytokine release, cerebral metabolic changes and mismatch with neurovascular supply, and disruption of the blood brain barrier. It is unclear if TBI triggers cortical spreading depression or has similar effects on the brain, but the outcome seems to trigger the same final pathway. Functional imaging studies have shown changes in metabolism and cerebral blood flow that can persist for weeks and even months after concussive injury, so this may be another potential cause of PTH. In addition, the action of neuropeptides that are involved in migraine, like CGRP and PACAP, are altered after head injury in animal models. This offers exciting therapeutic targets for PTH given the recent approval of CGRP antibodies treatments and CGRP antagonists. The influence of the cervical nerve roots on the trigeminocervical complex may also contribute to the pathophysiology of PTH. Like migraine, there are many different pathways involved in the generation of PTH and hypothalamic/thalamic and higher cortical centers in pain amplification and maintenance, likely have a role.[13]

Risk factors: Several factors have been associated with prolonged recovery from concussion, these include female sex, adolescent age, high number of symptoms immediately following concussion, migrainous symptoms following concussion, diagnosis of migraine or mental health problems prior to injury, and prior concussion with persistent symptoms.[9, 14, 15] There are few studies of pediatric PTH specifically, but it appears that the risk factors for persistent PTH are similar to those for persistent symptoms following concussion overall.[16] While it may seem that those with more severe brain injury would be at higher risk for prolonged or severe PTH, this does not appear to be true. In fact, those with moderate or severe TBI may have a lower risk of PTH than those with mild TBI, and neither loss of consciousness nor amnesia has been consistently associated with the risk of persistent symptoms or headache following TBI. Thus, for concussed individuals with PTH who have several of the risk factors noted above, one may consider early intervention for PTH following concussion to optimize headache management with little risk. This would include working on appropriate sleep, return to appropriate low-risk exercise, adequate hydration, and acute pain management (see Chapters 21–23), and then perhaps starting a low risk preventive treatment if headaches don't improve after a few weeks of conservative management. Mental health problems should also be addressed as part of the treatment process.

Evaluation: The initial evaluation of a child with PTH should include assessment of headaches and other symptoms, including mental and physical health issues, which were present prior to injury. After assessing premorbid conditions, then proceed to the injury history to understand how the injury occurred, what symptoms and disabilities were present immediately following the concussion, and how symptoms have changed since the injury. It is also important to learn what the patient and their family are most worried about, as they may have concerns that are unanticipated, and if these are not discussed, it will be difficult to provide satisfactory treatment. The exam should include vital signs, (including orthostatic HR and BP if there are complaints of orthostatic intolerance), palpation and movement of the head and neck (looking for any focal tenderness or signs of neuropathic pain), fundoscopic exam, and a neurological exam, looking for evidence of asymmetry, abnormal eye movements, balance problems, or other new deficits. If there are new focal deficits, or if headaches are increasing over time, neuroimaging should be considered. If there are signs of other systemic illness that could be contributing to headaches, these potential diagnoses should be worked up as appropriate.[17]

Initial management: Once the initial evaluation is complete and you have determined that your patient has PTH, rather than another primary or secondary headache syndrome, one can go forward with active headache management. Unfortunately, there is very little data on the ideal management of PTH for adults or children. The most typical approach to managing PTH is to use interventions appropriate to the "headache phenotype." In addition, it has become clear that prolonged, complete rest following a simple concussion is not beneficial, and actually has been associated with prolonged recovery.[18] Most individuals with PTH should begin "active recovery" or "subthreshold exercise," low-level aerobic exercise that does not exacerbate symptoms, sometime in the first week or two following injury.[19] In a formal subthreshold exercise program, patients complete a graded aerobic treadmill test to identify the level of exertion that provokes symptom worsening, and then they participate in a program that promotes exertion at 80% of the maximum heart rate achieved. Ideally, they will do this subthreshold exercise regime 5–7 days/week using a heart rate monitor, often supervised by a physical therapist who can help to advance exercise time and intensity as appropriate. In trials, after treatment for 3 weeks, patients reported improved symptoms as well as improvement in peak heart rate without symptom exacerbation.[18, 20, 21] We hope that most communities would have a physical therapist or athletic trainer who is familiar with the subthreshold exercise techniques that are recommended after concussion, so they can work together with the patient, family, and primary care provider as a team to help return the youth with PTH back to school and then back to athletic activities.

We also recommend following the typical lifestyle management strategies for headache regarding appropriate sleep, meals, hydration, and stress management (see Chapters 21–23). This can be more complex when patients have significant sleep disruption or mood changes related to head injury, so one may consider active management of these problems with medications or other treatments. Dealing with these challenges is essential to move forward with headache control, as poor sleep, active anxiety, or depression will lead to exacerbation of headache.

School and PTH: Most pediatric patients are going to require adjustments to the school day after a concussion.[22, 23] For those with persistent PTH, concussion accommodations may be extended by developing a 504/IEP plan. These plans can help the student manage the school environment with the persisting pain, environmental stimuli exacerbation, and slowed processing/cognitive speeds. The goal is for kids with PTH to attend school as regularly as possible, as extended absence may also lengthen recovery time.[22] It is important to discuss what types of activities/environments are worsening the headache to customize accommodations. General accommodations could include modified class schedule, ability to use sunglasses or tinted glasses, earplugs, the ability to skip noisy assemblies, have lunch with a friend in a quiet place, and extra time for assignments and tests. Patients may benefit from short rests in a quiet place if headache is worsening in class. Options to use a note taking services/audio recording instead of looking up and down at the board or screens can be helpful to reduce visually triggered headache. Sometimes it may be necessary to develop a plan that gradually increases school time and cognitive demands.[24] The CDC "Heads Up" program provides a template for "return to school" letter for children with concussion, including those with PTH that lists several options for accommodations (https://www.cdc.gov/traumaticbraininjury/pdf/pediatricmtbiguidelineeducationaltools/mTBI_ReturntoSchool_FactSheet-Pin.pdf).

Medications: Abortive therapy should be considered to control acute headaches following concussion. Ibuprofen may be more effective than acetaminophen for the management of PTH,[25] and ibuprofen or naproxen can be considered for acute management of headache once intracranial hemorrhage has been excluded by exam or imaging. There are case studies reporting that triptans can be effective for the management of PTH with migrainous features,[26] so their use can be considered in appropriate circumstances (see Chapter 12). However, opiates should not be used for the treatment of persistent or acute PTH following mild TBI or concussion, and providers and families should avoid overusing any abortive therapy to prevent rebound or medication overuse headaches following TBI.[27]

If the child has persistent migrainous PTH, particularly if they have a strong personal or family history of migraine, one might consider using preventive treatments that are used for migraine management. As a primary care provider, start with safe, well-tolerated supplements such as magnesium, which has shown some benefits in experimental models of TBI,[28] or melatonin for sleep induction. It is also important to recognize and treat anxiety and depression that co-occur with PTH. We let patients and families know that "stress" of all different kinds can make pain feel worse, and that addressing these issues is as important as any other therapy or testing. When PTH is disabling and persistent, it is reasonable to consider referral to a local headache or concussion specialist for further evaluation and treatment.

Information for the headache specialist

Comorbid conditions: In the evaluation of the headache patient who sustained head injury, it is important to understand some of the other physiological systems that may be affected in concussion, that can contribute to headaches including the vestibulo-ocular system, autonomic nervous system, and cervical paraspinal muscular system. It is helpful to know how to assess and address these systems to treat the patient appropriately. It is well known that concussion can cause vestibulo-ocular system dysfunction, and that this dysfunction can contribute to headaches. Concussion can disrupt the vestibular system function independently or when linked with ocular dysfunction. Vestibular dysfunction can cause movement induced headaches and motion sensitivity in addition to more typical vestibular signs like imbalance and vertigo. There are several balance screens that are easy to implement in an office setting, including the balance error scoring system (BESS)[29] as well as more advanced technologies if desired. Typically, vestibular therapy is used to recalibrate the vestibular system.[30] When vestibular dysfunction is identified, it is important to address these issues before starting aerobic physical therapy as the vestibular symptoms can prevent the patient from treadmill exercise.

Headaches that are worsened by visual tasks (reading/taking notes) or are accompanied by complaints of blurred vision or double vision should raise suspicion for visual dysfunction. Testing for ocular dysfunction should include an evaluation of smooth pursuits, saccadic movement, and convergence. There are several ways to do this. One quick standardized screen that can be used in the pediatric population is called the visual oculomotor screen (VOMS). The VOMS is easy to incorporate into your cranial nerve exam,[31] and there are videos online demonstrating its use in concussion. If ocular symptoms and signs are uncovered during your history and exam, you should consider visual therapy for the patient. Some vestibular therapists are familiar with certain visual exercises such as convergence strengthening. If a patient is having symptoms of vestibular and visual dysfunction, it is reasonable to start with vestibular therapy, as vestibular therapy is much more readily available and typically covered by insurance. Visual therapy is often an out of pocket expense. However, if vestibular therapy is not enough, the child can try a course of visual therapy as well. Vision therapy can provide a significant benefit for those with abnormalities of oculomotor system function. A retrospective analysis of children with concussion who underwent vision therapy for oculomotor dysfunction found that 90% had complete or marked improvement in their primary symptoms. Subsequent small studies have found that visual therapy improved saccades, fixation, and simulated reading as well as improved convergence and accommodation. Improvements in these vision measures were all associated with improvement in reading-related symptoms, including headache.[32–35]

Autonomic dysfunction, which has been associated with concussion, can lead to development of orthostatic dizziness and positional headaches (worse with standing). It can also lead to fatigue and exercise intolerance. Autonomic dysfunction can be identified on exam by noting a significant change in blood pressure or heart rate with change in position. Exercise, focusing on core and leg strengthening, is one of the best management techniques for autonomic dysfunction. In addition, ensuring proper electrolyte consumption, hydration, the use of compression stockings and medications to support blood pressure can be helpful. Liberating salt intake may improve headache in patients with autonomic dysfunction after concussion by increasing intravascular volume and making the patient thirsty.[36]

Cervicogenic headaches can arise from whiplash injury that leads to muscle spasm as well as misalignment of the cervical spine, in addition to activating the trigeminocervical complex. If headaches are occipital, occurring with neck movement, or exacerbated by activities that require prolonged neck stabilization the neck may be playing a role. Of note, cervicogenic headaches are not worsened by physical activity. On exam there may be tenderness or reproduction of the headache with pressure over the occipital groove or neck and there may be reduced range of motion. Clinical tests that evaluate the upper cervical spine, like the cervical flexion rotation test (CFRT), have been shown to have the highest accuracy and may be useful in identifying those with cervicogenic component to their headache.[30, 37, 38] For cervicogenic headache, therapeutic exercises and mobilization (a method of chiropractic treatment that does not involve quick high velocity movements) were equally effective. In addition, massage and acupuncture may provide benefit. A recent review concluded that the management of headaches associated with neck pain should include any or all these techniques to promote treatment of cervicogenic dysfunction[39–41] Greater occipital nerve injections have also been shown to relieve pain in PTH in children. Blocks are typically well tolerated by patients, have low risk of systemic side effects, and can provide quick and lasting relief[42] (see Chapter 16).

Collaborative care/wrap around care: For those with persistent PTH, one strategy that may be effective is "collaborative care intervention" providing the child with embedded cognitive-behavioral therapy, care management, and psychopharmacological consultation support.[43] Although this model may be difficult to replicate outside of a structured program, it indicates that close follow up, socio-emotional support, school intervention and support, and consideration of medication management together will play a role in the management of PTH. Thus, assuming many won't currently have access to this type of organized multidisciplinary care, it would be reasonable to consider at least one of these interventions when possible for those children with persistent PTH. Knowing community resources, one can create such a comprehensive plan while each member reports to the others.

Preventive medications: Medication may be used in children with PTH with the goal of decreasing headache frequency and severity and limiting disability. The timing of when to start preventive medication will vary depending on the patient, patient's family, and the provider's experience, as there is very little data on this topic. Children with significant disability, protracted symptoms, and a prior history of headache should be given the option of preventive medicine. It may be reasonable to consider earlier treatment for those with persistent headache and multiple risk factors for persistent symptoms following mild TBI.[9, 14] If the headache is migrainous it is very reasonable to follow the standard dosing and options used for migraine in children (see Chapter 15). A small retrospective study found that amitriptyline was helpful for 82% of those with PTH who were prescribed this treatment.[44] A prospective cohort study in children found that 64% had positive response to prophylactic medication, which included amitriptyline, melatonin, nortriptyline, flunarizine (not available in the United States), and topiramate. Of note, the topiramate group had the lowest response, and another retrospective study evaluating topiramate in chronic postconcussive headache found that only 16% of patients had greater than 50% reduction in headache.[3, 44] It is important to consider that topiramate may worsen cognitive function, so in a child with significant cognitive complaints it may be best to avoid topiramate. Medication overuse should be considered as well. A retrospective review of adolescent patients with concussion referred to a pediatric headache clinic identified 77 with PTH. Of those, 70% met the criteria for probable MOH from simple analgesics. After discontinuing the overused medications 68% had resolution of headaches or improvements to the preconcussion headache rate.[27]

Return to sport: One of the biggest challenges for those with posttraumatic headache is determining when it is okay to return to sport, particularly if the sport carries a high risk for concussion. There are no guidelines on retirement from contact sports following concussions. A physician guided family discussion should be held to discuss the ongoing risks of participating in the sport/activity with persisting headaches compared to the benefits the sport has on the child's physical and emotional health. In general, if there is a history of longer recovery with each successive concussion, reduced force required to elicit concussion, or significant sustained disability from the headaches, the recommendation to consider transitioning to a noncontact sport or no sport is typically made. Information to share with the family includes: the knowledge that if you have prolonged recovery from a concussion you are more likely to have prolonged recovery from the next concussion. If you have a prior concussion you are more likely to have headache as part of your next concussion. If you have baseline migraine or prior concussion, you are at greater risk of more severe headaches after the next concussion as well as more disability overall.[45, 46] There is a very nice guide published recently to highlight some of the nuances of this conversation written by Davis-Hayes.[47]

Also, for patients with preexisting migraine, it can be difficult to determine if they have sustained a concussion after an injury, if a head injury triggered status migrainosus, or they are simply at their baseline. For nonconcussed migraine patients, particularly those participating in high contact sports, keeping a diary of migraine frequency and treatments can be particularly helpful. In addition, we recommend doing a baseline assessment of balance, oculomotor function, as well as cognitive testing so you have baseline objective measures to use if they sustain a concussion in the future. There is some data to suggest that migraine patients may be at greater risk for sustaining a concussion[48] so it may be helpful to share this information with patients, particularly athletes with migraine, so that they understand when making decisions about sports participation.

References

1. Headache Classification Committee of the International Headache Society (IHS) the international classification of headache disorders, 3rd edition. *Cephalalgia*. 2018;38(1): 1–211.
2. Lucas S, Ahn AH. Posttraumatic headache: classification by symptom-based clinical profiles. *Headache*. 2018;58(6):873–882.
3. Kuczynski A, Crawford S, Bodell L, Dewey D, Barlow KM. Characteristics of posttraumatic headaches in children following mild traumatic brain injury and their response to treatment: a prospective cohort. *Dev Med Child Neurol*. 2013;55(7):636–641.
4. D'Onofrio F, Russo A, Conte F, Casucci G, Tessitore A, Tedeschi G. Post-traumatic headaches: an epidemiological overview. *Neurol Sci*. 2014;35(Suppl. 1):203–206.
5. Lucas S, Hoffman JM, Bell KR, Dikmen S. A prospective study of prevalence and characterization of headache following mild traumatic brain injury. *Cephalalgia*. 2013;34(2): 93–102.
6. Kontos AP, Elbin RJ, Lau B, et al. Posttraumatic migraine as a predictor of recovery and cognitive impairment after sport-related concussion. *Am J Sports Med*. 2013;41(7): 1497–1504.
7. Mihalik JP, Register-Mihalik J, Kerr ZY, Marshall SW, MC MC, Guskiewicz KM. Recovery of posttraumatic migraine characteristics in patients after mild traumatic brain injury. *Am J Sports Med*. 2013;41(7):1490–1496.

8. Barlow KM, Crawford S, Stevenson A, Sandhu SS, Belanger F, Dewey D. Epidemiology of postconcussion syndrome in pediatric mild traumatic brain injury. *Pediatrics.* 2010;126(2):e374–e381.

9. Zemek R, Barrowman N, Freedman SB, et al. Clinical risk score for persistent postconcussion symptoms among children with acute concussion in the ED. *JAMA.* 2016;315(10):1014–1025.

10. Eisenberg MA, Meehan III WP, Mannix R. Duration and course of post-concussive symptoms. *Pediatrics.* 2014;133(6):999–1006.

11. Ponsford J, Willmott C, Rothwell A, et al. Impact of early intervention on outcome after mild traumatic brain injury in children. *Pediatrics.* 2001;108(6):1297–1303.

12. Lumba-Brown A, Yeates KO, Sarmiento K, et al. Centers for disease control and prevention guideline on the diagnosis and management of mild traumatic brain injury among children. *JAMA Pediatr.* 2018;172(11), e182853.

13. Kamins J, Charles A. Posttraumatic headache: basic mechanisms and therapeutic targets. *Headache.* 2018;58(6):811–826.

14. Iverson GL, Gardner AJ, Terry DP, et al. Predictors of clinical recovery from concussion: a systematic review. *Br J Sports Med.* 2017;51(12):941–948.

15. Howell DR, O'Brien MJ, Beasley MA, Mannix RC, Meehan III WP. Initial somatic symptoms are associated with prolonged symptom duration following concussion in adolescents. *Acta Paediatrica.* 2016;105(9):e426–e432.

16. Blume HK, Vavilala MS, Jaffe KM, et al. Headache after pediatric traumatic brain injury: a cohort study. *Pediatrics.* 2012;129(1):e31–e39.

17. Blume HK, Szperka CL. Secondary causes of headaches in children: when it isn't a migraine. *Pediatr Ann.* 2010;39(7):431–439.

18. Leddy J, Hinds A, Sirica D, Willer B. The role of controlled exercise in concussion management. *PM R.* 2016;8(3 Suppl):S91–s100.

19. Chrisman SPD, Whitlock KB, Somers E, et al. Pilot study of the sub-symptom threshold exercise program (SSTEP) for persistent concussion symptoms in youth. *NeuroRehabilitation.* 2017;40(4):493–499.

20. Leddy JJ, Kozlowski K, Donnelly JP, Pendergast DR, Epstein LH, Willer B. A preliminary study of subsymptom threshold exercise training for refractory post-concussion syndrome. *Clin J Sport Med.* 2010;20(1):21–27.

21. Ellis MJ, Leddy J, Willer B. Multi-disciplinary management of athletes with postconcussion syndrome: an evolving pathophysiological approach. *Front Neurol.* 2016;7:136.

22. Purcell LK, Davis GA, Gioia GA. What factors must be considered in 'return to school' following concussion and what strategies or accommodations should be followed? A systematic review. *Br J Sports Med.* 2019;53(4):250.

23. Grubenhoff JA, Deakyne SJ, Comstock RD, Kirkwood MW, Bajaj L. Outpatient follow-up and return to school after emergency department evaluation among children with persistent post-concussion symptoms. *Brain Inj.* 2015;29(10):1186–1191.

24. Master CL, Gioia GA, Leddy JJ, Grady MF. Importance of 'return-to-learn' in pediatric and adolescent concussion. *Pediatr Ann.* 2012;41(9):1–6.

25. Petrelli T, Farrokhyar F, McGrath P, et al. The use of ibuprofen and acetaminophen for acute headache in the postconcussive youth: a pilot study. *Paediatr Child Health.* 2017;22(1):2–6.

26. Gawel MJ, Rothbart P, Jacobs H. Subcutaneous sumatriptan in the treatment of acute episodes of posttraumatic headache. *Headache.* 1993;33(2):96–97.

27. Heyer GL, Idris SA. Does analgesic overuse contribute to chronic post-traumatic headaches in adolescent concussion patients? *Pediatr Neurol.* 2014;50(5):464–468.

28. Cook NL, Corrigan F, van den Heuvel C. The role of magnesium in CNS injury. In: Vink R, Nechifor M, eds. *Magnesium in the Central Nervous System.* University of Adelaide Press; 2011. Adelaide (AU).

29. Riemann BL, Guskiewicz KM. Effects of mild head injury on postural stability as measured through clinical balance testing. *J Athl Train.* 2000;35(1):19–25.

30. Ellis MJ, Leddy JJ, Willer B. Physiological, vestibulo-ocular and cervicogenic post-concussion disorders: an evidence-based classification system with directions for treatment. *Brain Inj.* 2015;29(2):238–248.

31. Mucha A, Collins MW, Elbin RJ, et al. A brief vestibular/ocular motor screening (VOMS) assessment to evaluate concussions: preliminary findings. *Am J Sports Med.* 2014;42(10):2479–2486.

32. Ciuffreda KJ, Rutner D, Kapoor N, Suchoff IB, Craig S, Han ME. Vision therapy for oculomotor dysfunctions in acquired brain injury: a retrospective analysis. *Optometry.* 2008;79(1):18–22.

33. Thiagarajan P, Ciuffreda KJ. Versional eye tracking in mild traumatic brain injury (mTBI): effects of oculomotor training (OMT). *Brain Inj.* 2014;28(7):930–943.

34. Thiagarajan P, Ciuffreda KJ. Effect of oculomotor rehabilitation on accommodative responsivity in mild traumatic brain injury. *J Rehabil Res Dev.* 2014;51(2):175–191.

35. Thiagarajan P, Ciuffreda KJ. Effect of oculomotor rehabilitation on vergence responsivity in mild traumatic brain injury. *J Rehabil Res Dev.* 2013;50(9):1223–1240.

36. Middleton K, Krabak BJ, Coppel DB. The influence of pediatric autonomic dysfunction on recovery after concussion. *Clin J Sport Med.* 2010;20(6):491–492.

37. Ellis MJ, Cordingley DM, Vis S, Reimer KM, Leiter J, Russell K. Clinical predictors of vestibulo-ocular dysfunction in pediatric sports-related concussion. *J Neurosurg Pediatr.* 2017;19(1):38–45.

38. Rubio-Ochoa J, Benitez-Martinez J, Lluch E, Santacruz-Zaragoza S, Gomez-Contreras P, Cook CE. Physical examination tests for screening and diagnosis of cervicogenic headache: a systematic review. *Man Ther.* 2016;21:35–40.

39. Dunning JR, Butts R, Mourad F, et al. Upper cervical and upper thoracic manipulation versus mobilization and exercise in patients with cervicogenic headache: a multi-center randomized clinical trial. *BMC Musculoskelet Disord.* 2016;17:64.

40. Jull G, Trott P, Potter H, et al. A randomized controlled trial of exercise and manipulative therapy for cervicogenic headache. *Spine (Phila Pa 1976).* 2002;27(17):1835–1843 [discussion 43].

41. Varatharajan S, Ferguson B, Chrobak K, et al. Are non-invasive interventions effective for the management of headaches associated with neck pain? An update of the bone and joint decade task force on neck pain and its associated disorders by the ontario protocol for traffic injury management (OPTIMa) collaboration. *Eur Spine J.* 2016;25(7):1971–1999.

42. Dubrovsky AS, Friedman D, Kocilowicz H. Pediatric post-traumatic headaches and peripheral nerve blocks of the scalp: a case series and patient satisfaction survey. *Headache.* 2014;54(5):878–887.

43. McCarty CA, Zatzick D, Stein E, Wang J, Hilt R, Rivara FP. Collaborative care for adolescents with persistent postconcussive symptoms: a randomized trial. *Pediatrics.* 2016;138(4):e20160459.

44. Bramley H, Heverley S, Lewis MM, Kong L, Rivera R, Silvis M. Demographics and treatment of adolescent posttraumatic headache in a regional concussion clinic. *Pediatr Neurol.* 2015;52(5):493–498.
45. Ellis M, Krisko C, Selci E, Russell K. Effect of concussion history on symptom burden and recovery following pediatric sports-related concussion. *J Neurosurg Pediatr.* 2018;21(4): 401–408.
46. Register-Mihalik JK, Vander Vegt CB, Cools M, Carnerio K. Factors associated with sport-related post-concussion headache and opportunities for treatment. *Curr Pain Headache Rep.* 2018;22(11):75.
47. Davis-Hayes C, Baker DR, Bottiglieri TS, et al. Medical retirement from sport after concussions: a practical guide for a difficult discussion. *Neurol Clin Pract.* 2018;8(1):40–47.
48. Eckner JT, Seifert T, Pescovitz A, Zeiger M, Kutcher JS. Is migraine headache associated with concussion in athletes? A case-control study. *Clin J Sport Med.* 2017;27(3):266–270.

POTS and dysautonomia☆ 11

Juliana VanderPluym, MD, Madeline Chadehumbe, MD,
and Nicholas Pietris, MD

Postural orthostatic tachycardia syndrome (POTS) and headache

Introduction

POTS is a clinical syndrome that has heterogeneous causes and often manifests with multi-system complaints but are not limited to fatigue, lightheadedness, fainting, headaches, bloating, abdominal pain, nausea, and sleep disturbances. This entity has been described as early as 1935 where it was referred to as Postural Hypotension. It has also since been called Irritable Heart, Soldier's heart, Mitral Valve prolapse syndrome, Epidemic neuramyasthenia, Systemic Exertion intolerance disease, Dysautonomia, and Autonomic dysfunction syndrome.[1–3]

Postural Orthostatic Tachycardia Syndrome (POTS) is a clinical syndrome constituting: (a) frequent complaints of dizziness, lightheadedness, palpitations, tremor (shakiness), generalized weakness, blurred vision or loss of vision, exercise intolerance, and fatigue; (b) increase in heart rate of greater than or equal to *30 beats* per minute in adults (>19 years) or *40 beats* per minute in children (<18 years) when moving from a recumbent position to standing, the changes occur within 10 min of standing; and (c) the absence of orthostatic hypotension (drop in systolic blood pressure of more than 20 mmHg).[4] The accepted duration of symptoms requires a minimum length of 6 months.

☆Editor's note: There are lots of dizzy youngsters seen in a headache clinic. It is easy to fall into the trap of calling all dizzy kids POTS kids. The authors present a very rigorous approach to diagnosis, while suggesting work up to exclude secondary causes of POTS. I am reassured that the general advice we give to all headache sufferers apply to those with BP and HR manifestations. Staying hydrated, avoiding deconditioning, encouraging sleep habits, and getting kids back to school are cornerstones of good care. As with headache, the sicker the patient, the more involved is the care plan. When choosing medications, choose wisely in the headache patient with POTS to avoid making the situation worse.

Pediatric Headache. https://doi.org/10.1016/B978-0-323-83005-8.00023-9

Epidemiology

The current epidemiology of this condition is not known but there is spreading awareness of this condition. POTS is the most common form of orthostatic intolerance in the premenopausal age. It has an estimated prevalence of about 1%.[5] It predominantly affects women (ratio of 4:1) between the ages of 13–50 years.[6] There is a suspected predilection for whites, although referral bias may be at play.[7] The symptoms in this condition may be so disabling that about 25% are reported to be unable to work and there are strong correlates of having associated depression.[5,8]

Pathophysiology

The underlying mechanisms associated with this disorder include the impairment in the ability in having efficient venous return when assuming a recumbent position. Several theories exist as to the mechanisms involved but overall these are very poorly understood. These varied mechanisms provide for a varied clinical phenotype. There are no specific laboratory studies that are pathognomonic of this syndrome. Understanding the underlying mechanisms may be helpful in directing the treatment plan. Here are some of the proposed mechanisms:

1. *Abnormal autonomic regulation* due to increased or decreased sympathetic tone with poor peripheral sympathetic tone due to a neuropathy of the autonomic nerves.[9]

2. *Hypovolemic state* is seen in about 70% of patients with POTS. Some of these patients have been shown to have low levels of plasma renin and aldosterone which may suggest a neuroendocrine dysfunction within the kidney.[10]

3. *Autoimmune mechanism* is supported by the clinical history that may suggest the onset of symptoms after a febrile illness or vaccination. A few studies have shown the presence of various autoantibodies against cholinergic and adrenergic receptors.[11–13] The resolution of symptoms with some immune therapies may support this theory.[14]

4. *Mast cell disorders* - a subgroup of patients have facial flushing and face or extremity erythema in association with orthostatic intolerance. Elevation of methylhistamine has been documented in some of these patients.[15] The mechanism is unclear but perhaps the sympathetic activation leads to mast cell degranulation.

5. *Hyperadrenergic state* is seen in about half of the patients with a more gradual onset. These patients may have elevation in norepinephrine levels and may have clinical signs that support heightened adrenergic activation such as tremor, excessive sweating, and anxiety.[8] It is thought that 50% of patients have this hyperadrenergic subtype of POTS. These patients may have elevation in their systolic blood pressure.[4] Some of these patients have a loss of function mutation with resultant norepinephrine transporter (NET) deficiency.

6. *Connective tissue disorders and joint hypermobility* is yet another mechanism. Ehlers-Danlos syndrome (EDS) is an inherited connective tissue disorder with subtypes with fragile connective tissue and skin and joint hypermobility. The joint hypermobility subtype has high association with POTS.[16] About 18% of patients with POTS are thought to meet criteria for EDS.[17] The laxity is thought to contribute to increased venous pooling and associated orthostatic intolerance. The hypermobile joints predispose to frequent subluxations, chronic injury, and chronic pain.[18]

Clinical features common to headache disorders and POTS

There is significant overlap in clinical features of POTS and various primary and secondary headache disorders (Table 1). The majority of pediatric patients with POTS are adolescents but some have been diagnosed as young as 5 years old.[7,22]

Table 1 Clinical features of POTS compared to various primary and secondary headache disorders.

POTS feature	Description	Headache conditions to consider
Postural symptoms[19]	By definition, patients with POTS should have symptoms of chronic orthostatic intolerance, of which headache may be one	Headache attributed to spontaneous intracranial hypotension[20,21] Head and/or neck pain attributed to orthostatic (postural) hypotension[20]
Multi-system symptoms	General (fatigue, temperature intolerance/regulation difficulties, weakness, pain, sleep dysregulation) Cardiovascular (lightheadedness, tachycardia, chest pain, palpitations, exercise intolerance, syncope, acrocyanosis, diaphoresis, pallor, flushing) Gastrointestinal (nausea/vomiting, abdominal pain, dysmotility) Respiratory (dyspnea, hyperpnea) Neurologic (headaches, paresthesias, unsteadiness, vertigo, visual symptoms, tremor)	Migraine (particularly Chronic Migraine)[20] Episodic syndromes that may be associated with migraine (Ex. Cyclical Vomiting Syndrome or Abdominal Migraine)[20] Vestibular migraine[20]

Continued

Table 1 Clinical features of POTS compared to various primary and secondary headache disorders—*cont'd*

POTS feature	Description	Headache conditions to consider
Symptom onset	Neuropsychological (cognitive symptoms, brain fog, anxiety) Some patients with POTS have clearly remembered sudden onset of persistent, daily symptoms, sometimes preceded by events such as infection, surgery, immunization, etc.	New Daily Persistent Headache[20]

Greater than 80% are female.[23] Among adolescent patients presenting with headache and lightheadedness in a pediatric headache clinic, 53% had POTS.[24] Conversely among patients with POTS, 27.6%–95.8% report headache.[22,25–30] By definition, patients with POTS should have symptoms of chronic orthostatic intolerance combined with excessive upright tachycardia in the absence of postural hypotension. Symptoms of orthostatic intolerance can include those relating to cerebral hypoperfusion (lightheadedness, dizziness, presyncope, blurred vision, generalized weakness, and cognitive difficulties) or sympathoexcitation (palpitations, chest pain, shortness of breath, tremulousness, nausea, diarrhea, pallor, sweating, and coldness of the extremities); these symptoms can worsen when upright and resolve or improve with recumbency. Patients with POTS can also have many non-orthostatic symptoms.

Evaluation

Clarifying the extent to which autonomic conditions, such as POTS, have the potential to contribute to symptom burden in headache disorders is critical, especially in patients with chronic headache disorders or those refractory to standard headache therapies. This requires considering the possibility that a patient may have POTS. Unfortunately, misdiagnosis or delayed diagnosis of POTS is common.[7,31]

The diagnostic evaluation of suspected POTS starts with confirming the presence of postural symptoms and excessive postural tachycardia. For individuals aged 12–18 years, a heart rate increment of at least 40 beats per minute must be demonstrated.[32,33] Diagnostic criteria have not been established for younger children. Because POTS is a syndrome, it is also important to evaluate for conditions that have the potential to cause, be associated with, exacerbate or mimic disorders of the autonomic nervous system. Conditions within the differential of POTS include mastocytosis, spontaneous intracranial hypotension or CSF leak, adrenal insufficiency, anemia, pheochromocytoma, paraganglioma, carcinoid, thyroid disease, deconditioning, cardiomyopathy, inappropriate sinus tachycardia, mitochondrial disorders, median arcuate ligament syndrome, Chiari malformation, tethered cord syndrome, narcolepsy with cataplexy, vertebral artery dissection, cerebral venous sinus thrombosis, and anxiety disorder.[34,35] Table 2 outlines the components of POTS evaluation including history, clinical examination, and diagnostics. Note there is not a single test that is exclusively diagnostic of POTS.

Table 2 Evaluation of POTS: History, clinical examination and diagnostics.

History	
Presenting Symptoms	Documentation of symptoms of chronic orthostatic intolerance is required. Refer to Table 1 for a list of commonly reported multi-system symptoms of POTS
Timing of symptoms	Acute (<1 month), Subacute (1–3 months), Insidious (>3 month)
Mechanism of symptom onset	Antecedent symptoms suggestive of a viral infection with a prolonged course (ex. infectious mononucleosis) are noted in up to 50% of cases. Previous stressors, such as pregnancy, immunization, head trauma, or surgery, have also been reported; the remainder of patients develop symptoms insidiously. Inflammatory or autoimmune mechanisms may also be responsible[36-38]
Autonomic review of symptoms	A careful review of symptoms is necessary to establish the extent of autonomic system involvement: • Adrenergic (Postural lightheadedness, Near-syncope, Syncope) • Gastrointestinal (Dysphagia, Early satiety, Abdominal bloating, Nausea, Vomiting, Abdominal pain, Constipation, Diarrhea) • Genitourinary (Increased frequency, Difficulty initiating urination, Nocturnal enuresis, Incomplete bladder emptying) • Pupillomotor (Sensitivity to bright light, Trouble focusing vision) • Sudomotor (Hyperhidrosis, Hypohidrosis, Anhidrosis, Heat/Cold intolerance, Limb color changes) • Secretomotor (Dry eyes, Dry mouth)
Conditions that may be associated with POTS **Note comorbidity does not denote causation**[27]	Joint Hypermobility/Ehlers Danlos Syndrome (EDS)[39,40] • Inquire about hypermobile joints, "double-jointedness," joint dislocations, and clicking joints. Hypermobility 5-point questionnaire[41]

Continued

Table 2 Evaluation of POTS: History, clinical examination and diagnostics—*cont'd*

History	
	Autoimmune[42] • Celiac disease, Hashimoto's thyroiditis, Sjögren syndrome, Systemic lupus erythematosus, Antiphospholipid antibody syndrome Headache • Refer to Table 1 Gastrointestinal[43,44] • Gastroparesis, Gastrointestinal dysmotility, Irritable Bowel Syndrome Gynecologic[35,45] • Dysmenorrhea, Menorrhagia, Metrorrhagia, Polycystic ovarian syndrome Mast cell activation syndrome (MCAS)[15] • Inquire about flushing, hives, diarrhea, itchy skin, and urinary irritability Psychiatric[46] • Anxiety, Depression, Brain fog
Exacerbating factors	Dehydration, heat, food ingestion, menses, physical exertion, alcohol, insomnia, deconditioning
Medication History	Medications that might mimic or exacerbate POTS include[47]: • Angiotensin-converting enzyme inhibitors, stimulant medications, α and β blockers, calcium channel blockers, diuretics, serotonin and norepinephrine reuptake inhibitors, tricyclic antidepressants, monoamine oxidase inhibitors, and phenothiazines
Family History	A family history of orthostatic intolerance has been reported in 12.5%[25]
Clinical examination	
Vitals	Supine and standing heart rate and blood pressure Note: Validation of a standing test for POTS exists for adults but not yet for children, for whom the tilt table is standard[48]
Cardiac	To exclude structural heart disease or dysrhythmia
MSK	Joint hypermobility may be quantified by calculating a Beighton score[41]
Dermatologic	Sweat Output • Excessive resting sweat on the palms and feet may suggest hyperhidrosis or excessive sympathetic activation

Table 2 Evaluation of POTS: History, clinical examination and diagnostics—*cont'd*

Clinical examination	
	• Dry skin and dry oral mucosa may indicate secretomotor impairment from medication effect or with Sjögren syndrome Vasomotor instability • Blotchy, marbled, mauve or purple skin MCAS • Flushing of the face and upper chest and hives Antiphospholipid syndrome • Livedo reticularis EDS • Soft or velvety skin, mild skin hyperextensibility, unexplained striae, bilateral piezogenic papules of the heel, and atrophic scarring of at least two sites[41]
Neurologic	Neurologic exam in patients with POTS should generally be normal. Special considerations: • Pupillary response-if absent or sluggish, consider autonomic neuropathy • Sensory exam - if diminished pinprick or temperature sensation in the extremities, consider small fiber neuropathy

Diagnostic Evaluation
** Not all diagnostic studies need to be done for all patients. This should serve as a guide for test selection in particular clinical circumstances**

| Autonomic
** Autonomic and vasoactive drugs should be stopped for at least 5 half-lives before testing** | Consider in cases of suspected POTS to confirm the diagnosis and provide more precise categorization into different pathophysiologic POTS subtypes:
 • Tilt-table testing (TTT) at 60° for at least 10 min[49]
    • Excessive increase in heart rate of 40 bpm when younger than age 20, or a heart rate of >120 bpm when standing

May consider an autonomic reflex screen including:
 • Assessment of cardiovagal reflexes- analysis of heart rate variability with deep breathing and the Valsalva ratio
 • Assessment of sudomotor function- quantitative sudomotor axon reflex testing (QSART) or thermoregulatory testing (TST) |
| Laboratory
** Extent of laboratory testing should be influenced by the duration, severity, and treatment responsiveness of the patient's condition** | Consider in suspected POTS patients[34]:
 • Complete blood count, Thyroid cascade, Vitamin B12, AM cortisol, Serum and urine metanephrines, celiac testing, Antinuclear antibody, Sjogren antibody (ssa, ssb), Lyme, Ferritin, Urine drug screen |

Continued

Table 2 Evaluation of POTS: History, clinical examination and diagnostics—*cont'd*

	Consider in POTS patients with chronic, refractory symptoms (particularly those with autonomic neuropathy or GI dysmotility)[34]: • Dysautonomia autoantibodies: voltage gated potassium channel complex, N-type calcium channel antibodies, P/Q-type calcium channel antibodies, ganglionic AChR antibodies • Antiphospholipid antibodies: lupus anticoagulant, anticardiolipin antibodies, beta-2-glycoprotein antibodies • Complement: total, C3, C4 • Supine and standing catecholamines (May help show baroreflex sympathoexcitation and provide evidence of hyperadrenergic POTS) • For MCAS- Serum tryptase, 24h urine studies: n-methylhistamine, 11-beta prostaglandin F2, leukotriene E4
Cardiac	Consider in suspected POTS patients: • Electrocardiogram, echocardiogram, and 24-h Holter monitoring.
Other	MRI brain with and without contrast • Consider in patients with chronic headache, orthostatic headache (to rule out spontaneous intracranial hypotension), and new daily persistent headache Nerve conduction studies and needle electromyography • Consider in patients with symptoms and signs of large fiber peripheral neuropathy Epidermal skin punch biopsy • Consider in patients with symptoms (numbness, tingling, and burning extremity) and signs of small fiber peripheral neuropathy • Abnormal testing may indicate a neuropathic form of POTS
	Given the multi-system symptoms of POTS, evaluations with Gastroenterology, Cardiology, Rehabilitation medicine, Allergy, Urology, Gynecology, Sleep and Psychiatry may be considered

Treatment

As previously noted, there are many medical conditions and medication side effects that may masquerade as "POTS." As noted above, it is imperative that the differential diagnosis is considered and potential causes of symptoms fully ruled out during the evaluation and management of POTS. Once there is certainty of the diagnosis, it is reasonable for primary care physicians to manage most patients with the help and guidance of an expert. If there are atypical signs or symptoms, or if there is lack of improvement, then evaluation by a specialist is warranted.[50]

Management of POTS is often difficult given the various mechanisms that lead to the clinical symptomatology seen in patients. There are no gold standard therapies with complete efficacy and it will often take frequent reevaluations early on, in the clinical course to see improvement. Furthermore, a multidisciplinary approach is often useful in complex patients. This team may include the primary care physician, neurologist, cardiologist, gastroenterologist, psychologist/psychiatrist, physical therapist, and social worker. In addition to the medical team, it is crucial to have a patient and family who adhere to the plan.[51]

While there are several medications utilized in management of POTS, the optimal strategy is to start with a conservative management approach. This includes cessation of any medications that might be causing or exacerbating symptoms, such as norepinephrine transport inhibitors. Compression garments may be used to decrease venous pooling.[52]

Volume expansion

It is important to ensure there is adequate hydration. Patients should aim to drink 2–3 L of water daily. In order for optimal fluid retention, dietary sodium should be increased. This may be accomplished via dietary means with a goal of 10–12 g/day. If patients are unable to take in adequate dietary sodium through consumption of high sodium foods alone, salt tablets may be used. It is also important to avoid prolonged fasts, dehydration, or anything that leads to hypovolemia. It is important to ensure that there are no underlying conditions that may be leading to hypovolemia such as gastrointestinal disease or eating disorders. A rare condition, median arcuate ligament syndrome has been seen in patients presenting with symptoms of POTS.[52,53]

Physical activity

Physical activity is important in the nonpharmacologic management in patients with POTS. As one of the presenting symptoms may be fatigue, increasing physical activity may seem daunting when discussed with patients and their families. Rather than set unattainable goals, it is helpful and empowering to start slow but consistent, as there is evidence that demonstrates a significant improvement in symptoms after a period of regular, graduated activity. As patients see progress this often creates even further drive to adhere to an exercise program.[52,54]

Sleep

Sleep serves an important role in regulating many physiologic processes. Primary sleep disorders may be seen in patients with autonomic dysfunction as well as those with headaches.[55,56] A sleep study may be helpful in ruling out a primary sleep disorder in patients with evidence of autonomic dysfunction and/or chronic fatigue. Having a normal sleep study, however, does not indicate that a patient is having adequate sleep. We are seeing an increase in sleep deprivation. This has also been linked to increased incidence of complaints of chronic fatigue and POTS.[57] A good sleep history should be obtained and recommendations regarding proper sleep hygiene should be given. There may be obvious modifiable causes for lack of sleep, such as excessive or late night screen time prior to falling asleep or even use throughout the night leading to disrupted sleep.

Identifying and managing triggers

While it is important for patients to adhere to the previously discussed recommendations, it is also important to identify potential triggers that may increase symptoms. This may include avoiding over-exertion, exposure to heat, prolonged standing, dehydration, stressors, or any other suspected triggers that have historically been challenging for the patient. If there is a planned exposure (i.e., sports tournament on a hot weekend), additional plans to increase hydration, sodium intake, and maintenance of thermoregulation may be helpful. It is also helpful to have a plan in place and open communication for accommodations as needed with a patient's coaches, teachers, etc., to avoid missing family events, academic, or extra-curricular activities.

Medical therapy

Addition of medications may be a reasonable option for those patients with persistent symptoms. The tenets of nonpharmacologic treatment should still be adhered to as there is evidence of success with these strategies. Medical therapy will not be as effective if there are ongoing causes for symptoms such as hypovolemia, sleep deprivation, or deconditioning.

There are few clinical trials evaluating medications in pediatric patients with POTS. There are several medications that are utilized with some success. Many medications used in pediatric populations are considered off-label and use is derived from adult studies.[50,52,58]

When there are indications for blood pressure support, consider salt tablets, fludrocortisone, midodrine, desmopressin, erythropoietin, or octreotide. Similarly, when there are indications of tachycardia intolerance, consider beta blockers like propranolol, ivradabine, or clonidine. If the patient exhibits sleep difficulties, consider clonidine, amitriptyline, or cyproheptadine. If the patient has fatigue or brain fog, stimulant medications like modafinil may be in order. When headache is severe enough to require medical interventions, consider the nutraceuticals like magnesium and riboflavin, tricyclic antidepressants, topiramate, and cyproheptadine. Please try to avoid headache medicines that tend to lower blood pressure such as candesartan.

Prognosis

There is a paucity of data regarding outcomes in pediatric patients with POTS. Symptoms typically tend to resolve in late adolescence or early adulthood. Nonpharmacologic strategies are most efficacious at reducing the symptoms. For those with ongoing symptoms, pharmacologic therapies may also aid in management. It is important to encourage patients to continue activities that they enjoy, while acknowledging that their schedule with school or sports may require accommodations at times. It is also important for providers and families to avoid reinforcing or enabling negative behaviors that could lead to a vicious cycle of avoidance and further deconditioning which may have negative psychological effects. Therefore, a multidisciplinary team is often helpful in managing complex patients with autonomic dysfunction and headache syndromes.[51,52,59]

References

1. Croll WF, Duthie RJ. Postural hypotension: report of a case. *Lancet*. 1935;0140-6736. 225(5813):194–198. https://doi.org/10.1016/S0140-6736(00)56563-5. http://www.sciencedirect.com/science/article/pii/S0140673600565635.
2. Twisk FNM. A critical analysis of the proposal of the Institute of Medicine to replace myalgic encephalomyelitis and chronic fatigue syndrome by a new diagnostic entity called systemic exertion intolerance disease. *Curr Med Res Opin*. 2015;31 (7):1333–1347. https://doi.org/10.1185/03007995.2015.1045472.
3. Adkisson WO, Benditt DG. Syncope due to autonomic dysfunction: diagnosis and management. *Med Clin N Am*. 2015;0025-7125. 99(4):691–710. https://doi.org/10.1016/j.mcna.2015.02.002. ISBN 9780323391054 http://www.sciencedirect.com/science/article/pii/S0025712515000358.
4. Sheldon RS, Grubb BP, Olshansky B, et al. 2015 Heart rhythm society expert consensus statement on the diagnosis and treatment of postural tachycardia syndrome, inappropriate sinus tachycardia, and vasovagal syncope. *Heart Rhythm*. 2015;1547-5271. 12(6): e41–e63. https://doi.org/10.1016/j.hrthm.2015.03.029. http://www.sciencedirect.com/science/article/pii/S1547527115003288.
5. Garland EM, Celedonio JE, Raj SR. Postural tachycardia syndrome: beyond orthostatic intolerance. *Curr Neurol Neurosci Rep*. 2015;15(9):60.
6. Robertson D. The epidemic of orthostatic tachycardia and orthostatic intolerance. *Am J Med Sci*. 1999;317:75.

7. Boris JR, Bernadzikowski T. Demographics of a large paediatric postural orthostatic tachycardia syndrome program. *Cardiol Young.* 2018;28:668–674.

8. Grubb BP. Postural tachycardia syndrome. *Circulation.* 2008;117:2814–2817.

9. Peltier AC, Garland E, Raj SR, et al. Distal sudomotor findings in postural tachycardia syndrome. *Clin Auton Res.* 2010;20:93–99.

10. Nagiub M, Moskowitz W, Fortunato J. Systematic literature review of pathophysiology of postural orthostatic tachycardia syndrome (angiotensin II receptore subtype imbalance theory). *Prog Pediatr Cardiol.* 2018;50:50–61.

11. Ruzieh M, Batizy L, Dasa O, Oostra C, Grubb B. The role of autoantibodies in the syndromes of orthostatic intolerance: a systematic review. *Scand Cardiovasc J.* 2017;5:243–247.

12. Vernino S, Low PA, Fealey RD, Stewart JD, Farrugia G, Lennon VA. Autoantibodies to ganglionic acetylcholine receptors in autoimmune autonomic neuropathies. *N Engl J Med.* 2000;343:847–855.

13. Yu X, Stavrakis S, Hill MA, et al. Autoantibody activation of beta-adrenergic and muscarinic receptors contributes to an "autoimmune" orthostatic hypotension: receptor autoantibodies in orthostatic hypotension. *J Am Soc Hypertens.* 2012;6:40–47.

14. Gibbons CH, Vernino SA, Freeman R. Combined immunomodulatory therapy in autoimmune autonomic ganglionopathy. *Arch Neurol.* 2008;65:213–217.

15. Shibao C, Arzubiaga C, Roberts LJ, et al. Hyperadrenergic postural tachycardia syndrome in mast cell activation disorders. *Hypertension.* 2005;45:385–390.

16. Wallman D, Weinberg J, Hohler AD. Ehlers-Danlos syndrome and postural tachycardia syndrome: a relationship study. *J Neurol Sci.* 2014;340(1–2):99–102.

17. Hakim A, O'Callaghan C, De Wandele I, et al. Cardiovascular autonomic dysfunction in Ehlers-Danlos syndrome-hypermobile type. *Am J Med Genet C Semin Med Genet.* 2017;175(1):168–174.

18. Grigoriou E, Boris JR, Dormans JP. Postural orthostatic tachycardia syndrome (POTS): association with Ehlers-Danlos syndrome and orthopaedic considerations. *Clin Orthop Relat Res.* 2015;473(2):722–728.

19. Leep Hunderfund AN, Mokri B. Orthostatic headache without CSF leak. *Neurology.* 2008;71:1902–1906.

20. The international classification of headache disorders, 3rd edition. *Cephalalgia.* 2018;38(1):1–211.

21. Kato Y, Hayashi T, Arai N, Tanahashi N, Takahashi K, Takao M. Spontaneous intracranial hypotension associated with postural tachycardia syndrome. *Intern Med.* 2019;58:2569–2571.

22. Li J, Zhang Q, Hao H, Jin H, Du J. Clinical features and management of postural tachycardia syndrome in children: a single-center experience. *Chin Med J.* 2014;127(21):3684–3689.

23. Stewart JM. Chronic orthostatic intolerance and the postural tachycardia syndrome (POTS). *J Pediatr.* 2004;145(6):725–730. 15580191.

24. Heyer GL, Fedak EM, LeGros AL. Symptoms predictive of postural tachycardia syndrome (POTS) in the adolescent headache patient. *Headache.* 2013;53(6):947–953. 23574111.

25. Thieben MJ, Sandroni P, Sletten DM, et al. Postural orthostatic tachycardia syndrome: the Mayo Clinic experience. *Mayo Clin Proc.* 2007;82:308–313.

26. Ojha A, Chelimsky TC, Chelimsky G. Comorbidities in pediatric patients with postural orthostatic tachycardia syndrome. *J Pediatr.* 2011;158:20–23.

27. Deb A, Morgenshtern K, Culbertson CJ, Wang LB, Hohler AD. A survey-based analysis of symptoms in patients with postural orthostatic tachycardia syndrome. *Proc (Baylor Univ Med Cent).* 2015;28:157–159.
28. Khurana RK, Leisenberg L. Orthostatic and non-orthostatic headache in postural tachycardia syndrome. *Cephalalgia.* 2010;31(4):409–415.
29. Mack KJ, Johnson JN, Rowe PC. Orthostatic intolerance and the headache patient. *Semin Pediatr Neurol.* 2010;17(2):109–116. 20541103.
30. Piovesan EJ, Sobreira CF, Scola RH, et al. Episodic migraine associated with postural orthostatic tachycardia syndrome and vasovagal syncope: migraine triggers neuromediated syncope. *Arq Neuropsiquiatr.* 2008;66(1):77–79. 18392420.
31. Stiles L. http://www.dysautonomiainternational.org/pdf/PhysicianPatientInteraction InPOTS.pdf.
32. Freeman R, Wieling W, Axelrod FB, et al. Consensus statement on the definition of orthostatic hypotension, neutrally mediated syncope and the postural tachycardia syndrome. *Auton Neurosci.* 2011;161:46–48.
33. Singer W, Sletten DM, Opfer-Gehrking TL, et al. Postural tachycardia in children and adolescents: what is abnormal? *J Pediatr.* 2012;160:222–226.
34. Goodman BP. Evaluation of postural tachycardia syndrome (POTS). *Auton Neurosci.* 2018;215:12–19.
35. Boris JR. Postural orthostatic tachycardia syndrome in children and adolescents. *Auton Neurosci.* 2018;215:97–101.
36. Benarroch EE. Postural tachycardia syndrome: a heterogeneous and multifactorial disorder. *Mayo Clin Proc.* 2012;87(12):1214–1225. 23122672.
37. Raj SR. Postural tachycardia syndrome (POTS). *Circulation.* 2013;127(23):2336–2342. 23753844.
38. Vernino S, Stiles LE. Autoimmunity in postural orthostatic tachycardia syndrome: current understanding. *Auton Neurosci.* 2018;215:78–82.
39. Gazit Y, Nahir AM, Grahame R, Jacob G. Dysautonomia in the joint hypermobility syndrome. *Am J Med.* 2003;115(1):33–40. 12867232. CrossRefPubMedWeb of Science.
40. Kanjwal K, Saeed B, Karabin B, Kanjwal Y, Grubb BP. Comparative clinical profile of postural orthostatic tachycardia patients with and without joint hypermobility syndrome. *Indian Pacing Electrophysiol J.* 2010;10(4):173–178. 20376184.
41. Malfait F, Francomano C, Byers P, et al. The 2017 International classification of the Ehlers–Danlos syndromes. *Am J Med Genet C: Semin Med Genet.* 2017;175C:8–26.
42. Chelimsky G, Kovacic K, Nugent M, Mueller A, Simpson P, Chelimsky TC. Comorbid conditions do not differ in children and young adults with functional disorders with or without postural tachycardia syndrome. *J Pediatr.* 2015;167(1):120–124. 25917768.
43. Chelimsky G, Hupertz VF, Chelimsky TC. Abdominal pain as the presenting symptom of autonomic dysfunction in a child. *Clin Pediatr (Phila).* 1999;38(12):725–729. 10618765CrossRefPubMed.
44. Chelimsky G, Boyle JT, Tusing L, Chelimsky TC. Autonomic abnormalities in children with functional abdominal pain: coincidence or etiology? *J Pediatr Gastroenterol Nutr.* 2001;33(1):47–53. 11479407.
45. Peggs KJ, Nguyen H, Enayat D, Keller NR, Al-Hendy A, Raj SR. Gynecologic disorders and menstrual cycle lightheadedness in postural tachycardia syndrome. *Int J Gynaecol Obstet.* 2012;118(3):242–246.
46. Raj V, Haman KL, Raj SR, et al. Psychiatric profile and attention deficits in postural tachycardia syndrome. *J Neurol Neurosurg Psychiatry.* 2009;80(3):339–344.

47. Agarwal AK, Garg R, Ritch A, Sarkar P. *Postgrad Med J*. 2007;83:478–480.

48. Plash WB, Diedrich A, Biaggioni I, et al. Diagnosing postural tachycardia syndrome: comparison of tilt testing compared with standing haemodynamics. *Clin Sci (Lond)*. 2013;124(2):109–114.

49. Stewart JM, Boris JR, Chelimsky G, et al. Pediatric disorders of orthostatic intolerance. *Pediatrics*. 2018;141. https://doi.org/10.1542/peds.2017-1673 [Epub 2017 Dec 8].

50. Bryarly M, et al. Postural orthostatic tachycardia syndrome: JACC focus seminar. *J Am Coll Cardiol*. 2019;73(10):1207–1228.

51. Bruce BK, Weiss KE, Harrison TE, et al. *J Clin Psychol Med Settings*. 2016;23:147. https://doi.org/10.1007/s10880-015-9438-3.

52. Sheldon RS, Grub BP, Olshansky B. 2015 HRS expert consensus statement on the diagnosis of POTS, IST and vasovagal syncope. *Heart Rhythm*. 2015;12:e41–e57.

53. Huynh DTK, et al. Median arcuate ligament syndrome and its associated conditions. *Am Surg*. 2019;85.10:1162–1165.

54. Winker R, et al. Endurance exercise training in orthostatic intolerance: a randomized, controlled trial. *Hypertension*. 2005;45.3:391–398.

55. Ferini-Strambi L, Galbiati A, Combi R. Sleep disorder-related headaches. *Neurol Sci*. 2019;40(1):107–113.

56. Miglis MG. Autonomic dysfunction in primary sleep disorders. *Sleep Med*. 2016;19: 40–49.

57. Kizilbash SJ. Et al. adolescent fatigue, POTS, and recovery: a guide for clinicians. *Curr Probl Pediatr Adolesc Health Care*. 2014;44(5):108–133.

58. Miller AJ, Raj SR. Pharmacotherapy for postural tachycardia syndrome. *Auton Neurosci*. 2018;215:28–36.

59. Sieberg CB, Williams S, Simons LE. Do parent protective responses mediate the relation between parent distress and child functional disability among children with chronic pain? *J Pediatr Psychol*. 2011;36:1043–1051.

Ways other people can help me get better

IV

Treatments for when symptoms are acting up

Acute medications ☆

Irene Patniyot, MD and William Qubty, MD

Treatments for when symptoms are acting up
What patients and families need to know about acute treatments

Non-medication options

There are non-medication strategies to stop or reduce the severity of symptoms associated with a migraine attack. The goal is to get back to normal functioning while minimizing the risk of side effects. Drinking water, eating something healthy, resting, and addressing triggers can be helpful. These things may prevent the symptoms from escalating. Please see the chapters on Self-Care strategies. Natural treatments such as aromatherapy or ginger can be used to relieve nausea. Patients commonly ask if acupuncture, chiropractic, or massage could be helpful. Please refer to the chapter on Nonpharmaceutical Options for more information. The field of "neuromodulation" devices is growing, and can provide beneficial non-pharmacologic treatment of migraine associated symptoms. Please see the chapter on Devices.

Medication options

Headache pain is a common and disabling symptom in migraine children. Acute treatment refers to medication which can be given to relieve the pain and discomfort associated with a migraine attack. These medications can help lessen or stop a migrane from progressing. Ideally, they can be given whether the child or adolescent is at home, at school or on the go as they are most helpful when taken earlier in a migraine, before the pain is severe. First line treatments involve over the counter medications such as ibuprofen, naproxen, and acetaminophen. Ibuprofen or other medications in the same category have been found to be more effective than

---

☆Editor's Note: The acute treatment of migraine is a fine balancing act. If one waits too long, the attack becomes harder to treat. If one overreacts each time, there is the possibility of medication overuse. For patients with episodic headaches, prompt attention with medication and rest is the answer. For patients with chronic headache, it is more challenging knowing how best to treat headache exacerbations. This chapter deals primarily with the approach to the youngster with an acute attack who does not have daily headache. Incorporation of behavioral interventions can be helpful in deescalating the attack.

Pediatric Headache. https://doi.org/10.1016/B978-0-323-83005-8.00003-3

acetaminophen and are more commonly used. In young children, dosing is based on a child's weight, and can be found on the medication label. A dose which is too low may not help your child's pain and may require more frequent dosing. If the medication is given too frequently (typically ≥ 15 days per month), it may lead to medication overuse headache. This phenomenon can cause an increase in headaches, decreased effectiveness of medication, and depending on the medication, result in side effects such as stomach upset or liver abnormalities.

Some children also experience other symptoms such as nausea or vomiting with their migraine attacks. These symptoms contribute to discomfort and place them at risk for dehydration. If nausea is often a bothersome symptom, talk to your child's doctor about prescribing a nausea medication such as ondansetron.

Sometimes over the counter medications together with rest and hydration may not be helpful for your child's pain. In these cases, your child's doctor may be able to prescribe a migraine specific medication. Triptans are medications developed to stop pain associated with migraines. There are several different triptans, and depending on the medication, are available in dissolving and non-dissolving tablet, nasal spray, and injectable forms. Several of them are approved for use in the pediatric and adolescent population and can take effect in as little as half an hour. They are safe to use together with various other acute medications and often work better when taken with ibuprofen or other medications in the same class. If a medication is tried for one migraine attack and is not helpful, it is recommended to retry the medication for at least 2–3 migranes to fully assess how helpful it is. For acute medications that are well tolerated, families are encouraged to discuss with the school and their doctor that these medications should be available for administration at school if needed.

We hope that this information gives you the tools to help your child through their migraines. It is important to remain in communication with your child's doctor, as sometimes it takes a few trials to find the best acute treatment regimen for your child's migraine symptoms.

What primary care providers need to know about acute medication treatments

The majority of children and adolescents with migraine will be evaluated and treated first by their primary care provider (PCP). Many communities have significant waiting time for child neurology/headache specialist consultation, and thus there is a significant opportunity for PCPs to address their patient's pain in the interim before it becomes a more chronic and disabling disorder.

A commonly encountered scenario is a young, otherwise healthy teen with worsening migraine control, provoked by the onset of a new school year or viral upper respiratory infection. Once it is determined the issue is a primary and not secondary headache, it is not unusual for patients to be instructed to utilize acetaminophen and/or ibuprofen until the headache pattern improves. Unfortunately, when simple analgesics are overused, some patients may develop medication overuse headache

(MOH). MOH is diagnosed when a patient with a primary headache disorder develops headache occurring at least 15 days per month for over 3 months in the setting of an overused acute medication. It is the author's opinion that it may take less than 3 months for this issue to develop in some cases. Approximately one third to half of adolescents with chronic migraine have MOH.[1] Table 1 illustrates common classes of medications that result in medication overuse headache.[2]

The potential consequences of MOH are increased headache frequency, reduced efficacy of acute and preventive medications, dependence and tolerance to the overused medication, and side effects such as gastrointestinal upset or liver dysfunction depending on the medication. The chance for developing medication overuse headache can be mitigated by preemptively educating patients and their families on the potential for MOH, scheduling close follow-up and not prescribing too many doses and refills for medications with a strong potential for this condition.

Acute treatment options

Many patients during a severe migraine prefer to rest in a dark, cool, and quiet room until the intensity subsides. The goal of acute treatment is to provide rapid relief of migraine symptoms with little to no side effects. Treatment is dictated by the features and severity of the attack. Treating early, rather than later in an attack, may expedite the resolution of symptoms. For example, if a patient has a severe migraine and is already having emesis, an oral treatment such as an over the counter analgesic may have little to no efficacy. The clinician should guide the patient to treat this level of migraine more aggressively at onset rather than treating gradually or stepwise and allowing the migraine to intensify.

Acute treatment options include simple analgesics such as acetaminophen and non-steroidal anti-inflammatory drugs (NSAIDs) as well as triptans and antiemetics. In one of the few randomized double-blinded placebo-controlled trials for pediatric acute migraine treatment, ibuprofen (OR 2.9, 95% CI 1.0–8.1) was more likely than acetaminophen (OR 2.2, 95% CI 1.1–4.0), which was still more likely than placebo to reduce headache severity by at least 2 points on a 5-point scale.[3] The author prefers the use of longer acting NSAIDs such as naproxen, with limited evidence suggesting it may reduce the likelihood of transformation from episodic to chronic migraine. It also has been studied with concurrent triptan use for acute migraine and appears combined treatment provides more benefit use than using either treatment alone.[4] The author finds naproxen to be particularly helpful when used as short term "bridge therapy" when headache frequency flares in the setting of typical exacerbating triggers such as viral illness, mild head injury, or perimenstrually.

Triptans were the first class of medications designed specifically for acute migraine treatment. Triptans are 5-hydroxytryptamine (5-HT$_{1B/1D}$) receptor agonists. They have been shown to reduce levels of the nociceptive neuropeptide calcitonin gene-related peptide (CGRP), which as discussed in the prior chapter *Pathophysiology of Migraine*, becomes elevated during a migraine attack. Seven triptans are on the market; however, only four have Food and Drug Administration (FDA) approval for pediatric migraine use. For patients aged 12 years and older, FDA approved triptans include sumatriptan/naproxen, zolmitriptan nasal spray, and almotriptan while rizatriptan is approved for patients aged 6–17 years.[5] Triptans are contraindicated in patients with a history of cardiovascular disease or cardiac accessory conduction pathway disorders. Triptans are per the FDA still contraindicated for use with hemiplegic aura or migraine with brainstem aura. The 2019 American Academy of Neurology pediatric acute treatment of migraine guidelines emphasize this concern was based on an antiquated understanding of migraine pathophysiology, suggesting it may be safe for use in these patients.[5] The counter argument states that these drugs were never tested for these conditions so they should not be used. Triptans are generally well tolerated and should be offered to pediatric and adolescent patients with migraine. Oral triptans should be considered for most patients except those with a fairly rapid onset of peak migraine pain or emesis. In these cases, the nasal sprays or subcutaneous injections have a quicker onset of action and avoid the GI route for absorption.

What a headache specialist needs to know about acute medication treatments

Treatment of acute headache symptoms is multi-factorial. A headache specialist may emphasize hydration and rest, in addition to providing anti-emetics if nausea is present and other migraine rescue medication options. The most frequently studied and used medications for the acute treatment of headaches include NSAIDs, triptans, and dopamine receptor antagonists. The role of NSAIDs was discussed in the previous section on treatment of headache by the primary care provider. Anti-emetics will not be discussed in detail, except as a potential benefit of dopamine receptor antagonists.

Triptans

By the time a patient presents to a headache specialist's office, they have most likely tried NSAIDs and possibly one or more triptans. Triptans are serotonin $5HT_{1B,1D}$ receptor agonists that block the release of vasoactive peptides at the trigeminal nucleus caudalis. While triptans do not shorten aura duration, in one-third of people they can curtail a migraine attack within 2 hours of administration.[6] They are most effective if taken when the pain is still mild, which tends to be earlier in attack. Triptans are, however, contraindicated in patients with cardiovascular disease, uncontrolled hypertension, stroke, and in pregnancy. The low incidence of these contraindications in the pediatric and adolescent population make triptans a suitable acute therapy option.

There are seven triptans; three triptans and a fourth triptan/NSAID combination have been approved by the Food and Drug Administration for acute migraine therapy

Table 1 Medication overuse headache.

Drug class	Frequency resulting in medication Overuse Headache (in days)
Simple analgesics (e.g., acetaminophen, ibuprofen)	≥15
Triptans (e.g., sumatriptan, rizatriptan)	≥10
Opioids[a] (e.g., oxycodone, hydrocodone)	≥10
Combination analgesics (e.g., acetaminophen with butalbital or codeine) with adjuvants (e.g., caffeine)	≥10

[a]*Not indicated for pediatric acute migraine management.*

in the pediatric population. These approved triptans include (Table 2) almotriptan in 12- to 17-year olds (6.25 or 12.5 mg oral), rizatriptan in 6- to 17-year olds (5 mg MLT for 20–39 kg, 10 mg MLT for ≥40 kg), zolmitriptan NS in ages 12–17 years (2.5 or 5 mg), and sumatriptan 10 mg combined with naproxen 60 mg in ages 12–17 years (with an option to increase dosage to 85 mg sumatriptan combined with 500 mg naproxen). Other triptans which do not have the pediatric and adolescent FDA approval, but may still be effective when used off-label, include eletriptan, naratriptan, and frovatriptan. The most effective triptans include rizatriptan 10 mg, eletriptan 80 mg, and almotriptan 12.5 mg.[6, 7]

There are challenges in picking the most appropriate triptan. It makes the most sense to start with a triptan that is FDA-approved for use in the pediatric and adolescent population, as insurance is more likely to cover these medications. Sumatriptan is often a first line triptan covered by most insurance providers. If pain escalates very quickly, or significant nausea or emesis occurs with the attacks, then choosing a nasal spray formulation (sumatriptan, zolmitriptan), or injection (sumatriptan) would be appropriate. If side effects occur, using triptans with a slower onset of action and lower side effect profile (naratriptan, frovatriptan) can be considered. If a patient reports ineffectiveness, they can try taking the triptan together with an NSAID, in particular a longer acting agent such as naproxen. Providers should also be mindful of prescribing the appropriate dosing, as increasing the dose at onset is more advisable than repeating after 2 h. As with all rescue medications, the goal is to abort the headache to prevent lingering symptoms, so aim to use the highest dose tolerated to break the headache quickly.

Parents and primary care providers are sometimes concerned about potential medication side effects, and thus prescribing providers should educate patients and their parents about potential side effects of triptans such as heaviness or tightness of the chest, throat, or jaw, flushing or feeling a hot, burning sensation, fatigue, dizziness, and nausea. The incidence of triptan side effects varies among studies, and ranges from less than 2 to over 20%.[8] Patients should also be made aware of potential medication interactions, in particular not combining triptans with ergotamine containing medications such as dihydroergotamine (DHE) during a migraine attack. Usual advice is to refrain from administering triptans and DHE within a minimum of 24 h of each other. This caution is particularly important when patients present to the emergency department after failure of acute home medications.

There has been debate over the concern for serotonin syndrome while taking triptans and other serotonergic drugs such as selective serotonin reuptake inhibitors (SSRIs) and atypical antipsychotics. In 2006, the FDA warned about the risk of serotonin syndrome in patients taking triptans concurrently with SSRIs or SNRIs. It is important to note that triptans do not interact with the same serotonin receptor as SSRIs or SNRIs (the $5HT_2$ receptor), and the American Headache Society has concluded that inadequate data are available to determine the risk of serotonin syndrome with the addition of a triptan to SSRIs/SNRIs or with triptan monotherapy.[9] It is the authors' practice to prescribe triptans to patients on concurrent SSRI or SNRI therapy; however, caution patients against the theoretical risk of serotonin syndrome and ask them to look out for new tremor as a herald sign.

Dopamine receptor antagonists

Dopamine receptor antagonists are another class of medication useful in treating head pain and concurrent nausea. They can be used in cases where triptans are contraindicated, or as a next line agent if headaches are persisting after triptan use. The three classes include: phenothiazines (prochlorperazine, chlorpromazine, and promethazine), butyrophenones (droperidol and haloperidol), and metoclopramide. The butyrophenones are not commonly used due to the risk of Torsades de pointes. Prochlorperazine has been the most widely studied agent of this class in the pediatric population, and is available in IV, oral tablet, and suppository formulations. Chlorpromazine can also be beneficial in IV or oral forms; however, there is a risk of postural hypotension which can be mitigated with pretreatment with fluids. Promethazine has been studied in the pediatric population as an adjunct migraine medication with antiemetic properties[10] and is not typically recommended solely for acute migraine management. Metoclopramide is also commonly used for acute migraine treatment and antagonizes both dopamine and $5HT_3$ receptors, however at least in adult studies has not shown the same efficacy as prochlorperazine at lower doses.[11, 12]

Dopamine receptor antagonists have the potential to prolong QTc intervals, and if used on a regular basis consideration should be given to obtaining a baseline electrocardiogram. Other side effects can include the antihistaminic and anticholinergic side effects of drowsiness, in addition to antidopaminergic side effects of akathisia and dystonia. It is the author's practice to advise diphenhydramine pre-medication prior to administration, to prevent occurrence of side effects. Diphenhydramine has a mild dopaminergic effect and providers may be cautious of co-administration due to the potential to counteract the benefits of an antidopaminergic medicine. Studies in the pediatric and adolescent population on acute migraine management with prochlorperazine and diphenhydramine pre-medication, however, have noted efficacy rates of up to 94%.[13, 14] Thus, an effort should be made to limit potential extrapyramidal side effects of dopamine receptor antagonists with diphenhydramine pre-medication, as side effects may limit future use of a potentially beneficial medication.

Gepants

Gepants are a new class of medication, the first of which was FDA-approved for acute migraine treatment in 2019. See chapter on treatments targeting CGRP for more information.

References

1. Gelfand AA, Goadsby PJ. Medication overuse in children and adolescents. *Curr Pain Headache Rep.* 2014. https://doi.org/10.1007/s11916-014-0428-1.
2. (IHS) C of the IHS. Headache classification the international classification of headache disorders, 3rd edition. *Cephalalgia.* 2018. https://doi.org/10.1177/0333102417738202.
3. Hämäläinen ML, Hoppu K, Valkeila E, Santavuori P. Ibuprofen or acetaminophen for the acute treatment of migraine in children: a double-blind, randomized, placebo-controlled, crossover study. *Neurology.* 1997. https://doi.org/10.1212/WNL.48.1.103.
4. Law S, Derry S, Moore RA. Sumatriptan plus naproxen for the treatment of acute migraine attacks in adults. *Cochrane Database Syst Rev.* 2016. https://doi.org/10.1002/14651858.CD008541.pub3.
5. Oskoui M, Pringsheim T, Holler-Managan Y, et al. Practice guideline update summary: acute treatment of migraine in children and adolescents. *Neurology.* 2019. https://doi.org/10.1212/WNL.0000000000008095.
6. Ferrari MD, Roon KI, Lipton RB, Goadsby PJ. Oral triptans (serotonin 5-HT1B/1Dagonists) in acute migraine treatment: a meta-analysis of 53 trials. *Lancet.* 2001. https://doi.org/10.1016/S0140-6736(01)06711-3.
7. Xu H, Han W, Wang J, Li M. Network meta-analysis of migraine disorder treatment by NSAIDs and triptans. *J Headache Pain.* 2016. https://doi.org/10.1186/s10194-016-0703-0.
8. Ferrari MD, Goadsby PJ, Roon KI, Lipton RB. Triptans (serotonin, 5-HT1B/1D agonists) in migraine: detailed results and methods of a meta-analysis of 53 trials. *Cephalalgia.* 2002. https://doi.org/10.1046/j.1468-2982.2002.00404.x.
9. Evans RW, Tepper SJ, Shapiro RE, Sun-Edelstein C, Tietjen GE. The FDA alert on serotonin syndrome with use of triptans combined with selective serotonin reuptake inhibitors or selective serotonin-norepinephrine reuptake inhibitors: American headache society position paper. *Headache.* 2010. https://doi.org/10.1111/j.1526-4610.2010.01691.x.
10. Sheridan DC, Meckler GD. Inpatient pediatric migraine treatment: does choice of abortive therapy affect length of stay? *J Pediatr.* 2016. https://doi.org/10.1016/j.jpeds.2016.08.050.
11. Jones J, Pack S, Chun E. Intramuscular prochlorperazine versus metoclopramide as single-agent therapy for the treatment of acute migraine headache. *Am J Emerg Med.* 1996. https://doi.org/10.1016/S0735-6757(96)90171-0.

Table 2 *Triptans*[6].

Triptan	Formulations	Dosing	Notes
[a]Sumatriptan Suma/naproxen (Treximet)	Oral, NS, SQ, nasal powder	25 mg, 50 mg, 100 mg tabs; 5 mg, 20 mg NS; 4 mg or 6 mg SQ; sumatriptan 10 mg/naproxen60 85 mg/naproxen 500 mg	– available for the longest time (sumatriptan only)
Eletriptan	Oral	40 mg, 80 mg tabs	– higher 2 h response rate – low recurrence – limit grapefruit
[a]Rizatriptan	Oral, dissolvable	5 mg MLT for 20–39 kg, 10 mg MLT for ≥40 kg	– highest 2 h freedom rate – rapid onset – consider reducing dose to 5 mg in patients on propranolol
[a]Almotriptan	Oral	6.25 mg, 12.5 mg	– higher 2 h response rate – fewer side effects (three different routes of metabolism)
[a]Zolmitriptan	Oral, dissolvable, nasal spray	2.5 mg, 5 mg	– found effective when repeated for persistent headache – nasal spray works 10–15 min
Naratriptan		1 mg, 2.5 mg tabs	– slower onset – longer half-life – fewer side effects
Frovatriptan		1 mg, 2.5 mg tabs	– used in menstrual migraine – slower onset – longer half-life – fewer side effects

[a]*Denotes FDA approval in pediatric and adolescent populations. NS=nasal spray; SQ=subcutaneous; MLT=meltaway.*

12. Friedman BW, Esses D, Solorzano C, et al. A randomized controlled trial of prochlorperazine versus metoclopramide for treatment of acute migraine. *Ann Emerg Med.* 2008. https://doi.org/10.1016/j.annemergmed.2007.09.027.

13. Trottier ED, Bailey B, Dauphin-Pierre S, Gravel J. Clinical outcomes of children treated with intravenous prochlorperazine for migraine in a pediatric emergency department. *J Emerg Med.* 2010. https://doi.org/10.1016/j.jemermed.2008.08.012.

14. Trottier ED, Bailey B, Lucas N, Lortie A. Prochlorperazine in children with migraine: a look at its effectiveness and rate of akathisia. *Am J Emerg Med.* 2012. https://doi.org/10.1016/j.ajem.2010.12.020.

Acute behavioral headache management ☆

13

Dina Karvounides, PsyD, Maya Marzouk, MA, Alexandra C. Ross, PhD, Scott Powers, PhD, and Elizabeth Seng, PhD

Acute exacerbations in headache are often overwhelming and difficult to cope with for children. Medications may not always be effective and it can take time before children feel their impact. Problematically, the inherent stressful nature of pain may serve to intensify symptoms. Anxiety related to headache triggers sympathetic arousal, subsequently magnifying the child's experience of pain and making it more difficult to distract from active symptoms. Simultaneously, the pain experience itself may trigger the same sympathetic arousal response, eliciting further anxious thoughts. As these cognitive, emotional, behavioral, and physiological experiences build off one another, the child can feel trapped and overwhelmed by a cycle of fear and pain. The child and their family may feel helpless during these episodes, making it even more difficult to cope.

To address this cycle, the following chapter will introduce a set of evidence-based cognitive-behavioral strategies for children to actively cope with headache attacks and maintain a sense of autonomy in management of symptoms. Many of the active coping strategies are also discussed in Chapter 17, preventive behavioral headache management, and details regarding their practice may be found there. The skills presented in this chapter as well as resources and parent education as part of a good coping plan can be applied at home, in school, or during clinic procedures that might elicit acute pain, such as Botox injections or nerve blocks. Skills introduced include distraction, clinical hypnosis, relaxation strategies, mindfulness, biofeedback, and cognitive reframing.

Distraction

Distraction, as described by limited attentional capacity theory, is the act of redirecting attention away from pain, with the goal of reducing the cognitive resources the child has available for pain perception.[1, 2] This form of active coping encourages a

---

☆ Editor's note: In this chapter, the authors give practical advice on ways to cope during a migraine. Equally valuable is a section that advises parents and caregivers how to help their child while acknowledging the helplessness a parent might feel, while their child is in pain.

Pediatric Headache. https://doi.org/10.1016/B978-0-323-83005-8.00009-4

patient to immediately engage in an activity at the onset of a headache to help redirect attention away from presenting symptoms.

Efficacy of distraction in pediatric acute pain

In experimental paradigms, employing distraction strategies during an induced pain episode significantly reduces participants' reported pain intensity scores.[3] While there is little research specifically looking at the use of distraction during headaches, it is a central component of acute pediatric pain management using a cognitive behavioral (CBT) intervention framework. CBT meets the Chambless criteria for "empirically supported" treatment for acute pediatric procedural pain management.[4–6] Notably, this mechanism may not be applied as successfully when factors such as pain catastrophizing (worst-case scenario thinking) or clinically significant levels of anxiety co-occur during these episodes.[2]

How to support your patients with distraction

To support children in using distraction during a headache attack, the provider is encouraged to help their patient recall a time when they naturally used distraction to cope with pain. For example, you might ask, "Was there ever a time you were having so much fun playing soccer/laughing with your friends/drawing that maybe your headache did not go away, but you noticed it a little less?" It is possible to use these same skills during a painful headache attack. Anxiety and pain experiences can interfere with memory during a headache attack. Therefore, it is recommended that the child create a list of distraction techniques in advance for use in the moment, during difficult times.

This distraction list may take the form of *internal* mechanisms or *external* mechanisms.[2] *Internal* mechanisms include counting breaths, reciting a song, or imagining the sensory experience of visiting a favorite place (see guided imagery in the preventative behavioral intervention chapter). *External* mechanisms include accessing a "go to" playlist of music, list of writing topics, or a creative art project. Many patients have also endorsed identifying and downloading phone applications (e.g., mindfulness or relaxation apps with visual images and calming sounds) for easy access during a headache attack as very useful. Encouraging a "go to" positive self-statement or mantra to focus on such as "I can get through this" may also be an effective mechanism to distract from acute symptoms. Some patients may opt for social distraction, reaching out to a friend or family member and asking them to tell a funny story or engage in conversation as a way to redirect attention. All of these methods of engagement, while sounding quite simple, utilize different senses (audio, visual) to redirect attention away from pain, supporting the patient through a headache attack until symptoms stabilize.

Clinical hypnosis

Clinical hypnosis is broadly defined as a narrowing of attention and suspension of critical judgment during a relaxed state through the use of therapeutic suggestions that help the patient shift sensory perceptions and experience of their physiological state.[7] Although many aspects of clinical hypnosis involve relaxation, what makes this intervention unique is the deliberate use of therapeutic suggestions (i.e., "this relaxing place is where you are in control of how you want to feel") to help the child create their own sensory experience.[7] Working with a trained professional, the child learns how to access their natural ability to use imagery and other senses to elicit a relaxed state and cope through a headache. Through this process, the child maintains a sense of control over *how* they want to feel in that moment. For example, one child viewed her pain experience as "a roller coaster" and developed her own way of changing this experience by imagining pulling a lever to slow down the pain. Children can be taught how to build this skill independently and use it whenever they experience a headache attack.

Efficacy of hypnosis in pediatric acute pain

Although there are limited studies on the use of hypnosis with a pediatric migraine population, one retrospective record review of children referred for recurrent headaches over a 13-year period revealed that, for 144 patients, those who learned self-hypnosis reported a reduction in headache frequency from an average of 4.5 per week to 1.4 per week, as well as a reduction in intensity and average duration. Study methodology suggests that patients were taught hypnotic suggests for use during a headache and were encouraged to practice regularly.[8] The effectiveness of hypnosis has also been demonstrated in the management of other types of acute pain in children, including post-surgical pain,[7] pain during various dental and medical procedures,[9–12] and pain associated with oncological treatments.[13, 14] Although headaches can be comprised of a multitude of symptoms, the utilization of this intervention is helpful to reduce acute pain during these episodes. Clinical hypnosis can also be implemented during procedures that elicit acute pain such as Botox or nerve blocks. Anecdotally, patients have verbalized the utility of this intervention during these specific procedures in clinic.

How to support your patients with clinical hypnosis

Hypnosis is a helpful strategy to add to a patient's repertoire of skills. When describing the benefits of hypnosis, it is recommended to note the importance of this intervention being taught by a provider who has received training in pediatric clinical hypnosis, such as a psychologist, therapist, or primary care physician. Training in pediatric hypnosis can be found through the National Pediatric Hypnosis Training Institute (https://www.nphti.org/).

Relaxation strategies, mindfulness, and biofeedback

In addition to distraction, relaxation, and mindfulness strategies may be implemented during headache attacks to build the child's parasympathetic response (slowing heart rate, slowing breathing, relaxing muscles), counteracting sympathetic arousal (muscle tension, shallow breathing, increased heart rate) and downregulating their pain experience.[15] Strategies described in more detail in the chapter for preventative headache management (Chapter 17) can be applied during a headache attack as well: mindful breathing/exercises (e.g., "thought bubbles," "10 breaths"), diaphragmatic breathing, guided imagery, and progressive muscle relaxation.

Notably, it is important for the child to develop and practice these strategies outside of acute episodes in order to better access these skills quickly and competently when needed. As with preventative treatment, practice of these skills can be reinforced through biofeedback-assisted therapy. As discussed under "Distraction" section, it is useful to encourage the patient to identify a "relaxation list" that can easily be referenced in times of acute need.

Cognitive reframing

Cognitive reframing is another skill that children will learn as a part of cognitive behavioral therapy for preventative headache management that can also be applied during a headache attack. Given the role of anxious thoughts in perpetuating autonomic arousal and the pain-stress cycle, the development of this skillset to identify and reframe unhelpful thoughts is vital in increasing self-efficacy and interrupting this unhelpful cycle.

Efficacy of cognitive reframing in acute pain episodes

Prior research has demonstrated a child's cognitions about the pain experience directly influences his or her experience of pain.[16] Cognitive reframing is a central component of CBT, which as previously mentioned, is an evidence-based intervention for both acute and chronic pain.[5, 17]

How to support your patients with cognitive reframing

When referring your patient for cognitive behavioral treatment, it is useful to describe the types of cognitive skills they will be learning. In brief, typical thoughts during acute pain episodes tend to, understandably, be catastrophic in nature, such as, "It will never stop" or "It's going to keep getting worse and worse and I'll never feel better." These thoughts can directly magnify negative emotions, increase focus on pain, and due to the aforementioned pain-stress cycle, enhance the child's pain experience. This cycle serves to magnify the response to an acute episode and anticipation of these symptoms can trigger the same sympathetic response that pain triggers.[15] Learning ways to stop, breathe and reframe these thoughts (e.g., "Is there another way to look at this?" "Is this thought helping me?" "Have I been able to get through these episodes in the past?") with the help of positive self-statements increases the child's sense of autonomy and allows them to work towards increased coping in moments that might feel impossible to bear.

Parent education and family interactions

Pediatric headache not only affects the child but the entire family system. Parents often endorse elevations in anxiety and frustration during these episodes, wanting to understandably "take their child's pain away" but feel helpless in their efforts. Parental education, therefore, is a key component in treating pediatric headache. During a headache attack, parents are encouraged to validate their child's experience and reinforce active versus passive coping strategies.

Efficacy of parental education

The literature in pediatric pain indicates parental emotional and behavioral responses to their child's symptoms can play a role in their child's experience of pain.[18, 19] Specifically, parenting behaviors such as solicitous responses (i.e., frequently attending to pain symptoms), catastrophic thinking regarding their child's pain as well as highly protective behaviors are related to increased disability in children with pain.[18, 20, 21] Therefore, parents are encouraged to identify their own response during these stressful times and find ways to modify their behavior to disrupt the cycle of anxiety and pain during a headache attack.

In a Cochrane review looking at problem-solving skills training for parents of children with chronic conditions, this intervention was found to be effective in decreasing distress when parenting a child with a chronic illness.[22] Therefore, incorporating parent education is vital to treating pediatric headache.

How to support families helping their child

Scott Powers has identified parent guidelines to help encourage parents to respond adaptively to their child's pain.[17] These include encouraging your child to manage their pain independently and engage in normal daily activities, as well as eliminating status checks to help reduce the focus on pain. Parenting guidelines can be found at: https://www.cincinnatichildrens.org/research/divisions/b/psychology/labs/powers.

These recommendations are often a counterintuitive and challenging shift in perspective and behavior for parents. We encourage the provider to educate parents on the long-term benefits of reinforcing active and independent coping of headaches, building the child's sense of confidence in managing their own symptoms and promoting healthy identity development. The parent praising their child's efforts regardless of pain reduction shifts the focus from the headache itself to the implementation of a proactive behavior, reducing helplessness for both the child and parent.

Lastly, encouraging the patient to verbalize how their parent can best help them during a headache attack supports improved communication, identifies the child as the lead of their own headache coping plan, provides the parent concrete strategies to assist their child, and aims to allow the family working together to move through a headache attack successfully.

Conclusion

In summary, a patient's utilization of independent, active coping skills can feel difficult in the moment of a headache attack but sets a precedent for long-term benefit and increased self-efficacy. Active headache coping skills include distraction techniques, mindfulness exercises, clinical hypnosis, diaphragmatic breathing, imagery, progressive muscle relaxation, and cognitive reframing. Encouraging parents to reinforce active coping and to focus on what their child can control including other aspects of who they are (e.g., being a good friend, extacurricular interests) promote healthy identity development and positive coping behaviors. In your role as the patient's healthcare provider, you have the potential to positively influence patients and their families to develop an adaptive coping approach to managing acute headaches.

References

1. Shah RD, Sawardekar A, Suresh S. Pediatric acute pain management. In: *Practical Management of Pain: Fifth Edition.* Elsevier Inc; 2013:304–311.
2. Birnie KA, Chambers CT, Spellman CM. Mechanisms of distraction in acute pain perception and modulation. *Pain.* 2017;158(6):1012–1013.
3. Kohl A, Rief W, Glombiewski JA. Acceptance, cognitive restructuring, and distraction as coping strategies for acute pain. *J Pain.* 2013;14(3):305–315.

4. Chambless DL, Ollendick TH. Empirically supported psychological interventions: controversies and evidence. *Annu Rev Psychol*. 2001;52(1):685–716.

5. Powers SW. Empirically supported treatments in pediatric psychology: procedure-related pain. *J Pediatr Psychol*. 1999;24(2):131–145.

6. Blount RL, Piira T, Cohen LL. Management of pediatric pain and distress due to medical procedures. In: Roberts M, ed. *Handbook of Pediatric Psychology*. 3rd ed. New York: Guilford; 2003:216–233.

7. Kuttner L. Pediatric hypnosis: pre-, peri-, and post-anesthesia. *Pediatr Anesth*. 2012;22 (6):573–577.

8. Kohen DP, Zajac R. Self-hypnosis training for headaches in children and adolescents. *J Pediatr*. 2007;150(6):635–639.

9. Gokli MA, Wood AJ, Mourino AP, Farrington FH, Best AM. Hypnosis as an adjunct to the administration of local anesthetic in pediatric patients. *ASDC J Dent Child*. 1994;61 (4):272–275.

10. Butler LD, Symons BK, Henderson SL, Shortliffe LD, Spiegel D. Hypnosis reduces distress and duration of an invasive medical procedure for children. *Pediatrics*. 2005;115(1): e77–e85.

11. Oberoi J, Panda A, Garg I. Effect of hypnosis during administration of local anesthesia in six-to 16-year-old children. *Pediatr Dent*. 2016;38(2):112–115.

12. Accardi MC, Milling LS. The effectiveness of hypnosis for reducing procedure-related pain in children and adolescents: a comprehensive methodological review. *J Behav Med*. 2009;32(4):328–339.

13. Liossi C, White P, Hatira P. Randomized clinical trial of local anesthetic versus a combination of local anesthetic with self-hypnosis in the management of pediatric procedure-related pain. *Health Psychol*. 2006;25(3):307.

14. Richardson J, Smith JE, McCall G, Pilkington K. Hypnosis for procedure-related pain and distress in pediatric cancer patients: a systematic review of effectiveness and methodology related to hypnosis interventions. *J Pain Symptom Manag*. 2006;31(1):70–84.

15. Schaffer SD, Yucha CB. Relaxation & pain management: the relaxation response can play a role in managing chronic and acute pain. *Am J Nurs*. 2004;104(8):75–82.

16. Chen E, Joseph MH, Zeltzer LK. Behavioral and cognitive interventions in the treatment of pain in children. *Pediatr Clin N Am*. 2000;47(3):513–525.

17. Powers SW, Kashikar-Zuck SM, Allen JR, et al. Cognitive behavioral therapy plus amitriptyline for chronic migraine in children and adolescents: a randomized clinical trial. *JAMA*. 2013;310(24):2622–2630.

18. Palermo TM, Valrie CR, Karlson CW. Family and parent influences on pediatric chronic pain: a developmental perspective. *Am Psychol*. 2014;69(2):142.

19. Eccleston C, Crombez G, Scotford A, Clinch J, Connell H. Adolescent chronic pain: patterns and predictors of emotional distress in adolescents with chronic pain and their parents. *Pain*. 2004;108(3):221–229.

20. Claar RL, Simons LE, Logan DE. Parental response to children's pain: the moderating impact of children's emotional distress on symptoms and disability. *Pain*. 2008;138 (1):172–179.

21. Walker LS, Zeman JL. Parental response to child illness behavior. *J Pediatr Psychol*. 1992;17(1):49–71.

22. Eccleston C, Palermo TM, Fisher E, Law E. Psychological interventions for parents of children and adolescents with chronic illness. *Cochrane Database Syst Rev*. 2012;8, CD009660.

What should I expect when home therapy does not work ☆

14

Sharoon Qaiser, MD and Marielle Kabbouche, MD

Introduction to intravenous headache treatments for patients and families

A good acute treatment plan for migraine at home consists of quick hydration with electrolyte solution (sports drink) and appropriately dosed medicine (Anti-inflammatory medications such as Ibuprofen and or specific triptan migraine medications recommended by your physician) taken as soon as possible.

Despite a robust acute treatment plan and appropriate 2nd dose of NSAID and/or triptan taken within the allocated time, many children may still end up with a "stubborn" headache that refuses to go away. In this case, children may benefit from intravenous medications administered either in infusion center/inpatient or the emergency department. Intravenous medications are a group of medications administered through the vein and require needle insertion. An Emergency room or infusion center visit for intravenous medications may cause stress in both children and their caregivers. A basic knowledge regarding these medications may help to better prepare the children and their caregivers and may help relieve some stress. We will briefly discuss various intravenous medications used for intractable migraine when home therapy fails.

Intravenous Hydration: Over 60% of our body is made of water and electrolytes. Many children with attack of migraine experience nausea, vomiting, and decreased appetite resulting in dehydration and loss of electrolytes.[1] Many times, it is not possible to adequately hydrate our body by drinking electrolyte solution alone and intravenous hydration is warranted. The majority of children coming to emergency department require needle insertion for various reasons, hence we suggest intravenous fluid bolus depending upon degree of dehydration, age, and weight. A quick intravenous fluid bolus may replete essential fluid and electrolytes and prepares our body to safely handle other medications.

☆Editor's Note: When "nothing is working", there is often a feeling of desperation that pervades both the young person experiencing the headache and her family. In this chapter, the authors provide hope that there are still effective treatments that can bring the pain down to zero or back to previously managed levels. Before we had these treatments, all we could tell people was to wait it out.

Pediatric Headache. https://doi.org/10.1016/B978-0-323-83005-8.00026-4

Intravenous non-steroidal anti-inflammatory drugs (NSAIDs): Ketorolac: Ketorolac belongs to the same group of medicines as ibuprofen, naproxen etc. called non-steroidal anti-inflammatory drugs (NSAID). Once oral NSAIDs fail, you may respond to intravenous NSAIDs. A single dose of ketorolac is given along with intravenous fluid and dopamine antagonists. Together these are over 85% effective with good tolerance and minimal side effects.[2]

Intravenous dopamine receptor antagonists: Dopamine receptors are found to be important in initiation of attack of acute migraine so medicines targeted against those receptors in the brain may provide quick relief.[3] There are different medicines included in this group including metoclopramide, prochlorperazine, and chlorpromazine. In children, prochlorperazine (Compazine) is found to be more effective in relieving headache especially when combined with ketorolac and hydration.[2, 4] Prochlorperazine is usually tolerated well but around 5% children report side effects. Most common side effects include agitation or uneasiness, anxiety (akathisia) and muscle rigidity or tightness (dystonia). These side effects are dose dependent and may not occur in lower doses. These side effects resolve by oral or intravenous diphenhydramine (Benadryl). Those children who respond to prochlorperazine but have some side effect, may be given lower dose next time[4] or use a different medication that works on the same receptors.

Intravenous Steroids: Inflammation is an important part of acute migraine; steroids help to decrease inflammation. There is no evidence that oral steroids help in acute migraine, but intravenous steroids may help to decrease the relapse of acute headache in selected cases. Intravenous steroids may result in side effects including serious injury of joints and bones called avascular osteonecrosis. At present, not everyone is being offered intravenous steroids, but selected group of children may benefit with single intravenous steroid (dexamethasone) to reduce relapse of headache.[5]

Intravenous Dihydroergotamine (DHE): DHE is one of the oldest medicines used to treat intractable migraine not responding to usual intravenous treatments or migraine lasting >72h. DHE modulates the nerves carrying pain signals in the trigeminovascular system and also constricts blood vessels. DHE can be given in the ED as a single dose or in the inpatient setting where it is given every 8h for up to 15 doses. Most children respond after 5 doses. DHE is very effective in treating intractable migraine or migraine lasting >72h. DHE is tolerable in children aged 6 and above but is usually associated with nausea, and vomiting, so anti-nausea medications may be given prior to DHE. Some children may also experience chest tightness. The goal of DHE treatment is either to achieve headache freedom or reduce the pain back to the "usual" level. Once this goal is achieved, usually one extra dose of DHE is given for sustained response.[6–8]

Intravenous Valproic Acid infusion: Valproic acid is one of the anti-seizure medications which helps to resolve the acute migraine by acting at various ion channels in the brain. Valproic acid can be given either as single intravenous load or multiple loads including continuous infusion. In children it has been observed that valproic acid load, followed by continuous infusion for 24–48h may help to resolve attack of migraine lasting >72 h.[9, 10] It may also be given to those children who cannot take DHE or are unresponsive to DHE. The continuous infusion of valproic acid is tolerated well with similar risk profile as single dose. No major side effects are reported in various studies.[9, 10] It is suggested to check liver function tests, blood cell counts, and valproic acid levels while on the infusion. Youngsters of childbearing age need a pregnancy test, since valproic can cause defects in the fetus.

Novel Intravenous Drugs: CGRP antibodies. Calcitonin Gene Related Peptide (CGRP) is a small neuropeptide involved in the pathogenesis of migraine. There is a new class of drugs called CGRP antibodies which block the CGRP (molecule or receptor) and treat the migraine. Recently, an intravenous CGRP antibodies drug, eptinezumab, has been used to treat acute attack of migraine in adults and found to be effective[11]. The side effects are limited to injection site reactions only. Currently it is approved only for adults, but is being trialed in children. In the near future, intravenous CGRP antibodies may provide safe, efficient, and cost-effective way to treat acute migraine unresponsive to oral treatment. For more information please see chapter on Treatments that Target CGRP.

Other intravenous treatments: There are other intravenous medicines trialed in some cases of intractable migraine in children including different anesthetic drugs like propofol and lidocaine. At present there may be more risk than benefit and these medicines are usually not recommended for general use.

Other injectable treatments (not IV): Peripheral nerve blocks are injections of local anesthetic medicines over nerves in the scalp. Nerve blocks can be helpful to treat "stubborn" headaches. See more information in the chapter on Preventive Injections.

What to do when the headache does not respond to an infusion in the emergency room
Advice for the primary care clinician and headache specialist

About 7% of patients who receive the "Migraine cocktail" of Intravenous hydration, ketorolac, and an antidopaminergic medication, will still need further treatment. The next step would be to admit into a hospital bed for longer and more aggressive treatment.[1, 4] The main therapy used in an inpatient neurology service is dihydroergotamine (DHE). Treatment protocol and modality will be detailed in the following paragraphs.

The goal of the above intravenous treatments is to reduce the pain to 0/10 or to the patient's baseline pain level. Some patients function with a low-grade continuous headache and they call you because they are going through a severe exacerbation where the headache is disabling, and they are unable to function at school or at home. For these patients the goal for an ED visit is to get them to a functioning level which may not be a 0/10 level.

Migraine headache is mostly treated in outpatient setting. Headache specialists and primary care physicians usually focus on maximizing the outpatient treatment as reviewed in previous chapters in this book. Most of the outpatient treatments include a high dose of abortive medication (NSAID and/or triptan), combined with preventive approaches that may include preventive medication but also emphasizes healthy habits as well as coping skills and stress management.

Once in a while, an acute situation will occur where the usual outpatient plan will not work. This is frequent during teenager years especially in girls, but boys can have it too. When a headache lasts 72 h or more the patient is considered to be in status migrainosus and a more aggressive approach is necessary. So, when the headache gets bad, IV therapy should be discussed with the child and the family. If the headache is disabling, prolonged, and severe then the next step is to involve the youngster in the decision about coming into the ED. Usually children are agreeable if the headache is severe and disabling. The goal of treatment is not only to abort the acute disabling headache but to prevent it from becoming a chronic daily occurrence.

The child will need to be referred to the Emergency room (ED) or infusion center. Good communication with the center is very important. Staff in that facility need to be made aware of the specific instructions for appropriate treatment which should never include narcotics. A note can be faxed to them with recommendations with clear instructions of the treatment you recommend usually known as the "Migraine cocktail" (IV hydration, ketorolac, and an antidopaminergic medication).

(1) Intravenous hydration:

Intravenous hydration is essential in migraine headache due to the theory of an underlying inflammatory process occurring and fluid leakage. Also, most patients with an acute intractable headache are usually dehydrated and the fluids will help decrease the risk of any possible side effects of the abortive therapies that will be given during the visit.[1]

(2) The dopamine receptor antagonists

Different dopamine antagonists are used in the acute treatment of migraine. The most frequent medications used are Prochlorperazine (Compazine) and metoclopramide (Reglan). One pediatric study in the ED showed that these medications are both effective in treating an acute attack but Prochlorperazine had a much higher positive response.[4, 12] Both had a better response at 1–2 h when combined with ketorolac.[2] Dopamine antagonists are tolerated well but side effects may occur.

The most frequent antidopaminergic side effects are not limited to feeling anxious and restless (akathisia), but sometime patients will have a more prominent dystonic reaction including muscle spasms and "feeling stuck." This requires Diphenhydramine orally or IV depending on the severity of the reaction and the patient's comfort level. Diphenhydramine (Benadryl) should not be used as a preventive therapy since it blocks the effect of the antidopaminergic and eliminates its therapeutic effect on the migraine. It should only be used to treat a reaction only.

Another benefit of these medications is the control of the severe nausea and or the vomiting that frequently occur during a severe migraine.

(3)   Intravenous non-steroidal anti-inflammatory drug (NSAID)

A multi-center non-placebo double blind cross over study compared intravenous prochlorperazine (0.15 mg/kg; maximum 10 mg) with Ketorolac (0.5 mg/kg; maximum 30 mg) in patients simultaneously receiving an intravenous saline bolus of 10 mL/kg.[2] Patients who received both medications had a much higher response rate at 1 and 2 h. Based upon that, the usual recommendation is to use both IV ketorolac (0.5 mg/kg with maximum 30 mg) + IV prochlorperazine (0.15 mg/kg with 10 mg maximum) for an acute intractable attack of migraine that is unresponsive to home treatment. Ketorolac as you know is a parenteral non-steroidal anti-inflammatory medication with higher bioavailability acutely then over the counter medications when given through the IV for acute headache. It is widely used as part of the Migraine cocktail with limited side effects and contraindications such as bleeding disorders, or kidney disease.

Intravenous dihydroergotamine (DHE)

DHE is part of the ergot family. Ergot is a natural potent vasoconstrictor and has affinity for various serotonin, dopamine, and adrenergic receptors. DHE has an affinity for various serotonin receptor (5-HT) subtypes, but its anti-migraine effect is thought to be due to agonism at 5-HT_{1B} and 5-HT_{1D}. The 5-HT_{1B} receptors are widely distributed in cranial vessels and their stimulation leads to vasoconstriction. 5-HT_{1D} receptors are richly distributed in trigeminal nucleus caudalis and their stimulation leads to inhibition of inflammatory and vasoactive peptides including CGRP and Substance P. Thus, DHE may help to decrease vasogenic edema and block nociceptive pathways in the trigeminal vascular system. There is a lack of placebo-controlled studies for DHE but there is good evidence for tolerability, dosing, and efficacy in pediatric patients with an intractable attack of migraine. IV DHE is usually reserved for status migrainosus (migraine lasting >72 h) or an attack of migraine that has been refractory to outpatient and ED management including other IV therapies.[1, 4, 12]

Intravenous DHE is usually given to children and adolescents aged 6 years and above. Based on clinical experience and retrospective outcome studies, dosing, response, and tolerability of DHE in pediatric population has been established. Patients age ranging from 6–10 years (or <30 kg) are treated with 0.5 mg/dose up to 15 doses, while patients aged 10 years and above (or ≥30 kg) are given 1 mg/dose up to 15 doses. Doses are given at 8 h intervals. Patients usually receive 1 additional dose after reaching the goal of treatment. Most patients respond by the 5th dose of IV DHE, which may be a good time to evaluate overall response (Fig. 1), although a smaller patient group responded after 12th dose which may justify doses up to 15 mg.[2, 12]

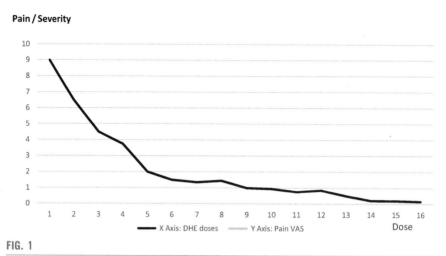

FIG. 1

DHE response chart by Kabbouche et al.

IV DHE is usually tolerated well in children but there may be acute worsening of their original headache after the initial administration of IV DHE. Acute worsening in headache after DHE administration does not predict ultimate outcome of the admission, so it should not cause termination of treatment.

One of the most common modifiable adverse effect of IV DHE is nausea and vomiting. Anti-emetics can be used as premedication to reduce this side effect. Common medications used include prochlorperazine, metoclopramide, chlorpromazine, and ondansetron. As noted before, prochlorperazine has better efficacy (especially when compared to metoclopramide) and it is a preferred first line prior to an IV DHE dose due to its dual effect as an antiemetic and migraine therapy. It is important to note that the prochlorperazine and metoclopramide act via similar pathways (dopamine antagonist) and may have cumulative side effects hence their usage should be limited to prevent an extrapyramidal reaction. Children should be reassessed after the third dose of antidopaminergic medication and different antiemetic may be considered (e.g., ondansetron). It is usually not recommended to give more than a total of three doses of antidopamine receptors during admission (counting the one received in the ED if given) to prevent any extrapyramidal side effects from these medications.

Since triptans can potentiate or alter vasoconstriction and the serotonin pathway, a triptan free period (based upon half-life) should be considered before IV DHE administration. For triptans, usually 8–24h drug free interval preceding IV DHE is recommended but it may be longer for long acting triptans. Similarly, a triptan should not be used for 24h after the last dose of DHE.

References

1. Karsan N, Prabhakar P, Goadsby PJ. Premonitory symptoms of migraine in childhood and adolescence. *Curr Pain Headache Rep*. 2017;21(7):34. https://doi.org/10.1007/s11916-017-0631-y.

2. Brousseau DC, Duffy SJ, Anderson AC, Linakis JG. Treatment of pediatric migraine headaches: a randomized, double-blind trial of prochlorperazine versus ketorolac. *Ann Emerg Med*. 2004;43:256–262.

3. Richer LP, Laycock K, Millar K, et al. Treatment of children with migraine in emergency departments: national practice variation study. *Pediatrics*. 2010;126(1):e150–e155. https://doi.org/10.1542/peds.2009-2337.

4. Kabbouche MA, Vockell A-LB, LeCates SL, Powers SW, Hershey AD. Tolerability and effectiveness of prochlorperazine for intractable migraine in children. *Pediatrics*. 2001;107:e62.

5. Cobb-Pitstick KM, Hershey AD, O'Brien HL, et al. Factors influencing migraine recurrence after infusion and inpatient migraine treatment in children and adolescents. *Headache*. 2015;55(10):1397–1403. https:/doi.org/10.1111/head.12654.

6. Frindinger S, Szperka C. Effectiveness of intravenous dihydroergotamine for pediatric headache: does headache diagnosis matter? *Neurology*. 2018;90(15 Suppl).

7. Kabbouche M. Pediatric inpatient headache therapy: what is available. *Headache*. 2015;55(10):1426–1429 [PubMed 26517974].

8. Kabbouche MA, Powers SW, Segers A, et al. Inpatient treatment of status migraine with dihydroergotamine in children and adolescents. *Headache*. 2009;49(1):106–109 [PubMed 19125879].

9. Cook Z, et al. Pharmacokinetics and clinical utility of valproic acid administered via continuous infusion. *CNS Drugs*. 2016;30(1):71–77. https:/doi.org/10.1007/s40263-015-0304-5.

10. Zafar, et al. Continuous intravenous valproate as abortive therapy for pediatric status migrainosus. *Neurologist*. 2018;23(2).

11. Ashina M, Saper J, Cady R, et al. Eptinezumab in episodic migraine: a randomized, double-blind, placebo-controlled study (PROMISE-1). *Cephalgia*. 2020;40(3):241–254.

12. Coppola M, Yealy DM, Leibold RA. Randomized placebo-controlled evaluation of prochlorperazine versus metoclopramide for emergency department treatment of migraine headache. *Ann Emerg Med*. 1995;26:541–546.

Treatments for trying to settle down frequency

Preventive treatments: Oral ☆

15

M. Cristina Victorio, MD

Introduction to preventive therapy

Preventive treatment is an important aspect in the management of migraine, whether in children, adolescents, or adults. Treatment options include pharmacologic interventions, nutraceuticals, neuromodulation devices, and nonpharmacologic treatments such as lifestyle modification and cognitive behavioral therapy. This chapter aims to provide clinicians with principles and strategies for implementing oral preventive pharmacologic treatments; and to guide patients who need preventive care.

INFORMATION FOR PATIENTS/FAMILIES: "Preventive" treatments are used with the goal of decreasing the frequency or intensity of headaches over time. They are recommended to patients when headaches are frequent or interfere with the ability to go to school or social activities. There are a variety of medication and non-medication options described in this chapter as well as the next few chapters. Some families prefer to start with treatments with the strongest evidence of benefit, whereas others prefer to start with treatments with the fewest side effects. It is important to discuss with your clinician which treatments are most likely to be helpful for you, and which you are comfortable trying.

Information for clinicians
Indications for preventive treatment

The 2019 practice guideline for pharmacologic treatment for pediatric migraine prevention by the American Academy of Neurology (AAN) and the American Headache Society (AHS) recommend discussing the potential role of preventive treatment in children and adolescents who have frequent migraine, migraine-related disability, or both; and those with medication overuse.[1] There was no specified

---

☆Editor's Note: This chapter covers the basics on prescription oral preventive treatments. It summarizes the most recent guidelines for the preventive treatment of headache in youth, as well as the available literature on treatments that did not have sufficient evidence to be included in the guidelines. It gives practical advice for clinicians and families about how to use preventive oral medications, as well as expectations for preventive treatments in general.

Pediatric Headache. https://doi.org/10.1016/B978-0-323-83005-8.00014-8

minimum headache frequency at which to have this conversation, however, pediatric clinical trials for migraine prevention have generally included patients with 4 headache days per month or more. In adults, headache frequency of more than 6 days per month is a risk factor for headache chronicity.[2] Migraine-related disability can be assessed using the Pediatric Migraine Disability Assessment (Ped-MIDAS) and a score of >30 indicates moderate to severe disability.

Cognizant of some similarities in the challenges of migraine treatment in children and adult, other points to guide clinicians when considering preventive treatment adapted from the US, Canadian, and European adult migraine guidelines are: failure of or contraindication to acute therapies, patient preference, and presence of uncommon and potentially frightening migraine conditions such as hemiplegic migraine.

Goals of preventive therapy

When starting a preventive therapy, the main goal is to reduce headache frequency. Consequently, this can reduce disability and improve function. Another clinically observed benefit of preventive therapy is potentially making acute therapy more effective.

When starting a preventive treatment, emphasis must be made on setting realistic goals of treatment and to inform patients that there is currently no cure for migraine. While it is reasonable in many cases to set the goal to reduction of headache frequency by 50%; and to reduce disability, it is also important to involve patients and parents in what they would consider to be a meaningful treatment outcome. Their participation in clinical decision making will improve adherence to and success of treatment. It is also important to counsel patients and families that it generally take 6–8 weeks in this age group to know whether a migraine preventive treatment will work.

Pharmacologic preventive migraine treatment

Compared to adults, there are fewer clinical trials on migraine prevention in children and adolescents. Many pediatric migraine clinical trials also failed to demonstrate statistical superiority over placebo, which may reflect the benefit of placebo and other contextual effects in migraine treatment in youth, at least among those who would have qualified for inclusion in the trials. Nonetheless, the 2019 pediatric migraine prevention guideline recommended that clinicians should discuss the evidence for the potential role of preventive medications for pediatric migraine as well as the effectiveness of placebo in pediatric migraine trials.[1]

In general, there are four medication classes that are commonly used in migraine prevention: antiepileptics, antidepressants, antihypertensives, and antihistamines. These medications are also used to treat other disorders. The exact mechanisms by which these medications prevent migraine is not understood in all cases. Potential mechanisms of action include raising the threshold to migraine activation by stabilizing a more reactive nervous system; enhancing nociceptive control; inhibition of cortical spreading depression; inhibiting peripheral and central sensitization; blocking neurogenic inflammation; and modulating sympathetic, parasympathetic, or serotonergic tone.[3] Table 1 summarizes the commonly used preventive medications for pediatric migraine.

Table 1 Medication treatment options for pediatric migraine prevention.

Drug	Dose	Side effects
Antiepileptics Topiramate	1–3 mg/kg/day Typical dose:50mg BID; Max dose: 200mg/day	Tingling in extremities, decreased appetite, weight loss, fatigue, upper respiratory tract infection, and memory/cognitive impairment. Serious side effects: renal stones and thoughts of suicide
Divalproex sodium	15–30mg/kg/day: Max dose: 2000 mg/day	Nausea, weight gain, dizziness, sleepiness, tremor, hair loss. Monitor for low platelets, low white blood cells, elevated liver enzymes. Serious side effects: pancreatitis, elevated ammonia level, hepatotoxicity
Gabapentin	300–1200mg TID Max dose: 3600mg/day	Dizziness, sleepiness, fatigue, weight gain, and swelling in the extremities
Zonisamide	4–10mg/kg/day Max dose:600mg/day	Sleepiness, decreased appetite, weight loss, tingling in extremities, dizziness, fatigue
Levetiracetam	125–750mg BID Max dose: 3000mg/day	Sleepiness, fatigue, irritability, behavior/mood change
Antidepressant Amitriptyline	0.25–2mg/kg/day (hs) Max dose: 100mg/day	Sleepiness, dizziness, dry mouth, and weight gain. May cause prolonged QTc on EKG
Antihypertensives Propranolol	1–3mg/kg/day Max dose: 120mg/day	Sleepiness, low blood pressure, low heart rate, and weight gain. May worsen depression and exercise-induced asthma
Flunarizine[a]	5–10mg hs Max dose: 10mg/day	Sleepiness, weight gain
Cinnarizine[a]	1.5mg/kg/day for <30kg; 50mg/day for >30kg max dose: 50mg/kg/day	Sleepiness, weight gain
Antihistamine Cyproheptadine	0.25–0.5mg/kg/day Max dose: 16mg/day	Sleepiness, increased appetite, and weight gain

[a]*Not available in the United States.*

Antiepileptic medications

The two most commonly used and studied antiepileptic medications for pediatric migraine are topiramate and divalproex sodium.

Topiramate is the only FDA approved medication for migraine prevention for youths 12 years and older. There were 4 class I studies in topiramate in the pediatric setting. All of these studies showed that there is reduction in the mean number of headache days at the end of treatment for those in the Topiramate group.[4–7] Two of these studies[5,7] showed that Topiramate was not superior to placebo in reducing migraine days and migraine related disability by 50%. In the clinical trials, the dose used was 1–3 mg/kg/day with typical target dose of 100 mg/day and a maximum allowed dose of 200 mg/day. Common adverse events were paresthesia, anorexia, weight loss, fatigue, upper respiratory tract infection, and memory impairment. Serious side effects such as renal stones and suicidal ideation are rare. Topiramate is also known cause increased risk of development of cleft lip and cleft palate in infants born to women on this medication during pregnancy; putting Topiramate in category D for teratogenic risk. At a higher dose (above 200 mg/day), it also lowers efficacy of estrogen containing contraceptives.

Divalproex sodium (combination of valproic acid and sodium valproate) is the other anti-epileptic drug that has FDA approval and level A evidence for migraine prevention in adults. A retrospective study comparing valproic acid with Topiramate showed that both medications are effective in reducing headache frequency, intensity, duration, and disability.[8] A small open label trial of sodium valproate in 15 pediatric patients showed similar results.[9] A prospective double-blind clinical trial comparing efficacy and tolerability of propranolol and sodium valproate also supported that both medications are effective in reducing headache frequency, severity, and duration.[10] The typical dose is 15–30 mg/kg/day and overall is well tolerated. Side effects include nausea, weight gain, dizziness, somnolence. Treatment using this medication needs close monitoring due its risk of hyperammonemia, pancreatitis, liver failure, thrombocytopenia, and other blood dyscrasias. Avoid using this in children younger than 5 years due to its hepatotoxic risk. It is also well known for its teratogenic effects particularly for neural tube defects, so must be used with caution in adolescent females.

Other anti-epileptic drugs that are currently used in clinical practice, although with very limited evidence, are gabapentin, levetiracetam, and zonisamide. Gabapentin is commonly used for neuropathic pain, fibromyalgia, and other pain syndromes in adults hence it is compelling to be used in migraine as well. However, a clinical trial for migraine in adults showed no significant difference between active treatment and placebo.[11] One retrospective study in children showed a >50% decrease in headache frequency and duration in 15 of 18 children aged 6–17 years. The effective dose used in this study is 15 mg/kg/day.[12] Common side effects are dizziness, sedation, fatigue, weight gain, and peripheral edema. One disadvantage of using this drug is its three times a day dosing.

An open-label study of 63 adult patients showed that Zonisamide is effective and well tolerated for migraine prevention in patient's refractory to topiramate. A small pediatric retrospective study ($N = 12$) also showed that Zonisamide with dosing of 4–10 mg/kg/day was effective with more than 50% reduction of headache frequency.[13] Side effects are similar to Topiramate although to a lesser degree.

Levetiracetam is a widely used anti-epileptic drug for generalized and focal seizures and its use in pediatric migraine is based on several small studies. A recent randomized controlled trial ($N = 31$ in Levetiracetam group and 30 in placebo group) showed both groups to have reduction in migraine frequency and intensity; with 68% of patients in the levetiracetam group having greater than 50% reduction of migraines compared to placebo.[14] A retrospective study on the efficacy and safety of levetiracetam in 19 pediatric patients also demonstrated that headache frequency decreased by 1.7 days per month from baseline. It also showed that it was well tolerated.[15] A small open label study similarly showed that 18 out of 20 patients had significant reduction in headache frequency and disability.[16] The typical dose in these trials was 125–750 mg BID. Levetiracetam is well tolerated however it is notorious for causing irritability, aggressive behavior, and mood change. This can be unfavorable for migraineurs who can have anxiety and depression as co-morbid conditions.

Antidepressants

Amitriptyline, a tricyclic anti-depressant, has a level B evidence for migraine prevention in adults. It is widely used for both pediatrics and adults not only for migraine but also for other pain syndromes. In pediatrics, the CHAMP study is the only randomized controlled trial on Amitriptyline. Its results showed that Amitriptyline reduced the number of headache days per month; headache frequency by 50% and headache disability, however, was not more effective than placebo.[7] The effective dose in adults is variable from 10 to 150 mg daily; and in the pediatric trial, a dose of 1 mg/kg/day was utilized. Clinical experience also suggests that even a low dose 0.25 mg/kg/day may be adequate to control migraines. Common side effects are sedation (hence it is recommended to be given as a night time dose), dizziness, dry mouth, and weight gain. At higher doses, it can cause cardiac arrhythmia with prolonged QTc. Due to its potential cardiac effects, some clinicians obtain EKG prior to starting this medication.

Antihypertensives

Beta blockers, particularly propranolol, metoprolol, and timolol, received level A evidence in the adult guidelines for migraine prevention. In children and adolescents, propranolol has long been used as migraine prevention and there have been no newer clinical trials on this medication. There were two double blind cross-over design studies on propranolol.[17, 18] Forsythe et al. performed the study on patients aged 9–15 years using a dose of propranolol 40 mg BID. It did not show any difference in reducing headache frequency, duration, or associated symptoms between propranolol and placebo. In the study in 1974, 28 children with migraine aged 7–16 years were randomized to propranolol treatment group or placebo. Propranolol dose was 20 mg TID for patients weighing less than 35 kg and 40 mg TID for those weighing above 35 kg. This study showed 71% of patients treated with propranolol had complete remission from headaches and another 10% had reduction of attacks to less than one third. In the second phase of the study, similar efficacy was observed.[17] Based on the magnitude of effect of this study, the 2019 pediatric guideline upgraded its level of evidence and concluded that children treated with propranolol are possibly more likely to have 50% reduction of headaches compared to those on placebo. Recommended dosing for propranolol is 1 mg to 3 mg/kg/day. Side effects are sedation, hypotension, bradycardia, and weight gain. Due to its effect on heart rate and blood pressure, and bronchospasm, caution must be used especially when prescribing to young athletes and those with asthma. Similar caution must be taken when prescribing to those with depression as this may worsen depressive symptoms. Propranolol, on the other hand, may benefit those with anxiety without depression and those with essential tremors.

Three calcium channel blockers, flunarizine, cinnarizine, and nimodipine, have been reviewed in the 2019 pediatric migraine prevention guidelines. Both flunarizine and cinnarizine are not available in the United Stated. The effectiveness of flunarizine for migraine prevention was based on one double blind placebo controlled cross-over design study in children with migraine aged 5–11 years of age. They were randomized to flunarizine group (dose of 5 mg/day) or placebo group. Result showed that headaches were reduced significantly in the flunarizine treated group than placebo.[19] Side effects reported were daytime sedation and weight gain. Cinnarizine, an anti-histamine and calcium channel blocker, has shown its efficacy in one double blind placebo-controlled parallel group study. There was reduction in headache frequency, achieved more than 50% reduction in month headaches and reduction in headache severity in the cinnarizine group compared to placebo. The dose used in this study was 1.5 mg/kg/day for those weighing less than 30 kg; and 50 mg/day for weights >30 kg). Drowsiness and weight gain were reported side effects.[20] One randomized controlled trial with crossover design was done on Nimodipine for migraine prevention in children. Headache frequency was reduced from a mean of ~2.7 attacks/month to ~1.9 vs. no change for placebo.[21] Abdominal discomfort was reported as a side effect.

Antihistamine

Cyproheptadine is a 5-HT2 antagonist with calcium channel blocking properties is widely used for migraine prevention especially in younger children.[22, 23] While there are no randomized clinical trials, clinical experience demonstrates its effectiveness in controlling migraine as well as recurrent abdominal pain. It is also the most commonly prescribed preventive medication among the youngest children with migraine.[24] Its availability in liquid and tablet formulations and tolerability in children makes Cyproheptadine a commonly prescribed preventive medication and preferred treatment option by parents of children with migraine. Typical dose is 0.25–1.5 mg/kg/day and based on clinical experience, rarely exceeds 12 mg/day. Common side effects are sedation, increased appetite, and weight gain. Due to its sedating effect, most clinicians recommend single dosing at bedtime.

How to implement preventive treatment in the clinical setting

Once a patient who requires preventive treatment is identified, several steps that include education and counseling, discussion of treatment options, side effects, duration of treatment, and screening for co-morbid conditions are needed to ensure successful treatment. Key elements to be discussed with patients are summarized in Table 2 based on the recommendations from the 2019 AAN and AHS practice guideline update on pharmacologic treatment for pediatric migraine prevention.

Table 2 Recommendations of the AAN and AHS 2019 practice guideline update: pharmacologic treatment for pediatric migraine prevention.

Level	Recommendation
Counseling and education for children and adolescents with migraine and their families	
Level B	Clinicians should counsel patients and families that lifestyle and behavioral factors influence headache frequency
Level B	Clinicians should educate patients and families to identify and modify migraine contributors that are potentially modifiable (i.e., being overweight, caffeine, and alcohol use, lack of physical activity, poor sleep habits)
Level B	Clinicians should discuss the potential role of preventive treatments in children and adolescents with frequent headache (minimum of 4 headache days per month and 3–4 migraines per month for at least 3 months) or migraine-related disability (PedMIDAS score > 30) or both
Level B	Clinicians should discuss the potential role of preventive treatments in children and adolescents with medication overuse
Starting preventive treatment	
Level B	Clinicians should inform patients and caregivers that in clinical trials of preventive treatments for pediatric migraine, placebo was effective and majority of preventive medications were not superior to placebo
Level B	Acknowledging the limitations of currently available evidence, clinicians should engage in shared decision making regarding the use of short-term trials (a minimum of 2 months) for those who could benefit from preventive treatment
Level B	Clinicians should discuss the evidence for amitriptyline combined with Cognitive Behavioral Therapy for migraine prevention, inform them of the potential side effects of amitriptyline including risks of suicide, and work with families to identify providers who can offer this type of treatment

Continued

Table 2 Recommendations of the AAN and AHS 2019 practice guideline update: pharmacologic treatment for pediatric migraine prevention—*cont'd*

Level	Recommendation
Level B	Clinicians should discuss the evidence for topiramate for pediatric migraine prevention and its side effects
Level B	Clinicians should discuss the evidence for propranolol for pediatric migraine prevention and its side effects
Counseling for patients of child bearing potential	
Level A	Clinicians must consider the teratogenic effect of topiramate and valproate in their choice of migraine prevention therapy recommendations to patients of child bearing potential
Level A	Clinicians who offer topiramate or valproate for migraine prevention to patients of child bearing potential must counsel these patients about potential effects on fetal-childhood development
Level A	Clinicians who prescribe topiramate for migraine prevention to patients of child bearing potential must counsel these patients about the potential of this medication to decrease the efficacy of oral combined hormonal contraceptives, particularly at doses over 200 mg daily
Level B	Clinicians who prescribe topiramate or valproate for migraine prevention to patients of child bearing potential should counsel patients to discuss optimal contraception methods with their health care provider during treatment
Level A	Clinicians must recommend daily folic acid supplementation to patients of child bearing potential who take topiramate or valproate
Monitoring and stopping medication	
Level A	Clinicians must periodically monitor medication effectiveness and adverse events when prescribing migraine preventive treatment
Level B	Clinicians should counsel patients and families about risks and benefits of stopping preventive medication once good migraine control is established.
Mental illness in children and adolescents with migraine	
Level B	Children and adolescents with migraine should be screened for mood and anxiety disorders because of the increased risk of headache persistence
Level B	In children and adolescents with migraine who have co-morbid mood and anxiety disorders, clinicians should discuss management options of these disorders

Adapted from the AAN Practice Guideline Summary for Clinicians.

It is equally important to have an individualized approach when starting a preventive regimen. All preventive treatments have potential side effects and patients must be informed of the common and rare side effects. An ideal treatment is one that is effective with minimal side effects, and one that does not interfere with other medications or worsen co-existing medical conditions. Also consider using one medication that can treat one or two co-morbid conditions; for example, a patient with seizure may benefit from use of Topiramate or valproate. It may also be worthwhile to use a medication whose side effects may benefit the patient such as cyproheptadine for a child who has a poor appetite or a picky eater. Once the medication is selected, start it at a low dose and go slow in incrementally titrating the dose, ideally over 4–12 weeks. Side effects are minimized and better tolerated with this approach. Emphasis should be made that treatment needs time to be effective, typically at least 2 months. In some patients, the first preventive treatment may fail. In such case, try another medication from another therapeutic class and re-evaluate for other potential causes such as nonadherence to healthy lifestyle, presence of medication overuse or emergence of a co-morbid condition such as depression. It is also important not to discontinue the medication abruptly, rather wean it off slowly.

Lastly, careful monitoring of improvement must be made by reviewing headache diaries and frequency of acute medications used. Reduction of headache disability as assessed by Ped-MIDAS is another method to assess success of treatment.

References

1. Oskui M, Pringsheim T, Holler-Managan Y, et al. Practice guideline update summary: pharmacologic treatment for pediatric migraine prevention. Report of the guideline development, dissemination, and implementation Subcommittee of the American Academy of neurology and the American headache society. *Neurology*. 2019;93:500–509.
2. Katsavara Z, Schneeweiss S, Kurth T, et al. Incidence and predictors for chronicity of headache in patients with episodic migraine. *Neurology*. 2004;62:788–790.
3. Silberstein SD, Lipton RB, Dodick DW. *Wolff's Headache and Other Head Pain*. 8th ed. Oxford University Press; 2008.
4. Lewis D, Winner P, Saper J, et al. Randomized, double blinc, placebo-controlled study to evaluate the efficacy and safety of topiramate for migraine prevention in pediatric subjects 12 to 17 years of age. *Pediatrics*. 2009;123:924–934.
5. Winner P, Pearlman EM, Linder SL, et al. Topiramate for migraine prevention in children: a randomized, double-blind, placebo-controlled trial. *Headache*. 2005;45:1304–1312.
6. Lakshmi CV, Singhi P, Malhi P, Ray M. Topiramate in the prophylaxis of pediatric migraine: a double blind placebo-controlled trial. *J Child Neurol*. 2007;22:829–835.
7. Powers SW, Coffey CS, Chamberlin LA, et al. Trial of amitriptyline, topiramate, and placebo for pediatric migraine. *N Engl J Med*. 2017;376:115–124.
8. Unalp A, Uran N, Ozurk A. Comparison of the effectiveness of topiramate and sodium valproate in pediatric migraine. *J Child Neurol*. 2008;23:1377–1381.
9. Serdaroglu G, Erhan E, Tekgul H, et al. Sodium valproate for the prophylaxis of migraine in childhood migraine. *Headache*. 2002;42:819–822.
10. Bidabadi E, Mashouf M. A randomized trial of propranolol versus sodium valproate for the prophylaxis of migraine in pediatric patients. *Paediatr Drugs*. 2010;44:238–243.
11. Silberstein S, Goode-Sellers S, Twomey C, et al. Randomized, double-blind, placebo-controlled, phase II trial of gabapentin enacarbil for migraine prophylaxis. *Cephalalgia*. 2012;33(2):101–111.
12. Belman AL, Milazo M, Savatic M. Gabapentin for migraine prophylaxis in children. *Ann Neurol*. 2001;50(suppl 1):S109.

13. Bermejo PE, Dorado R. Zonisamide for migraine prophylaxis in patients refractory to topiramate. *Clin Neuropharmacol*. 2009;32(2):103–106.

14. Montazerlotfelahi H, Amanat M, Tavasoli AR, et al. Levetiracetam for prophylactic treatment of pediatric migraine: a randomized double-blind placebo-controlled trial. *Cephalalgia*. 2019;39(12):1509–1517.

15. Miller GS. Efficacy and safety of levetiracetam in pediatric migraine. *Headache*. 2004; 44(3):238–243.

16. Pakalnis A, Kring D, Meier L. Levetiracetam prophylaxis in pediatric migraine—an open-label study. *Headache*. 2007;43(3):427–430.

17. Ludgvigsson J. Propranolol used in prophylaxis of migraine in children. *Acta Neurol Scand*. 1974;50:109–115.

18. Forsythe WI, Gillies D, Sills MA. Propranolol ('Inderal') in the treatment of childhood migraine. *Dev Med Child Neurol*. 1984;26:737–741.

19. Sorge F, De Simone E, Marano E, et al. Flunarizine in prophylaxis of childhood migraine. A double-blind, placebo controlled, crossover study. *Cephalalgia*. 1988;8:1–6.

20. Ashrafi MR, Salehi S, Malamiri RA, et al. Efficacy and safety of cinnarizine in the prophylaxis of migraine in children: a double blind placebo-controlled randomized trial. *Pediatr Neurol*. 2014;51:503–508.

21. Battistella PA, Ruffilli R, Moro R, et al. A placebo-controlled crossover trial of nimodipine in pediatric migraine. *Headache*. 1990;30:264–268.

22. Bille B, Ludgvigsson J, Sanner G. Prophylaxis of migraine in children. *Headache*. 1977;17:61–63.

23. Peroutka SJ, Allen GS. The calcium antagonist properties of cyproheptadine: implications for an anti-migraine action. *Neurology*. 1984;34(3):304–309.

24. Johnson A, Bickel J, Lebel A. Pediatric migraine prescription patterns at a large academic hospital. *Pediatr Neurol*. 2014;51:706–712.

Preventive injections: onabotulinum toxin A and nerve blocks[☆]

16

Rebecca Barmherzig, MD and Christina L. Szperka, MD, MSCE

Injection strategies are important for clinicians and families alike to be aware of in the armamentarium of headache prevention. These are often considered when other natural, integrative, and oral medication preventive strategies have not yielded sufficient benefit; when a therapeutic treatment trial of oral medication cannot be tolerated due to side effects or contraindications; or in other specific circumstances including concern for medication interactions or polypharmacy, medical co-morbidities, or patient/family preference.[1]

Onabotulinum toxin A

Information for families

Onabotulinum toxin A is a medication which can be used to treat chronic migraine, meaning headache at least 15 days/month for at least 3 months, sometimes accompanied by migraine features like nausea or sensitivity to light and sound. It is injected in small amounts over several places on the face, head, neck, and shoulders. It is approved by the FDA for use in adults,[2] but is also used "off-label" in teens. We don't know exactly how onabotulinum toxin works to prevent headaches. One possibility is that the medicine works by tracking back through the nerves that carry pain messages to turn off pain signals in the brainstem. Since the onabotulinum toxin works near the site of injection, it does not usually cause side effects like sleepiness, thinking problems, or mood changes.

To use onabotulinum toxin A, your headache specialist will inject a very small amount of medicine into 30 or more spots. These will be spread over the forehead, sides of the head, back of the head, neck, and shoulders. The benefits can start 1 week after injections, and usually last until about 10–12 weeks after the injections. The

---

[☆]Editor's note: While it may initially sound scary to use injections on the head to treat headaches, injection therapies can be very helpful. The discomfort of the procedure is short-lived, and the benefits can be substantial. This chapter reviews both onabotulinum A injections and nerve blocks for the treatment of headaches.

Pediatric Headache. https://doi.org/10.1016/B978-0-323-83005-8.00006-9

injections are repeated every 12 weeks until headaches are well-controlled. If the onabotulinum toxin does not help on the first try, it is usually recommended to repeat the injections once 12 weeks later. Some patients who were not helped the first time do see benefit after repeated injections.

Side effects are generally mild. Some people are very anxious about the injections; it will be important to discuss this with your doctor. There is usually minimal discomfort associated with the injections, but if the headache is severe the injections may feel more painful. This initial discomfort lasts just a few minutes. Some patients will experience a worsening of head and neck pain for the first few days after the injections. To prevent this, your child may use ice and an anti-inflammatory medication such as ibuprofen or naproxen for a few days after the procedure and should avoid carrying a backpack until the neck/shoulder pain is resolved. Many patients find that their forehead muscles don't move while the medicine is active. Other side effects can include droopy eyelid and weakness of chewing muscles or neck muscles, which is rare when the medication is administered by an experienced injector. Even when present, these side effects are usually mild, and wear off when the medication wears off at 12 weeks. Any injection carries a small risk of bleeding or infection. There have been rare cases of more serious breathing or swallowing problems when onabotulinum toxin A was used for tight muscles or salivary problems in children with cerebral palsy.

Some insurance companies will cover onabotulinum toxin A medicine and injections for children or teens. They usually require a diagnosis of chronic migraine, and documentation that the child has not had much benefit from at least 2 or 3 classes of preventive prescription medications. Some insurance companies will not cover it for patients under 18 years at all. If it is covered, two authorizations are needed in the United States. The insurance company has to authorize the procedure to inject the medicine. The insurance company's specialty pharmacy has to approve the medicine. It can take weeks to obtain these authorizations. The portion of the total treatment cost which must be paid by the family depends on the details of the insurance plan.

Information for primary care clinicians

Onabotulinum Toxin A is approved for the preventive treatment of chronic migraine in adults aged >18.[2] It is used "off-label" in pediatric chronic migraine, as well as in other chronic headaches that can have overlapping symptoms with migraine including new daily persistent headache (NDPH)[3] and persistent headache attributed to traumatic head injury,[4] which is often referred to as post-traumatic headache. It is not entirely clear how onabotulinum toxin works to help prevent headaches. One hypothesis is that onabotulinum toxin helps to disrupt nerve signaling in the pain pathways in the peripheral trigeminovascular neurons, which are implicated in the initiation of a migraine. The largest trial evaluating onabotulinum toxin for headache was the PREEMPT (Phase III Research Evaluating Migraine Prophylaxis Therapy) trial, which included only adults with chronic migraine. Onabotulinum toxin was found to be well-tolerated and effective, with a significant reduction in both head-ache frequency and severity. In this trial, 155 units of onabotulinum toxin were deliv-ered as a series of 31 intramuscular injections over predefined points on the face, scalp, neck, and upper back. Injections were repeated on a 12-weekly cycle.[2]

The evidence for onabotulinum toxin in the treatment of migraine in children and adolescents is more limited. Several pediatric studies, mostly case series, have described benefit with the use of onabotulinum toxin injections for children with medically-intractable migraine and daily headache.[5–10] Randomized-controlled data has been mixed.[11, 12] Pediatric headache specialists may recommend onabotulinum toxin injections as a preventive treatment for children and adolescents with chronic migraine after other natural, integrative, and oral preventive therapies have been trialed without success. Most headache specialists will follow the adult PREEMPT dosing and injection protocol[2] in adolescents and teens being treated with onabotulinum toxin.

Information for headache specialists

Onabotulinum toxin A is a neurotoxin derived from Clostridium botulinum, which has been a well-established therapeutic intervention for a wide variety of FDA-approved indications including the treatment of cervical dystonia, spasticity, bleph-arospasm, and neurogenic bladder, among others. Open-label studies have described long-term tolerability[13, 14] as well as benefit in adults with chronic migraine with and without daily headache,[15] with and without allodynia,[16] and in those with new daily persistent headache[3] and persistent post-traumatic headache.[4] The exact mechanism of onabotulinum toxin in modulating headache pain is unknown. The primary hypothesis is that onabotulinum toxin inhibits nociception in peripheral trigemino-vascular neurons. Trigeminal and meningeal nociceptors are implicated in the initi-ation of a migraine via fusion of mechanosensitive ion channels in the nerve terminal membrane, and onabotulinum toxin may exert a preventive benefit by preventing the fusion of these channels.[2]

The PREEMPT trial, which included only adults with chronic migraine, demon-strated a 50% or better reduction in total headaches days per month by the second injection cycle in about half of the patients included.[2] The injections as per PRE-EMPT are repeated on a 12-weekly cycle. Some patients may be quicker metaboli-zers of the onabotulinum toxin and begin to notice "wear-off" effect earlier. In these patients, consideration may be given towards moving up the injection cycles by no less than 10-week intervals.

The PREEMPT protocol divides the head/neck into seven specific regions: pro-cerus (5 units over 1 site); corrugator (10 units over 2 sites); frontalis (20 units over 4 sites); temporalis (40 units over 8 sites, 4 on each side); occipitalis (30 units over 6 sites, 3 on each side); the cervical paraspinal muscles (20 units over 4 sites, 2 on each side); and the trapezii (30 units over 6 sites, 3 on each side). As a point of practicality, given that onabotulinum toxin vials come in units of 50, in order to provide the standard 155 unit dose, a 200-unit vial would have to be used. With these additional units, neurologists have considered the option of increasing the dose at certain injection sites or adding additional injection sites based on the individual's specific pain pattern, as elicited by myofascial pain via palpation of the head/neck regions. This has become known as the follow-the-pain protocol,[2] which many clinicians now use in adjunct to the standard PREEMPT protocol.

Several pediatric case series have described benefit with the use of onabotulinum toxin injections for children with medically-intractable migraine and daily headache.[5–10] One parallel-design randomized trial of a single treatment of onabotulinum toxin 155 units versus 74 units versus placebo in adolescents with chronic migraine did not demonstrate benefit of onabotulinum toxin over placebo injections.[11] However, parallel-design randomized trials of therapies for migraine in children are known to have high rates of placebo response, making it difficult to demonstrate efficacy of active therapy over placebo.[17] A more recent double-blinded placebo-controlled trial compared onabotulinum toxin 155 units to placebo over a 48-week period in adolescents with chronic migraine.[12] Study results supported tolerability and efficacy for onabotulinum, with decreased headache frequency, severity, and function-related disability scores. Given the possible benefit suggested in limited pediatric trials, and the established benefit and safety in adults, many pediatric headache specialists use onabotulinum toxin injections as a preventive treatment for children and adolescents with chronic migraine. This therapy is typically considered when there has not been sufficient benefit achieved despite therapeutic treatment trials of multiple preventives including oral prescription medications and/or cognitive behavioral therapy.

Injection training materials are available at headache and neurology conferences, and through the company that makes the toxin.

Nerve blocks including sphenopalatine ganglion blocks
Information for families

A peripheral nerve block is a procedure that uses local anesthetic (numbing) medicines to block messages coming from sensory nerves. Nerve blocks have been shown to help adults with several different types of headaches. In children and teens, nerve blocks can help with migraine, headache after concussion, and new daily persistent headache.

Numbing medicines (like lidocaine and/or bupivacaine) are injected with a very small needle. It is very similar to the injection that a dentist uses to numb the mouth before filling a cavity. Injections are done over the nerves that control sensation in the area that hurts. For example, if pain is on one side at the back of the head then 1 or 2 injections will probably control that pain. Sometimes injections on the side or front of the head are done as well.

Think of a computer that glitches. Often turning it off, waiting, and turning it back on again can help get things back to normal. Think of your nerves in the same way. At first, these anesthetics block sensation, so there will be numbness together with decreased pain. The numbness only lasts for a few hours before sensation is restored. However, that brief break in nerve transmission may allow the pain nerve an opportunity to reset. The goal is that the pain relief will last much longer than the numbness, sometimes many days or even a few weeks.

A peripheral nerve block procedure is often performed in a regular examination room, and usually takes only a few minutes. There may be some discomfort when the medication is first injected, which feels like a brief pressure or pulling sensation (like tugging on the hairs at the base of your scalp for a few seconds). The medication may cause a temporary bump until it is absorbed by the skin and may cause redness. These usually goes away after a few minutes but for some can last for hours. Some people report that their head feels "spacey" or that they feel nauseated while their head feels numb. Some people become very anxious about the procedure. Anxiety can make the headache more severe, and rarely can cause fainting. Among those people whose pain returns within a few days, some report that the pain feels more severe. There are low risks of itching, rash, allergic reaction, and bleeding. There are very low risks of infection and damage to the nerves.

In certain cases, your headache specialist may consider a different type of nerve block, called a sphenopalatine ganglion (SPG) block. The SPG is a collection of nerve cells located just behind the bones of the nose on either side. This ganglion has a close relationship to the trigeminal nerve, which is one of the main nerve networks involved in headache. The SPG contains both sensory and autonomic nerve fibers. Autonomic nerves are specialized nerves involved in controlling the automatic parts of our body's function, such as heart rate and blood pressure. In the SPG, the autonomic nerve fibers help regulate tears in the eyes and congestion in the nose.

The SPG has connections to the brainstem, which is where the signals for many types of headaches are generated. The SPG also has connections to the pain-sensitive tissues covering the brain, via the trigeminal nerve. When your brain is making a headache, pain receptors are activated in the brainstem which send signals through the trigeminal nerve. These signals eventually make their way to the sensory area of the brain and let your brain know you are having pain. In migraine and cluster headache, nerves carrying these pain signals pass through the SPG. This is why, with these types of headaches, there can sometimes be symptoms such as eye tearing or nasal congestion.

The clinician may use a cotton swab or a device called a catheter to perform the SPG block. The catheter technique involves placing a very thin plastic tube into the nose to insert numbing medication in and around the SPG. During the procedure, there may be mild pressure and you may feel like sneezing. Some patients also experience a quick burning sensation or have a bad taste in the mouth. Sucking on a piece of candy during the procedure can help provide a distraction taste. Tearing and a brief temperature change may occur on the side of the nostril where the medication has been applied. For some, there is an immediate reduction in head and/or facial pain, but results can take anywhere from 15 min to a few hours to occur. The risks of the procedure are typically minimal. They include discomfort during and after the procedure, numb sensation in the back of the throat if any medication drips down, bitter taste, bleeding from the nose, and light-headedness. These side effects are typically mild and resolve within minutes to a few hours.

Information for primary care clinicians

Peripheral nerve blocks are an interventional procedure in which local anesthetic medication (typically lidocaine, bupivacaine, or a combination of the two) is injected over branches of the occipital and trigeminal nerves.[18] The medication infiltrates the soft tissue and is taken up by the nerve endings, effectively anesthetizing the nerve territory. While this period of anesthesia is relatively short-lived (*usually 2–6 h, depending on the anesthetic used and individual metabolism*), the analgesic effect can be more sustained.[19]

Similar to restarting a computer, anesthetizing the nerves perpetuating the headache pain forces them to reboot. Forcing the nerves to briefly "turn off" allows for the interruption of nociception, thereby disrupting pain processing through the network, and providing an opportunity for the nerves to reset their signaling frequency. This is why the benefit for pain reduction continues even after the medication wears off and the nerves come back online.

There are several nerves involved in processing headache pain that can be targeted with nerve block injections, including the greater and lesser occipital nerves, the auriculotemporal nerves, and the supratrochlear and supraorbital nerves. The occipital nerves are the most commonly targeted for peripheral nerve blocks. The occipital nerves communicate with the other nerves of the head and neck through the pain relay center in the brainstem, the trigeminal nucleus caudalis (TNC).[20] Think of the occipital nerves as the "on-ramp" to the pain signaling highway, and the pain signaling as traffic. If you can block the on-ramp, you can interrupt the traffic.

Given the broad mechanism of action, nerve blocks can be considered for a number of different headaches. Retrospective, uncontrolled pediatric case series have described benefit from nerve blocks as both acute and preventive treatment for migraine, including chronic migraine, and post-traumatic headache, as well as for new daily persistent headache (NDPH).[21–24] Occipital nerve blocks are also used for cluster headache, hemicrania continua, occipital neuralgia, and cervicogenic headache[25, 26]—although these conditions are far less common in pediatrics. In the presence of myofascial pain, trigger point injections (TPIs) may be considered alongside peripheral nerve blocks.[25] The presence of active trigger points, in both primary and secondary headaches, may be associated with greater intensity and longer duration of headache.[27] Although the exact mechanism is unknown, trigger points may be formed in part as a result of abnormal endplate potentials leading to excessive acetylcholine release in the neuromuscular junction, resulting in the formation of a taut band.[28]

Another target for possible nerve blockade is the sphenopalatine ganglion (SPG). Also called the pterygopalatine ganglion, the SPG is an extra-cranial parasympathetic ganglion found in the pterygopalatine fossa posterior to the middle nasal turbinate. The ganglion has both sensory and autonomic (sympathetic and parasympathetic) components.[29] The autonomic pathway is activated during many different types of headaches including migraine. This activation may manifest with a variety of symptoms including lacrimation, nasal congestion, rhinorrhea, forehead/facial sweating, conjunctival injection, nausea, emesis, diarrhea, and polyuria.[29, 30] Clinical trials have supported the efficacy and tolerability of SPG blocks for both acute and chronic migraine in adults.[31, 32] SPG blocks have also been evaluated for the treatment of other primary and secondary headaches, including the trigeminal autonomic cephalalgias (cluster headache, paroxysmal hemicrania); trigeminal neuralgia; atypical facial pain; and headache attributed to temporomandibular joint disorder.[33–40]

Information for headache specialists

The indications for nerve blocks are reviewed above in the *primary care clinician's* section. Our own retrospective study of nerve blocks, in which injections were tailored to the individual response of teenagers with headaches unresponsive to prior treatments, found that 86% of those with acute headache flare had at least transient improvement in pain severity.[24] Despite the lack of controlled trials, nerve blocks and trigger point injections are used commonly among pediatric headache specialists. A survey of the Pediatric & Adolescent Section of the American Headache Society (AHS) found that 80% of respondents either perform or refer patients for peripheral nerve blocks.[26] There is wide variability in the medication used, site(s) injected, and in the use of repeated injections. Additional information regarding injection methodology and recommended technique is available for interested clinicians, based on expert consensus review.[18, 25]

The indications for SPG blocks are reviewed above in the *primary care clinician's* section. As an acute intervention, SPG blocks may block sensory afferent sensory fibers projecting to the trigeminal nucleus caudalis (TNC). As a preventive intervention, repeated SPG blocks may disrupt the autonomic pain cycle, reducing pain over time by changing processing through the TNC via afferent blockage of the SPG.[29, 30] Clinical trials have supported the efficacy and tolerability of SPG blocks for both acute and chronic migraine in adults.[29–33, 35–40] As a preventive treatment, SPG blocks can be performed twice a week over 6 weeks period.[32]

The traditional transnasal topical approach for SPG blocks involves using a cotton tipped applicator soaked in lidocaine, applied posteriorly to the middle nasal turbinate on the nasopharyngeal mucosa. More recently, transnasal devices have recently been made available for administration to accommodate varying anatomy and ensures that the anesthetic more reliably reaches the ganglion. These devices are minimally invasive and the procedure can be performed as quickly as 10 s on each side.

The three devices currently FDA-cleared and commercially available are the SphenoCath (*Dolor Technologies, Salt Lake City, UT*); Allevio SPG Nerve Block Catheter (*Jet Medical, Schwenksville, PA*); and the Tx360 (*Tian Medical, Lombard, Il, USA*). Studies comparing the efficacy of all the three devices are lacking.

In pediatrics, SPG blocks have been studied for the acute treatment of migraine.[40] A retrospective review of a total of 489 SPG blocks performed in patients aged 6 to 26 years with migraine or status migrainosus demonstrated complete technical success for all procedures, and a significant reduction in pain scores. No immediate or acute complications were reported. SPG blocks appear to be a safe and relatively minimally-invasive treatment approach. Although further pediatric studies are needed, SPG blocks may be a viable treatment approach in refractory headache, as an alternative to the need for IV medication, hospital admission, or prolonged use of oral pain medication with risk of medication overuse headache.

References

1. Schulman E. Refractory migraine—a review. *Headache*. 2013;53(4):599–613.
2. Dodick DW, Turkel CC, DeGryse RE, et al. OnabotulinumtoxinA for treatment of chronic migraine: pooled results from the double-blind, randomized, placebo-controlled phases of the PREEMPT clinical program. *Headache*. 2010;50(6):921–936.
3. Ali A, Kriegler J, Tepper S, Vij B. New daily persistent headache and OnabotulinumtoxinA therapy. *Clin Neuropharmacol*. 2019;42(1):1–3.
4. Yerry JA, Kuehn D, Finkel AG. Onabotulinum toxin a for the treatment of headache in service members with a history of mild traumatic brain injury: a cohort study. *Headache*. 2015;55(3):395–406.
5. Kabbouche M, O'Brien H, Hershey AD. OnabotulinumtoxinA in pediatric chronic daily headache. *Curr Neurol Neurosci Rep*. 2012;12(2):114–117.
6. Ali SS, Bragin I, Rende E, Mejico L, Werner KE. Further evidence that Onabotulinum toxin is a viable treatment option for pediatric chronic migraine patients. *Cureus*. 2019;11(3), e4343.
7. Ahmed K, Oas KH, Mack KJ, Garza I. Experience with botulinum toxin type a in medically intractable pediatric chronic daily headache. *Pediatr Neurol*. 2010;43(5):316–319.
8. Chan VW, McCabe EJ, MacGregor DL. Botox treatment for migraine and chronic daily headache in adolescents. *J Neurosci Nurs*. 2009;41(5):235–243.
9. Marcelo R, Freund B. The efficacy of botulinum toxin in pediatric chronic migraine: a literature review. *J Child Neurol*. 2020;35(12):844–851.
10. Shah S, Calderon MD, Wu W, Grant J, Rinehart J. Onabotulinumtoxin A (BOTOX®) for ProphylaCTIC treatment of pediatric migraine: a retrospective longitudinal analysis. *J Child Neurol*. 2018;33(9):580–586.
11. Winner PK, Kabbouche M, Yonker M, Wangsadipura V, Lum A, Brin MF. A randomized trial to evaluate Onabotulinumtoxin A for prevention of headaches in adolescents with chronic migraine. *Headache*. 2020;60(3):564–575.
12. Shah S, Calderon M, Crain N, et al. Effectiveness of onabotulinumtoxinA (BOTOX) in pediatric patients experiencing migraines: a randomized, double-blinded, placebo-controlled crossover study in the pediatric pain population. *Reg Anesth Pain Med*. 2021;46:41–48.

13. Winner PK, Blumenfeld AM, Eross EJ, et al. Long-term safety and tolerability of Ona-botulinumtoxinA treatment in patients with chronic migraine: results of the COMPEL study. *Drug Saf.* 2019;42(8):1013–1024.

14. Vikelis M, Argyriou AA, Dermitzakis EV, Spingos KC, Makris N, Kararizou E. Sustained onabotulinumtoxinA therapeutic benefits in patients with chronic migraine over 3 years of treatment. *J Headache Pain.* 2018;19(1):87.

15. Young WB, Ivan Lopez J, Rothrock JF, et al. Effects of onabotulinumtoxinA treatment in chronic migraine patients with and without daily headache at baseline: results from the COMPEL study. *J Headache Pain.* 2019;20(1):12.

16. Young WB, Ivan Lopez J, Rothrock JF, et al. Effects of onabotulinumtoxinA treatment in patients with and without allodynia: results of the COMPEL study. *J Headache Pain.* 2019;20(1):10.

17. Lewis DW, Winner P, Wasiewski W. The placebo responder rate in children and adolescents. *Headache.* 2005;45(3):232–239.

18. Blumenfeld A, Ashkenazi A, Napchan U, et al. Expert consensus recommendations for the performance of peripheral nerve blocks for headaches—a narrative review. *Headache.* 2013;53(3):437–446.

19. Afridi SK, Shields KG, Bhola R, Goadsby PJ. Greater occipital nerve injection in primary headache syndromes—prolonged effects from a single injection. *Pain.* 2006;122:126–129.

20. Bartsch T, Goadsby PJ. Stimulation of the greater occipital nerve induces increased central excitability of dural afferent input. *Brain.* 2002;125:1496–1509.

21. Gelfand AA, Reider AC, Goadsby PJ. Outcomes of greater occipital nerve injections in pediatric patients with chronic primary headache disorders. *Pediatr Neurol.* 2014;50(2):135–139.

22. Dubrovsky AS, Friedman D, Kocilowicz H. Pediatric post-traumatic headaches and peripheral nerve blocks of the scalp: a case series and patient satisfaction survey. *Headache.* 2014;54:878–887.

23. Seeger TA, Orr S, Bodell L, Lockyer L, Rajapakse T, Barlow KM. Occipital nerve blocks for pediatric posttraumatic headache: a case series. *J Child Neurol.* 2015;30(9):1142–1146.

24. Mumber H.E., Szperka C.L. Retrospective study of nerve blocks for the treatment of headaches in children & adolescents. In: American Headache Society 58th Annual Scientific Meeting 2016. Headache 56 (S1), 37.

25. Ashkenazi A, Blumenfeld A, Napchan U, et al. Peripheral nerve blocks and trigger point injections in headache management—a systematic review and suggestions for future research. *Headache.* 2010;50:943–952.

26. Szperka CL, Gelfand AA, Hershey A. Patterns of use of peripheral nerve blocks and trigger point injections for pediatric headache: results of a survey of the American Headache Society pediatric & adolescent section. *Headache.* 2016;56(10):1597–1607.

27. Fernández-de-Las-Peñas C, Alonso-Blanco C, Cuadrado ML, Gerwin RD, Pareja JA. Myofascial trigger points and their relationship to headache clinical parameters in chronic tension-type headache. *Headache.* 2006;46(8):1264–1272.

28. Robbins MS, Kuruvilla D, Blumenfeld A, et al. Trigger point injections for headache disorders: expert consensus methodology and narrative review. *Headache.* 2014;54(9):1441–1459.

29. Khan S, Schoenen J, Ashina M. Sphenopalatine ganglion neuromodulation in migraine: what is the rationale? *Cephalalgia.* 2014;34(5):382–391.

30. Levin M. Nerve blocks in the treatment of headache. *Neurotherapeutics.* 2010;7(2):197–203.
31. Cady R, Saper J, Dexter K, Manley HR. A double-blind, placebo-controlled study of repetitive transnasal sphenopalatine ganglion blockade with Tx360® as acute treatment for chronic migraine. *Headache.* 2015;55(1):101–116.
32. Cady RK, Saper J, Dexter K, Cady RJ, Manley HR. Long-term efficacy of a double-blind, placebo-controlled, randomized study for repetitive sphenopalatine blockade with bupivacaine vs saline with the Tx360® device for treatment of chronic migraine. *Headache.* 2015;55(4):529–542.
33. Ho KWD, Przkora R, Kumar S. Sphenopalatine ganglion: block, radiofrequency ablation and neurostimulation—a systematic review. *J Headache Pain.* 2017;18(1):118.
34. Láinez MJ, Marti AS. Sphenopalatine ganglion stimulation in cluster headache and other types of headache. *Cephalalgia.* 2016;36(12):1149–1155.
35. Maizels M, Scott B, Cohen W, Chen W. Intranasal lidocaine for treatment of migraine: a randomized, double blind, controlled trial. *JAMA.* 1996;27:319–321.
36. Piagkou M, Demesticha T, Troupis T, et al. The pterygopalatine ganglion and its role in various pain syndromes: from anatomy to clinical practice. *Pain Pract.* 2012;12(5):399–412.
37. Jenkins B, Tepper SJ. Neurostimulation for primary headache disorders, part 1: pathophysiology and anatomy, history of neuromodulation in headache treatment, and review of peripheral neuromodulation in primary headaches. *Headache.* 2011;51:1254–1266.
38. Martelletti P, Jensen RH, Antal A, et al. Neuromodulation of chronic headaches: position statement from the European Headache Federation. *J Headache Pain.* 2013;14(1):86.
39. Schoenen J, Jensen RH, Lantéri-Minet M, et al. Stimulation of the sphenopalatine ganglion (SPG) for cluster headache treatment. Pathway CH-1: a randomized, sham-controlled study. *Cephalalgia.* 2013;33(10):816–830.
40. Mousa MA, Aria DJ, Mousa AA, Schaefer CM, Temkit MHH, Towbin RB. Sphenopalatine ganglion nerve block for the treatment of migraine headaches in the pediatric population. *Pain Physician.* 2021;24(1):E111–E116.

Preventive behavioral headache management☆

17

Alexandra C. Ross, PhD, Maya Marzouk, MA, Dina Karvounides, PsyD, Elizabeth Seng, PhD, and Scott Powers, PhD

Behavioral headache management is central to a comprehensive care plan for children and adolescents with primary headaches. In fact, The American Academy of Neurology and American Headache Society practice guidelines recommend behavioral headache treatment as a *first line preventive intervention* for pediatric headache.[1] Behavioral treatment goals are numerous, including: reducing the frequency and severity of headache pain; increasing the patient's sense of control of their headaches; reducing related disability and symptoms; and for some patients, limiting reliance on ineffective, poorly tolerated, and/or unwanted medications.[2]

To support medical providers in securing these valuable services for their patients, this chapter has two primary aims: First, we will overview the evidence-base for integration of four commonly used behavioral headache management interventions (cognitive behavioral therapy, relaxation training, biofeedback, and mindfulness) into a pediatric neurology or primary care practice. Second, we will provide concrete recommendations and resources to support medical providers in making behavioral headache management resources available to this patient population. Notably, in this chapter, neurology and primary care provider (PCP) recommendations will be reviewed simultaneously as there are relatively few differences between these specialties in approaching behavioral headache intervention.

☆Editor's note: This is probably our favorite chapter in the book. Medicines alone will not help most of our patients. There are some simple steps all headache suffers can do, there are more sophisticated techniques in the realm of the headache psychologist and there are tricks for the primary care giver. I have learned to teach people deep breathing exercises in just 2 min. You can too. Feel free to incorporate whatever you can. It makes a tremendous difference!

Pediatric Headache. https://doi.org/10.1016/B978-0-323-83005-8.00002-1

Describing behavioral headache intervention to families

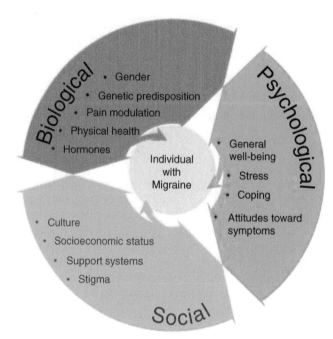

Bio-psycho-social model of migraine.

When introducing the concept of behavioral intervention to patients with headache and their families, it is critical to first normalize behavioral strategies as a central, evidence-based component of headache treatment. Optimal headache management occurs when all providers on a team utilize a biopsychosocial model. This model recognizes that biological, psychological, and social/environmental factors all play an interactive role in the trajectory of symptom development, progression, and treatment.[3] Importantly, evidence in broader pediatric pain populations suggests families' adoption of a biopsychosocial understanding relates to an increased receptivity to behavioral pain management strategies.[4] It is therefore incumbent upon referring providers to foster a biopsychosocial disease model of migraine in patients and their families prior to initiating a referral to behavioral medicine.

Due to negative past experiences (for example, a prior provider not believing the patient's pain experience) and the invisible nature of headache, when first hearing the terms "behavioral," "psychology," or "therapist," a family may inadvertently internalize the message that their provider views the child's headache as "psychologically based" or "in their head." To place behavioral intervention within the framework of treating the patient's neurological disorder, a referring provider may give an overview of the role of autonomic nervous system dysregulation in headache symptoms. The assumption is *not* that stress causes symptoms (that is, the child does not have a headache *because* they are more anxious than their peers). Rather, the experience of chronic headache symptoms inherently places the body in a state of stress, contributing to an overactive sympathetic nervous system, subsequently amplifying the headache problem.[5] Furthermore, typical life stressors (e.g., social and academic stress) can contribute to the child's physiological arousal, feeding a problematic cycle of physical, cognitive, behavioral, and emotional symptoms. The goal of behavioral headache management is to disrupt this cycle, improving the child's functioning across the aforementioned domains.[6]

In our conversations with families about the importance of behavioral intervention in pediatric headache management, we typically introduce the role of sympathetic arousal in symptom maintenance through a description of "the fight or flight response." As a classic example, if the child saw a bear in the forest, the sympathetic response (rapid heart rate, increased respiration, and tightened muscles) would adaptively prepare their body for action, such as to run away or fight the bear. However, when this automatic response is triggered in reaction to day-to-day stressors (for example, when the child is taking a difficult exam or experiencing an aura and thinking about the consequences of their impending headache), the fight or flight response no longer serves a protective function and instead serves as a "false alarm" to the body. This physiological activation can then, problematically, exacerbate or trigger a headache.

When describing these processes, the referring provider is encouraged to emphasize that behavioral headache management *does not imply the child's pain is not real*. Instead, these strategies are a standard component of headache treatment: In behavioral headache treatment, the patient will learn how to identify situations where the "false alarm" may be triggered and develop a set of skills they can employ to activate a parasympathetic response or "calm their nervous system." Importantly, taking the time to teach the patient and their parents these concepts prior to making a therapy referral serves as an intervention in itself, illustrating the ways in which the child *does* have the ability to control certain aspects of their body in the context of a disorder that often feels scary and outside of their control.

Summary of evidence-base

To date, research has demonstrated Level A evidence (established efficacy with at least two Class I trials) for the following behavioral pediatric headache interventions in preventive headache management: cognitive behavioral therapy (CBT); relaxation training; thermal biofeedback combined with relaxation training; and electromyographic (EMG) biofeedback. Additionally, Level B evidence (probably effective with one Class I or two Class II studies) is established for behavioral therapy combined with preventive drug therapy to achieve additive clinical improvement for migraine.[7, 8] In this chapter, we will overview the above therapies. We will additionally provide information on mindfulness, given the potential benefits of incorporating this intervention to better cope with functional disability (that is, the impact of headache on the child's day to day functioning) and the popularity/availability of mindfulness-based interventions.[9–11]

Cognitive behavioral therapy (CBT)

Cognitive behavioral therapy (CBT) is a brief (typically 6–8 sessions), skills-based psychotherapy intervention with considerable empirical support in the treatment of children and adolescents with headache.[12] This intervention is also effective in addressing a range of other disorders including anxiety, depression, insomnia, and chronic pain.[13, 14] CBT is built on interrelationships between thoughts, emotions, behaviors, and physiological responses, illustrated in the "CBT cycle" below. As suggested by its name, cognitive behavioral therapy (CBT) includes the instruction of both thought-related "cognitive" strategies (to address anxious, negative thoughts) and action oriented "behavioral" strategies (to address daily stressors and general self-care).

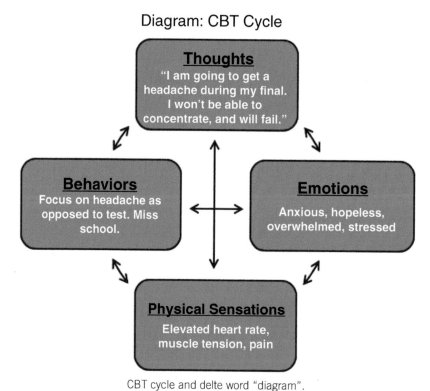

Diagram: CBT Cycle

Thoughts
"I am going to get a headache during my final. I won't be able to concentrate, and will fail."

Behaviors
Focus on headache as opposed to test. Miss school.

Emotions
Anxious, hopeless, overwhelmed, stressed

Physical Sensations
Elevated heart rate, muscle tension, pain

CBT cycle and delte word "diagram".

Cognitive CBT strategies

Cognitive CBT strategies teach the child to identify and challenge negative "self-talk" statements, enhance their belief in their own self-efficacy, and build an internal locus of control. For example, a child who is anxious about the onset of a migraine secondary to prolonged focused concentration during an upcoming school examination may generate anxious thoughts such as "I am going to get a headache during my final. I won't be able to concentrate and will fail." This thought may serve as a self-fulfilling prophecy, creating an anxious emotional response, triggering sympathetic arousal, and subsequently a migraine, which impairs the child's test performance just as predicted. Using a strategy called "cognitive reframing" the therapist will help the child learn to shift their focus away from this unhelpful thought to the factors that they *can* control in the situation. This intervention does not aim to teach the child to be artificially positive ("I will probably never get a headache again!") or simply to push the thought away, but instead to focus on *realistic* and *helpful* ways of thinking. For example, this child may learn to generate the coping statement: "If I use the coping skills I have learned in therapy and take breaks during this test, I can manage a headache and get through this test. I might not do perfect but I do know the material and studied hard so I will probably do OK." Cognitive reframing improves a child's self-efficacy in managing anxiety and headache as they choose how to respond to a negative self-talk statement as opposed to automatically reacting to it.

Behavioral CBT strategies

Behavioral CBT strategies in headache treatment may include: identifying behaviors that precipitate, increase, or maintain headaches (including modifying triggers and teaching problem-solving skills to adaptively manage daily stressors such as school stress described in the example above), teaching self-regulation skills that help decrease physiological arousal and increase relaxation and wellbeing (described in detail in the "Relaxation" section), and setting up a structured behavioral plan to promote healthy lifestyle habits such as regular sleep, hydration, meals, and exercise (described in detail in other chapters of this book).

Notably, a skilled child and adolescent therapist will adapt CBT strategies to the developmental level of the patient, making this intervention applicable to a wide age range. Parents and school staff will be incorporated in treatment as is appropriate.

Efficacy of CBT in pediatric headache

Numerous meta-analyses demonstrate the benefit of cognitive behavioral therapy in reducing the intensity of pain in pediatric chronic headache.[12, 15] Furthermore, a randomized clinical trial of 135 youth aged 10–17 demonstrated that supplementing amitriptyline with cognitive behavior therapy resulted in a greater reduction in days with headache and headache related disability as compared to a control group of amitriptyline with headache education after 20 weeks (11.5 headache day reduction for CBT supplementation vs 6.8 headache day reduction for headache education supplementation[16]). This study emphasizes the added benefit of CBT even when children are improving with pharmacotherapy. Prior randomized controlled trials also indicate efficacy of multiple modalities of CBT for headache including therapist-administered group therapy and home-based self-help[17] and a 4-week computerized CBT program as a supplement to medical care.[18] Taken together, these data suggest that specific CBT training can be recommended based on accessibility and individual preference, with the expectation of clinically significant improvement in headache days and disability.

How to support your patients in accessing CBT
Helping your patient access a therapist
- Depending on the volume of headache patients in your clinic it may be warranted to consider pursuing access to funding to integrate a behavioral health specialist into your clinical care team. A neurology provider may argue the evidence-base for cognitive behavioral therapy for headache specifically.[12, 15] There is also a national push for improved access to behavioral health in a primary care setting.[19]
- If you do not have access to an embedded psychology provider, encourage your patients to search for a therapist who (A) has experience working with children and adolescents and (B) is trained in Cognitive Behavioral Therapy (CBT). Expertise in pain management or health psychology specifically is wonderful – however in many locations a pain specialist may not be accessible. A therapist who specializes in anxiety will have an applicable skillset.

Electronic resources
- *WebMAP Mobile:* a program from Seattle Children's Hospital designed to help teens cope with chronic pain and increase their ability to do things that are important to them.

Books for interested families
- "Managing Your Child's Chronic Pain" by Tonya Palermo, PhD[20]
- "When Your Child Hurts: Effective Strategies to Increase Comfort, Reduce Stress, and Break the Cycle of Chronic Pain" by Rachel Coakley, PhD[21]
- "The Chronic Pain & Illness Workbook for Teens: CBT & Mindfulness-Based Practices to Turn the Volume Down on Pain" by Rachel Zoffness, PhD[22]

Relaxation strategies
Relaxation strategies are skills that decrease sympathetic arousal and help the patient gain a sense of efficacy and mastery over a specific aspect of their body's functioning. As noted above, relaxation strategies are an important component of CBT. These

strategies, however, also have a strong evidence-base in preventive headache treatment as an independent intervention.[23] Evidence-based relaxation strategies reviewed in this section include diaphragmatic breathing, progressive muscle relaxation, and guided imagery. Of note, prior research suggests that these strategies work best when practiced daily and proactively (that is, in advance of having a headache), to help initiate the parasympathetic "relaxation response" and maintain autonomic balance.[24] When teaching relaxation strategies to children, it is important to emphasize the active practice of these skills and their benefit compared to simply relaxing passively (that is, watching television or taking a nap is not a relaxation strategy). Reinforcing daily practice is key to building the child's sense of self-efficacy and allowing these strategies to become automatic and naturally implemented.

Diaphragmatic breathing

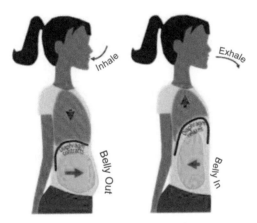

Diaphragmatic breathing is a simple breathing strategy taught to help induce the parasympathetic response in the body. When anxious or in pain, the child will naturally react by taking short and shallow breaths. When breathing diaphragmatically, the child learns to delineate between thoracic breathing ("chest"; typical of the body when it is in a state of chronic stress), versus diaphragmatic breathing ("belly"; indicative of relaxation). When practicing this skill, the diaphragm moves downward during inhalation, allowing the lungs to fill and moves upward during exhalation as the lungs empty.[25] Children are shown this technique by placing one hand on their upper chest and the other hand on their abdomen just below the rib cage at the bottom of the sternum while breathing in through the nose and out through the mouth at a slow steady pace. The goal is for the child to move the lower "belly" hand along with the breath while keeping the upper "chest" hand as still as possible.

Diaphragmatic breathing can be taught in combination with imagery (for example, a balloon filling and emptying with air), by simply counting between each breath cycle, or in conjunction with adopting a calming statement with each in-breath in and out-breath (e.g., "I am…calm"). For younger children, utilizing bubbles or a pinwheel to practice breathing in the office and at home can also be helpful.

Progressive muscle relaxation

Progressive muscle relaxation (PMR) involves a process of tightening and loosening muscle groups in a systematic way throughout the body. This practice aims to counteract a state of chronic muscle tension derived from pain-related sympathetic arousal by increasing the child's awareness of when their muscles are tense and when they are relaxed, subsequently promoting a relaxation response.

PMR can begin with the toes and slowly work through the larger muscles of the entire body such as the feet, calves, thighs, arms, hands, and neck. Children are directed to isolate and tense each muscle for approximately 5–10s while concentrating on the difference between that muscle feeling tense versus relaxed. Like diaphragmatic breathing, PMR can also incorporate imagery. Imagery is particularly important to engage younger children in PMR (e.g., "squeeze your hand like you are squeezing a lemon" or "relax your arms like they are made of spaghetti"). Once the patient has mastered PMR, they can apply this skill to more simple breath-guided or cue-controlled muscle relaxation that is not contingent on first tensing muscle groups.

Guided imagery

Guided imagery teaches children to implement their natural ability to create images to simultaneously distract their mind from a focus on pain and evoke their body's natural relaxation response.[25] During this intervention, children are encouraged to elicit an image that provides them with a sense of comfort and relaxation. When explaining the mechanism of using the brain to imagine a relaxing place, a metaphor of watching a scary movie can be used. Returning to the "fight or flight" discussion, the child is prompted to recall a time where they were watching a scary movie and what they saw on the screen elicited a sympathetic response (increased heart rate, shallow breathing). The images from the movie caused the body to respond as if the child were experiencing danger even while the child was aware they were in the safety of their home. In guided imagery, positive visualization is used by the child to create the opposing physiological response, relaxing the body and calming the nervous system.

Guided imagery can be conducted by using a formal script such as going to the beach or forest, or asking the patient to choose to travel to their own comforting place. The child is typically prompted to evoke all five senses to help deepen the imagery and experience while engaging children in this exercise. Such strategies can be very effective at not only reducing headache symptoms but, again, in increasing self-efficacy to independently cope.

Efficacy of relaxation in pediatric headache

Like CBT, the use of relaxation techniques in decreasing the frequency and severity of headache is well established with Level A evidence.[26] Particularly for children with migraine, significant reductions have been found compared to controls in both the frequency and intensity of headaches.[27] Working with an experienced clinician when learning these strategies appears to be of benefit: prior research has demonstrated superior efficacy when working with a dedicated and experienced clinician as opposed to a school nurse.[28, 29]

How to support your patients in accessing relaxation training

Helping Your Patient Access a Therapist: Many therapists provide relaxation training as a part of treatment. As noted above, relaxation training is often a component of CBT. Families may also simply ask a potential mental health provider if they have experience in the above modalities.

In Clinic Supports: Clinic staff, such as nurses, can be trained by experienced therapists to teach these skills to patients even at an initial neurology or primary care appointment.

Electronic Resources: Phone applications designed to assist with relaxation include: *Calm; Stop, Breathe, and Think; iBreathe; The Breathing App; Headspace; Relax Melodies.*

Books for interested families

"The Relaxation and Stress Reduction Workbook for Teens" by Michael A. Tompkins & Jonathan Barkin.[30]

Biofeedback

In biofeedback, a clinician will use precise sensors to measure the physiologic effects of a relaxation exercise on the child's body, enhancing the child's understanding of the physiological impact of the relaxation skills they are learning. This instrumentation pairs changes in various types of physiological activity (heart rate, muscle tension, temperature, etc.) with visual or audio feedback and gives the child concrete data on changes to their body through relaxation practice. As the child practices over time, physiologic changes endure without continued use of the device.[31, 32]

There are several types of biofeedback interventions with an evidence base in pediatric headache including electromyographic (EMG) biofeedback (feedback of electrical activity from muscles, typically scalp or neck – aimed to teach patient to recognize and subsequently reduce muscle tension) for tension headaches and thermal biofeedback (feedback of skin temperature from a finger – aimed to teach patients to increase body temperature) for migraines. Additionally, while it does not have Level A evidence in headache specifically, heart rate variability (HRV) biofeedback (feedback of changes in heart rate aimed to teach patients to induce relaxation) has been demonstrated as efficacious in other pain populations as well as managing anxiety/stress more broadly[33, 34] and is often more available within the context of a hospital.

Efficacy of biofeedback in pediatric headache

A recent meta-analysis looking systematically at results from prospective, randomized controlled trials of biofeedback for migraine among children and adolescents found significant reductions in migraine frequency, average pain intensity, and headache duration compared to controls.[35] Like CBT, biofeedback demonstrates benefit even in a short course (1–2 sessions) of treatment.[36, 37]

How to support your patients in accessing biofeedback

Helping Your Patient Access a Therapist: Encourage your patients to look into the *Biofeedback Certification International Alliance website* (https://certify.bcia.org/) to search for a local provider.

Electronic Resources: The Food and Drug Administration (FDA) does not regulate many biofeedback devices marketed for home use. Qualitatively, in our experience patients have reported finding the following device to be useful:

- Heartmath InnerBalance App and Heart Rate Variability Sensor, $159 (https://store.heartmath.com/innerbalance)

Mindfulness

Mindfulness is awareness of the present moment and one's own experiences in that moment in a purposeful, non-judgmental manner.[38] This skill helps patients learn to improve areas of focused attention while practicing acceptance of "what is" without trying to change that experience.[39] In our practice, we have learned that some children may state they have tried mindfulness before and describe the experience that mindfulness is "just sitting and trying not to think." An active mindfulness exercise, such as "thought bubbles" (imagine placing a bubble around each thought as it arises), mindful breathing, or even focusing their attention on an activity such as eating a raisin or listening to a song may help the child learn to apply this skill proactively. These exercises are designed to help patients let go of what they cannot change in the moment, subsequently decreasing the stress and frustration that occurs when internally fighting with the chronicity of symptoms.

Efficacy of mindfulness in pediatric headache

In the adult literature, there is some support for mindfulness as effective in reducing pain intensity and headache.[40, 41] While evidence is limited in reducing pain in pediatric headaches, there does appear to be benefit of using mindfulness to decrease disability and symptom impact among children with chronic pain.[42] There is also data demonstrating mindfulness-related improvements in self-regulation and coping within the context of stress.[43] Therefore, introduction to mindfulness practice may be warranted for children with high levels of disability.

How to support your patients in accessing mindfulness training

Helping Your Patient Access a Therapist: Many therapists integrate mindfulness as a part of behavioral health treatment. Encourage a family to talk to their existing therapist about this skill or inquire if a potential new therapist has experience in mindfulness.

Mindfulness is also often taught in schools. The child may ask for extra instruction from a school counselor or you can simply encourage patients to practice the strategies they are already learning in class.

Electronic Resources: Apps to assist with mindfulness include: *Headspace, Stop Breathe and Think*, and *Calm*; One helpful website is: http://www.mindfulnessforteens.com.

Books for interested families

Teens:

- "The Mindful Teen: Powerful skills to help you manage stress one moment at a time" by Dzung Vo.[44]
- "The Stress Reduction Workbook for Teens: Mindfulness skills to help you deal with stress" by Gina M. Biegel.[45]

Older Elementary/Middle School Children:

- "Mindfulness for Kids" by Carole Roman and Robin Albertson-Wren.[46]
- "The Mindful Child" by Susan Kaiser Greenland.[47]

Young Children (4–8 years old):

- "A Handful of Quiet: Happiness in Four Pebbles" by Thich Nhat Hanh.[48]
- "Moody Cow Meditates" by Kerry Lee MacLean.[49]

Parental role in preventive behavioral headache management

It is strongly recommended that parents be involved in any of the therapies above to monitor and reinforce coping behaviors. The specifics of parents' role in supporting these strategies will be variable based on the developmental level of the child. As a medical provider, one brief but effective clinic-based intervention may include educating parents on well-intentioned parental actions that may unknowingly, reinforce and maintain their child's pain related disability. For example, frequent requests for pain ratings from parents aiming to support and understand their child, may redirect a distracted child's attention back to their headache. Problematically, this question often increases the child's focus on discomfort, enhancing the child's perception of pain, and making it more difficult for the child to engage in whatever activity is at hand[50] Therefore, it is suggested that the child take the lead on verbalizing their pain to their parent when they are in need of, empathetic support, assistance with coping or medication management. Details regarding supporting parents in optimizing parental management of headaches can be found in relevant treatment manuals.[16]

Conclusion

Overall, the literature suggests the use of cognitive behavioral therapy, relaxation strategies, and biofeedback to teach regulation of autonomic arousal as first line interventions in pediatric headache. Integration of parents into any treatment is additionally key to success. We recommend introduction to these techniques and, ideally, referral to a trained therapist for any patient whose headaches are impacting their day to day functioning, who experiences difficulty maintaining a positive regularity schedule, and/or who experiences stress as a migraine trigger. In fact, for both youth and adults with migraine, current evidence would suggest a behavioral treatment combined with medication is the most effective therapy. Additionally, if disability persists even with the incorporation of the discussed cognitive and behavioral interventions, introducing tenets of mindfulness and teaching specific exercises to add to the patient's repertoire of active coping skills can increase self-efficacy and better management of symptoms. While behavioral headache strategies do require motivation on the part of the patient and family, as well as the investment of time, once learned, these interventions are always accessible to the patient and can be typically implemented independently and privately. Furthermore, self-efficacy in coping with not only migraine symptoms but daily stressors more broadly may provide continued benefits over the course of a lifetime.

References

1. Oskoui M, et al. Practice guideline update summary: pharmacologic treatment for pediatric migraine prevention: report of the guideline development, dissemination, and implementation Subcommittee of the American Academy of neurology and the American headache society. *Neurology*. 2019;93(11):500–509.
2. Kabbouche MA, Gilman DK. Management of migraine in adolescents. *Neuropsychiatr Dis Treat*. 2008;4(3):535–548.
3. Powers SW, Gilman DK, Hershey AD. Headache and psychological functioning in children and adolescents. *Headache*. 2006;46(9):1404–1415.
4. Guite JW, et al. Pain beliefs and readiness to change among adolescents with chronic musculoskeletal pain and their parents before an initial pain clinic evaluation. *Clin J Pain*. 2014;30(1):27–35.

5. Sauro KM, Becker WJ. The stress and migraine interaction. *Headache*. 2009;49(9):1378–1386.
6. Palermo TM. *Cognitive-Behavioral Therapy for Chronic Pain in Children and Adolescents*. Oxford University Press; 2012.
7. Silberstein SD. Practice parameter: evidence-based guidelines for migraine headache (an evidence-based review): report of the quality standards Subcommittee of the American Academy of neurology. *Neurology*. 2000;55(6):754–762.
8. Penzien DB, et al. Well-established and empirically supported behavioral treatments for migraine. *Curr Pain Headache Rep*. 2015;19(7):34.
9. Hesse T, et al. Mindfulness-based intervention for adolescents with recurrent headaches: a pilot feasibility study. *Evid Based Complement Alternat Med*. 2015;2015:1–9.
10. Ludwig DS, Kabat-Zinn J. Mindfulness in medicine. *JAMA*. 2008;300(11):1350–1352.
11. Wells RE, et al. Meditation for migraines: a pilot randomized controlled trial. *Headache*. 2014;54(9):1484–1495.
12. Trautmann E, Lackschewitz H, Kröner-Herwig B. Psychological treatment of recurrent headache in children and adolescents-a meta-analysis. *Cephalalgia*. 2006;26(12):1411–1426.
13. Hofmann SG, et al. The efficacy of cognitive behavioral therapy: a review of meta-analyses. *Cogn Ther Res*. 2012;36(5):427–440.
14. Fisher E, et al. Systematic review and meta-analysis of psychological therapies for children with chronic pain. *J Pediatr Psychol*. 2014;39(8):763–782.
15. Fisher E, et al. Psychological therapies for the management of chronic and recurrent pain in children and adolescents. *Cochrane Database Syst Rev*. 2018;9:1–110.
16. Powers SW, et al. Cognitive behavioral therapy plus amitriptyline for chronic migraine in children and adolescents: a randomized clinical trial. *JAMA*. 2013;310(24):2622–2630.
17. Kroener-Herwig B, Denecke H. Cognitive–behavioral therapy of pediatric headache: Are there differences in efficacy between a therapist-administered group training and a self-help format? *J Psychosom Res*. 2002;53(6):1107–1114.
18. Connelly M, Rapoff MA, Thompson N, Connelly W. Headstrong: a pilot study of a CD-ROM intervention for recurrent pediatric headache. *J Pediatr Psychol*. 2006;31(7):737–747.
19. Foy JM, et al. Improving mental health services in primary care: reducing administrative and financial barriers to access and collaboration. *Pediatrics*. 2009;123(4):1248–1251.
20. Palermo TM, Law EF. *Managing Your Child's Chronic Pain*. USA: Oxford University Press; 2015.
21. Coakley R. *When Your Child Hurts: Effective Strategies to Increase Comfort, Reduce Stress, and Break The Cycle of Chronic Pain*. Yale University Press; 2016.
22. Zoffness R, Schader K. *The Chronic Pain and Illness Workbook for Teens: CBT and Mindfulness-Based Practices to Turn the Volume Down on Pain*. New Harbinger Publications; 2019.
23. Holden EW, Deichmann MM, Levy JD. Empirically supported treatments in pediatric psychology: recurrent pediatric headache. *J Pediatr Psychol*. 1999;24(2):91–109.
24. Benson H, Beary JF, Carol MP. The relaxation response. *Psychiatry*. 1974;37(1):37–46.
25. Williams SE, Zahka NE. *Treating Somatic Symptoms in Children and Adolescents*. Guilford Publications; 2017.
26. Faedda N, et al. Behavioral management of headache in children and adolescents. *J Headache Pain*. 2016;17(1):80.

27. Fichtel Å, Larsson B. Does relaxation treatment have differential effects on migraine and tension-type headache in adolescents? *Headache.* 2001;41(3):290–296.
28. Fichtel Å, Larsson B. Relaxation treatment administered by school nurses to adolescents with recurrent headaches. *Headache.* 2004;44(6):545–554.
29. Larsson B, et al. Relaxation treatment of adolescent headache sufferers: results from a school-based replication series. *Headache.* 2005;45(6):692–704.
30. Michael A, Tompkins JRB. In: Schaeder K, ed. *The Relaxation and Stress Reduction Workbook for Teens.* Oakland, CA: Instant Help Books: New Harbinger Publications, Inc.; 2018.
31. Yucha C, Montgomery D. *Evidence-Based Practice in Biofeedback And Neurofeedback.* Wheat Ridge, CO: AAPB; 2008.
32. Powers SW, Andrasik F. Biobehavioral treatment, disability, and psychological effects of pediatric headache. *Pediatr Ann.* 2005;34(6):461–465.
33. Stern MJ, Guiles RA, Gevirtz R. HRV biofeedback for pediatric irritable bowel syndrome and functional abdominal pain: a clinical replication series. *Appl Psychophysiol Biofeedback.* 2014;39(3–4):287–291.
34. Knox M, et al. Game-based biofeedback for paediatric anxiety and depression. *Ment Health Fam Med.* 2011;8(3):195.
35. Stubberud A, et al. Biofeedback as prophylaxis for pediatric migraine: a meta-analysis. *Pediatrics.* 2016;138(2), e20160675.
36. Blume HK, Brockman LN, Breuner CC. Biofeedback therapy for pediatric headache: factors associated with response. *Headache.* 2012;52(9):1377–1386.
37. Powers S, et al. A pilot study of one-session biofeedback training in pediatric headache. *Neurology.* 2001;56(1):133.
38. Kabat-Zinn J. *Wherever You Go, There You Are: Mindfulness Meditation in Everyday Life.* New York: Hyperion; 1994.
39. Perry-Parrish C, et al. Mindfulness-based approaches for children and youth. *Curr Probl Pediatr Adolesc Health Care.* 2016;46(6):172–178.
40. Gu Q, Hou J-C, Fang X-M. Mindfulness meditation for primary headache pain: a meta-analysis. *Chin Med J (Engl).* 2018;131(7):829.
41. Crowe M, et al. Mindfulness-based stress reduction for long-term physical conditions: a systematic review. *Aust N Z J Psychiatry.* 2016;50(1):21–32.
42. Ali A, et al. Mindfulness-based stress reduction for adolescents with functional somatic syndromes: a pilot cohort study. *J Pediatr.* 2017;183:184–190.
43. Perry-Parrish C, et al. Improving self-regulation in adolescents: current evidence for the role of mindfulness-based cognitive therapy. *Adolesc Health Med Ther.* 2016;7:101.
44. Vo DX. *The Mindful Teen: Powerful Skills to Help You Handle Stress One Moment at a Time.* New Harbinger Publications; 2015.
45. Biegel GM. *The Stress Reduction Workbook for Teens: Mindfulness Skills to Help You Deal with Stress.* New Harbinger Publications; 2017.
46. Roman CP, Albertson-Wren JR. *Mindfulness for Kids: 30 Fun Activities to Stay Calm, Happy, and in Control.* Emeryville, CA: Althea Press; 2018.
47. Greenland SK. *The Mindful Child: How to Help Your Kid Manage Stress and Become Happier, Kinder, and More Compassionate.* Simon and Schuster; 2010.
48. Hanh TN. *A Handful of Quiet: Happiness in Four Pebbles.* Parallax Press; 2008.
49. MacLean KL. *Moody Cow Meditates.* Simon and Schuster; 2009.
50. Walker LS, Garber J, Greene JW. Psychosocial correlates of recurrent childhood pain: a comparison of pediatric patients with recurrent abdominal pain, organic illness, and psychiatric disorders. *J Abnorm Psychol.* 1993;102(2):248.

Treatments that can act both acutely and preventively

Devices ✩

Samantha Lee Irwin, MB BCh, MS

Neuromodulation for migraine treatment

Neuromodulation is a nonmedication alternative for both migraine prevention and for the acute treatment of migraine. There are several devices with FDA clearance for such uses and these will be reviewed below. For a patient who has either not benefited from other treatments or prefers nonmedication-based treatments, neuro-modulation devices are reasonable alternatives. A common factor limiting use of these devices is cost, as insurance generally doesn't cover them. A further challenge is convenience, as these devices require various degrees of storage, charging, space, and time to use. Overall, efficacy appears to be similar to medications, although no head-to-head trials exist.

Transmagnetic stimulation (TMS)

Single Pulse Transcranial Magnetic Stimulation (sTMS), manufactured by eNeura, is FDA cleared for acute and preventive migraine treatment in both adolescents (2019) and adults (2013). sTMS is a simple, painless, and noninvasive transcranial electromagnetic induction device. It works by delivering a magnetic current at a certain frequency through the bone and soft tissue of the cranium. The magnetic current decreases "cortical spreading depression" (CSD), a process involved in migraine, and may decrease activation of central cortical areas involved in migraine, specifically, the thalamocortical projection neurons and corticothalamic networks. Evidence suggests that instead of having a direct effect on trigeminovascular neurons in the brainstem, however, sTMS likely works by modulating cortical excitability in a few key nonbrainstem areas of the migraine pathway.[1]

✩Editor's Note: No matter how hard we try to find medications that are well tolerated, there are a group of patients who either cannot tolerate medicine, or are loathe to use them. Thankfully we have new techniques for quieting migraine that involve decreasing spreading depression, overstimulating the trigeminal nerve Vagus Nerve, or Peripheral Nerve. These devices offer our patients the ability to control their pain at will and transfer locus of control back to them. Side effects are minimal, but cost is maximal.

Pediatric Headache. https://doi.org/10.1016/B978-0-323-83005-8.00019-7

For patients and families

sTMS does not cause discomfort and can be used for both prevention and for treating migraines acutely. However, it is a device that requires storage and charging and is relatively large, which can preclude use in those who travel frequently. It is also loud during use which may be problematic if prominent noise sensitivity is present. Practically, it is a reasonable option for those seeking nonmedication treatments and who prefer a device that can treat both acute attacks and be used for prevention. It is also ideal for someone who is sensitive to adhesives or gels or prefers a device that they don't have to "wear" and won't be able to feel on their head/neck during use.

For providers

Acute use efficacy was established in an adult trial that showed a 17% reduction in 2-h pain freedom with sTMS use compared to the sham device (39% vs. 22%, $p = 0.179$).[2] The open label ESPOUSE trial evaluated sTMS for migraine prevention and found that after 3 months of use, 46% of participants reported a greater than 50% reduction in the number of headache days per month and there was on average 2.8 less headaches days per month with use.[3] In pediatrics, a small open label prospective trial ($n = 12$) primarily looking at safety also noted an improvement in headache days from 13.3 at baseline to 8.8 after 3 months of daily use, an absolute reduction of -4.5 days.[4]

Typically, this device is recommended to be used for 4 pulses in the morning and 4 pulses at night (2 pulses, wait 15 min, 2 pulses) for prevention. Pediatric trial data however, seems to suggest that it is safe and just as effective to remove the 15 min pause between the 2 pulses.[4] For acute treatment, it is recommended to give three sequential pulses at onset of migraine, wait 15 min and then if needed treat again with 3 additional pulses. This can be repeated a 3rd time for a total of 9 acute pulses over a 30-min period.

There does not appear to be any significant or serious side effects with use of the device. Reported side effects from trials were seen in 13%–29% and included: dizziness or light-headedness, discomfort from noise, application site tenderness or tingling, and headache.[3,4] sTMS is contraindicated in those with epilepsy or a family history of epilepsy or in those with a history of stroke. Caution should be used in those with recent head injury or if a patient is on medications that can "lower" seizure threshold. It should not be used in those with any implanted metal devices in the head, neck and upper body including vagal nerve stimulators, pacemakers, or implanted cardioverter defibrillator (ICD). A full list of metal containing implants is listed on the company website. It should not be used in those with suspected or diagnosed heart conditions. Dental fillings appear to be safe. It has not been adequately studied in those who are pregnant or <12 years of age (Label insert, eneura.com).

Transcranial supraorbital nerve stimulator

Transcranial supraorbital nerve stimulation (tSNS), also known as Cefaly, is another FDA cleared device for the acute and preventive treatment of migraine in adults (2017). Although the pathophysiology is not fully elucidated, it appears to work by sending a painless electric current through the supra-orbital nerve, a branch of the trigeminal nerve (V1), which terminates in the trigeminal nucleus, an area of the brainstem that is implicated in migraine.[5] It may also modulate top-down cortical sites that regulate the migraine pain pathway, such as the anterior cingulate cortex.[6]

For patients and families

The tSNS device needs to be worn for 20 min daily for preventive use and can be used for up to 1 hour for the acute treatment of migraine. Patients often find it helpful to practice cognitive behavioral therapy, mindfulness, or biofeedback during the "downtime" while using the device. The tSNS device is helpful for those seeking non medication alternatives and ideal for those who like the idea of using the time required for treatment to practice various complementary medicine techniques. Limitations to use are that it does require one to spend 20 min daily with something affixed to their forehead, which may be unrealistic for some. Other limitations are that it may cause tingling in the forehead and it uses an adhesive that may cause a hyper-sensitivity reaction in vulnerable patients or in those with allergies.

For providers

tSNS was initially studied in a pilot study ($n = 10$) in patients with episodic migraine and was found to be effective in reducing monthly attack frequency by 1.3 days.[7] This led to a larger trial for migraine prevention in adults called PREMICE. In this randomized, sham-controlled trial of adult patients with episodic migraine ($n = 59$) who used the device for 20 min a day for 3 months, 38.2% had a 50% reduction in migraine days per month vs. 12.1% in the sham group ($p = 0.023$), a therapeutic gain of 26.1%. Migraine days per month reduced by 2.06 days in the active group and 0.32 days in the sham group, (6.94 to 4.88 for tSNS vs. 6.54 to 6.22 for sham) but this was not a statistically significant result.[8] The authors also noted a 36.7% reduction in acute medication use (vs. sham that experienced a 0.4% increase). In a trial evaluating the acute use of tSNS in migraine ($n = 109$), 63% of patients achieved >50% relief at 1 h (vs. 31% in the sham group, $p = 0.0017$) and 29% of patients reported pain freedom at 1 h (vs. 6% in the sham group, $p = 0.0016$).[9] In chronic migraine, tSNS for both prevention and acute treatment also seems to be favorable. In an open-label prevention trial in chronic migraine ($n = 19$), after 4 months of use 35% of patients had a 50% reduction in both headache days and acute medication use. Mean reduction of headache days was 57.9%.[10] In an open-label acute treatment trial in adults with chronic migraine ($n = 23$), 44% were pain free at 1 h with use of tSNS.[11]

The device is overall well tolerated with no serious adverse events reported. In a large post-marketing survey of 2313 users, 4.3% reported minor side effects including tingling in the area of the device, pain or intolerance, allergic reaction to device or gel, fatigue or headache.[12] No contraindication is noted for use in pregnancy. Contraindications include any implanted metallic devices or electronic devices, pacemakers, or ICD. Adherence may be a problematic for some considering tSNS, as compliance rates in one trial were noted to be only ~60%.[8]

Vagal nerve stimulation

Noninvasive vagal nerve stimulation (nVNS) is FDA cleared for the acute and preventive treatment of migraine for adults (acute 2018 and prevent 2020), and as of February 2021, FDA cleared for adolescents >12 years of age (label extension based on prior data[13]).[14] nVNS sends a signal through the skin to the vagus nerve. There are various cortical and subcortical end targets to nVNS stimulation, but specifically for migraine, it seems to block pain-induced activation of the trigeminovascular complex.[15]

For patients and families

This is a smaller device than the two mentioned above and may be ideal for those seeking a quick, nontablet-based treatment, but who need a smaller device to accommodate their lifestyle. It does, however, require the use of a gel at the application site and three-times-per day use for migraine prevention which may limit its convenience.

For providers

Efficacy was established for preventive use in chronic migraine in the prospective, randomized sham-controlled EVENT trial ($n=59$) where a nonsignificant reduction in headaches days was seen in the nVNS group vs. sham (-1.4 days vs. -0.2 days).[16] During the open-label extension of this trial, after 8 months of use, there was a significant mean change from baseline in headache days of -7.9 ($p \leq 0.01$). Acute treatment was evaluated in the PRESTO trial ($n=248$) with 30-min pain freedom rates of 12.7% in the nVNS group vs. 4.2% in the sham group ($p=0.012$). This extended to 21% vs. 10% by 60 min ($p=0.023$) and 30.4% vs. 19.7% at 120 min ($p=0.067$).[17]

nVNS use for migraine prevention involves three treatments (morning, mid-day and night. Each treatment consists of two consecutive 2-min stimulations (2-2-2)). For acute migraine treatment, it is used for two consecutive 2-min stimulations, followed by a 20-min wait and then if pain persists, two further 2-min stimulations and then, after a 2-h wait, if required a third treatment consisting of two consecutive 2-min stimulations (2-(20 min)-2-(2 h)-2) (package insert, gammacore.com).

The most commonly reported side effects included: neck discomfort and/or shoulder twitching/pain, facial/lip pulling, twitching or drooping, voice change, dizziness, and application site pain or skin irritation.[17–19] Despite vagal involvement in cardiac control, animal data suggests that the use of nVNS does not seem to effect cardiac function,[20] however, it should not be used in those with a history of hypertension, hypotension, bradycardia, or tachycardia. It should not be used if a person has an implantable medical device (pacemakers/defibrillators, hearing aid implant or any other implanted electronic medical device), an implanted metallic device in or near the neck, or if one is using another device at the same time (TENS unit, muscle stimulator, or mobile phone). Additionally, it should not be used if someone has been diagnosed with carotid atherosclerosis or has a history of cervical vagotomy. Use in children <12 and pregnancy has not been evaluated *(package insert, gammacore.com)*.

Remote electrical neuromodulation device

The remote electrical neuromodulation(REN) device, also known as Nerivio, works by stimulating pain fibers in the arm in a nonpainful way to induce a process called "conditioned pain modulation" (CPM) that uses the body's own pain mechanisms to activate the cortical descending pain inhibition pathways (inlcuding the periaqueductal gray) to "shut off" migraine genesis in the trigeminal cervical complex.[21] It is FDA cleared for the acute treatment of migraine in adults (2020) and, as of January 2021, also cleared for adolescents >12 years of age.[22]

For patients and families

The REN device is an acute use-only treatment device for migraine. It is a relatively affordable nonmedication option for the acute treatment of migraine that can be worn discretely under clothing and used at any time of the day. It connects remotely via the user's smartphone and doesn't require any wires, adhesives or gels for use once it is in place.

For providers

The first pilot trial for acute migraine treatment ($n=71$) showed pain reduction in 58% vs. 24% for placebo ($p=0.02$) and pain freedom in 30% vs. 6% ($p=0.004$).[23] In larger follow-up prospective acute trial in episodic migraine ($n=252$), significantly higher pain freedom was seen in the treatment vs. sham group (37.4% vs. 18.4%, $p=0.03$) at 2-h and significantly higher pain reduction was seen in the treatment vs. sham group (66.7% vs. 38.8%, $p<0.001$).[24] In chronic migraine, an open label pilot study ($n=42$) showed that 73.7% of participants achieved pain relief at 2-h in at least 50% of their treated attacks and 26.3% had pain freedom in at least 50% of treated attacks at 2-h. At 2-h, mean pain relief across subjects was 59.3%

and mean pain freedom across subjects was 25.9%.[25] In a follow up larger "real world" trial ($n = 4725$), pain relief was seen in 58.9% in those seen by headache specialists and 74.2% of those seen by nonheadache specialists in at least 50% of treated attacks. Pain freedom was seen in 20% of those in the headache specialists group and 35.6% of those in the nonheadache specialists group.[26]

The REN device appears to be very safe with device related adverse events occurring in <2% and the only consistently reported side effects being tingling, pain, redness or burning at the site of the device.[26]

References

1. Andreou AP, Holland PR, Akerman S, et al. Transcranial magnetic stimulation and potential cortical and trigeminothalamic mechanisms in migraine. *Brain*. 2016;139(Pt 7):2002–2014.
2. Lipton RB, Dodick DW, Silberstein SD, et al. Single-pulse transcranial magnetic stimulation for acute treatment of migraine with aura: a randomised, double-blind, parallel-group, sham-controlled trial. *Lancet Neurol*. 2010;9:373–380.
3. Starling AJ, Tepper SJ, Marmura MJ, et al. A multicenter, prospective, single arm, open label, observational study of sTMS for migraine prevention (ESPOUSE study). *Cephalalgia*. 2018;38(6):1038–1048.
4. Irwin SL, Qubty W, Elaine Allen I, Patniyot I, Goadsby PJ, Gelfand AA. Transcranial magnetic stimulation for migraine prevention in adolescents: a pilot open-label study. *Headache*. 2018;58(5):724–731.
5. Schwedt TJ, Vargas B. Neurostimulation for treatment of migraine and cluster headache. *Pain Med*. 2015;16:1827–1834.
6. Russo A, Tessitore A, Esposito F, et al. Functional changes of the perigenual part of the anterior cingulate cortex after external trigeminal neurostimulation in migraine patients. *Front Neurol*. 2017;8:282.
7. Gérardy PY, Fabry D, Fumal A, Schoenen J. A pilot study on supra-orbital surface electrotherapy in migraine. *Cephalalgia*. 2009;29:134.
8. Schoenen J, Vandersmissen B, Jeangette S, et al. Migraine prevention with a supraortibal transcutaneous stimulator: a randomized controlled trial. *Neurology*. 2013;80:697–704.
9. Chou DE, Shnayderman Yugrakh M, Wilnegarner D, et al. Acute migraine therapy with external trigeminal neurostimulation (ACME): a randomized controlled trial. *Cephalalgia*. 2019;39(1):3–14.
10. Di Fiore P, Bussone G, Galli A, et al. Transcutanous supraorbital neurostimulation for the prevention of chronic migraine: a prospective, open-label preliminary trial. *Neurol Sci*. 2017;38:s201–s206.
11. Di Fiore P, Galli A, D'Arrigo G, et al. Transcutaneous supraorbital neurostimulation for acute treatment of chronic migraine: open-label preliminary data. *Neurol Sci*. 2018;39:s163–s164.
12. Magis D, Sava S, d'Elia TS, et al. Safety and patients' satisfaction of transcutaneous supraorbital neurostimulation (tSNS) with the Cefaly(R) device in headache treatment: a survey of 2,313 headache sufferers in the general population. *J Headache Pain*. 2013;14:95.
13. Grazzi L, Egeo G, Liebler E, Padovan AM, Barbanti P. Non-invasive vagus nerve stimulation (nVNS) as symptomatic treatment of migraine in young patients: a preliminary

safety study. *Neurol Sci.* 2017;38(Suppl 1):197–199. https://doi.org/10.1007/s10072-017-2942-5. PMID: 28527086.

14. Gaul C, Diener HC, Silver N, PREVA Study Group, et al. Non-invasive vagus nerve stimulation for PREVention and acute treatment of chronic cluster headache (PREVA): a randomised controlled study. *Cephalalgia.* 2016;36(6):534–546.

15. Akerman S, Simon B, Romero-Reyes M. Vagus nerve stimulation suppresses acute noxious activation of trigeminocervical neurons in animal models of primary headache. *Neurobiol Dis.* 2017;102:96–104.

16. Silberstein SD, Calhoun AH, Lipton RB, et al. Chronic migraine headache prevention with noninvasive vagus nerve stimulation: the EVENT study. *Neurology.* 2016;87:529–538.

17. Tassorelli C, Grazzi L, de Tommaso M, et al. Noninvasive vagus nerve stimulation (nVNS) for the acute treatment of migraine: a randomised controlled trial. *Cephalalgia.* 2017;37(1 Suppl):319–374.

18. Silberstein SD, Mechtler LL, Kudrow DB, et al. Non-invasive vagus nerve stimulation for the acute treatment of cluster headache: findings from the randomized, double-blind, sham-controlled ACT1 study. *Headache.* 2016;56:1317–1332.

19. Goadsby PJ, de Coo IF, Silver N, et al. Noninvasive vagus nerve stimulation for the acute treatment of episodic and chronic cluster headache: a randomized, double-blind, sham-controlled ACT2 study. *Cephalalgia.* 2018;38.

20. Castoro MA, Yoo PB, Hincapie JG, et al. Excitation properties of the right cervical vagus nerve in adult dogs. *Exp Neurol.* 2011;227:62–68.

21. Rapoport AM, Lin T, Tepper SJ. Remote electrical neuromodulation (REN) for the acute treatment of migraine. *Headache.* 2020;60:229–234. https://doi.org/10.1111/head.13669.

22. Hershey AD, Lin T, Gruper Y, et al. Remote electrical neuromodulation for acute treatment of migraine in adolescents. *Headache.* 2020. https://doi.org/10.1111/head.14042. Published online December 21.

23. Yarnitsky D, Volokh L, Ironi A, et al. Nonpainful remote electrical stimulation alleviates episodic migraine pain. *Neurology.* 2017;88(13):1250–1255. https://doi.org/10.1212/WNL.0000000000003760.

24. Yarnitsky D, Dodick DW, Grosberg BM, et al. Remote electrical neuromodulation (REN) relieves acute migraine: a randomized, double-blind, placebo-controlled, multicenter trial. *Headache.* 2019;59:1240–1252. https://doi.org/10.1111/head.13551.

25. Nierenburg H, Vieira JR, Lev N, et al. Remote electrical neuromodulation for the acute treatment of migraine in patients with chronic migraine: an open-label pilot study. *Pain Ther.* 2020;9:531–543. https://doi.org/10.1007/s40122-020-00185-1.

26. Tepper SJ, Lin T, Montal T, Ironi A, Dougherty C. Real-world experience with remote electrical neuromodulation in the acute treatment of migraine. *Pain Med.* 2020;1–8. https://doi.org/10.1093/pm/pnaa299.

CGRP pathway treatments ☆

19

Amy A. Gelfand, MD

Introduction

Calcitonin gene-related peptide (CGRP) is a 37 amino acid long protein with a strong role in the pathophysiology of migraine.[1, 2] CGRP's other roles in the body include acting as a vasodilator (helping to widen blood vessels) and helping with bone formation.[3] Monoclonal antibodies to CGRP, or one of its receptors, have been developed and shown to decrease migraine frequency in adults, including those with chronic migraine and those who have not responded to previous preventive trials.[4–15]

CGRP pathway monoclonal antibodies for migraine prevention
For patients and families

As of early 2021, there are not yet randomized trials on the use of CGRP pathway monoclonal antibodies in children or adolescents. That said, since the first of these treatments, erenumab, was FDA approved for migraine prevention in adults in 2018, some U.S. pediatric headache specialists have been using CGRP pathway monoclonal antibodies "off label" to treat adolescents who have difficult to treat headaches that have not responded to other treatments. In deciding whether or not these treatments are right for you (or your child), the two main things to consider are (1) what are the possible side effects? and (2) what are the possible benefits, relative to how severe my/my child's headache problem is and what treatments have already been tried? In terms of side effects, the most commonly seen are constipation and injection-site reactions. Constipation can often be managed with diet changes, physical activity, or use of stool softeners and fiber supplements. The injection-site reactions are typically mild and short-lived. Rarely, new or worsened high blood pressure has occurred in adults treated with erenumab.[16]

☆Editor's note: Although the treatment of headache has improved dramatically since I started practicing in the late 1980s, there have been quantum leaps that have changed the lives of those with headaches, Triptans, offered in the mid-1990s, provided quick relief for migraine. CGRP treatments now provide outstanding acute and chronic treatment with few side effects.

Pediatric Headache. https://doi.org/10.1016/B978-0-323-83005-8.00004-5

Since these treatments have only been in use for a few years (as of the time of this writing), the main question when considering whether to use them in a young person might be, *Is there a risk to their use in young people that we don't yet know about?* Unfortunately, the only way to answer this question adequately is with careful observations made over the passage of time. In the meantime, in consultation with your/your child's clinicians, you will need to decide how much to weigh the theoretical risk of an unknown side effect against the real and likely (if you are considering these treatments) substantial impact and disability that headache is having on you/your child right now. How to weigh these things and integrate them into a treatment plan that is right for you/your child is a very personal decision and speaking with your/your child's headache specialist about your/your child's individual situation is highly advisable.

For primary care providers

Prescribing and managing CGRP pathway monoclonal antibodies in adolescents is probably best left to headache specialists (as least as of our current state of knowledge in 2021). However, having a basic familiarity with CGRP pathway monoclonal antibodies will be helpful in that, your patients may reach out to you for advice when considering whether to start one of these, and being familiar with them can inspire confidence. It is also helpful to understand how other treatments you may be prescribing or managing might interact with the CGRP pathway monoclonal antibody your patient is taking. Monoclonal antibodies are eliminated through the endothelial cells lining the blood vessels. They are not hepatically or renally metabolized, so typical "drug–drug" interactions are generally not a concern.[3] If constipation was already an issue for your patient, it may worsen when they go on a CGRP pathway monoclonal antibody and they may need more assistance with managing this. Constipation can also arise for the first time on these therapies. As CGRP is a vasodilator, the rare side effect of new or worsened hypertension that can be seen in adults treated with erenumab may also be possible in adolescents, and may also be possible with the CGRP pathway monoclonal antibodies other than erenumab. The author has not seen hypertension arise, or worsen, in adolescents treated with CGRP pathway monoclonal antibodies. However, for youth with pre-existing hypertension, it may be prudent to increase blood pressure monitoring if they do start one of these treatments. There have also been rare reports of hypersensitivity reactions as well.

It is prudent to avoid these treatments in people who are pregnant, or in those who have had a stroke or thromboembolic event.

For headache specialists

Given that the CGRP pathway monoclonal antibodies are still relatively new, relatively costly, and not yet formally studied in children and adolescents other than in retrospective chart review,[17] they are generally not considered first-line migraine preventive therapy in youth. However, pediatric headache experts have suggested that they be considered for adolescents with migraine who have significant

Table 1 When to consider prescribing a CGRP pathway monoclonal antibody.

- Patient is at least 12 years of age and ≥40 kg
- At least two other migraine preventive strategies have been tried and failed to bring relief (and/or caused intolerable side effects)
- Headache is present ≥15 days/month
- Headache related disability is moderate or severe (i.e., PedMIDAS score is ≥31)
- Patient does not have a history of severe constipation, or there is a plan in place for how to manage constipation if it worsens
- Patient does not have a history of hypertension, or there is a plan in place for how to monitor blood pressure if they do

headache-related disability and who have not responded to other preventive treatments.[3] In the table are some suggested criteria for when to consider offering these treatments. If the patient is also taking medications that predispose to constipation, such as tricyclic antidepressants, consider weaning these off if possible or at least giving good anticipatory guidance about constipation management (Table 1).

Once the decision to treat with a CGRP pathway monoclonal antibody has been made, the question then is which one to prescribe. Sometimes this decision comes down to which one the patient's insurance will cover, as these treatments are relatively costly (approximately $600/month out of pocket for the injectables, presumably more for the intravenous option). Erenumab blocks the canonical CGRP receptor but does not bind CGRP itself (i.e., the ligand).[4] It has been available in the U.S. the longest, hence there may be more clinical experience with its use in adolescents relative to the others.[17] The other three CGRP pathway monoclonal antibodies (fremanezumab, galcanezumab, and eptinezumab) bind to CGRP itself.[10,12,14] Erenumab, galcanezumab, and fremanezumab are given by subcutaneous injection, while eptinezumab is given by intravenous infusion. If a patient has a strong preference not to do subcutaneous injections at home, but is comfortable getting intravenous infusions, eptinezumab may be a good option. The dosing interval for the three injectable ones are every 28 days, although fremanezumab was studied both as 225 mg SC monthly and as 675 mg SC quarterly.[13] If the patient is going to be traveling abroad for several months, or going away to camp for the summer, quarterly dosing may be advantageous.

If a patient does not respond to one CGRP monoclonal pathway antibody, they may respond to another. How long a treatment trial has to be conducted before assessing for treatment efficacy is not empirically known. While adult trials with these agents suggest that benefit in the first month or two is possible, some may take more time to respond. It is important to note that, generally speaking, people with chronic migraine who are experiencing daily, continuous headache have been excluded from treatment trials. Therefore, how long it might take to know if a preventive is helpful in this population is unknown, and it may be longer than the duration needed in the migraine population overall. Whether to try a third or even fourth CGRP pathway monoclonal antibody if the first two did not work is also not known. On the one hand, it may seem futile. On the other hand, often patients who have gotten to this point in treatment have already had 9 or 10 preventive trials, as well as copious lifestyle advice and cognitive behavioral therapy and often nerve injections and headache-related hospitalizations. Whether it is "worth it" to try another one may depend on patient and family preference, as well as what other treatment options are still available for them to try. The box below shows one possible approach to choosing and progressing through CGRP pathway monoclonal antibodies in adolescents:

Possible approach to use of CGRP pathway monoclonal antibodies in adolescents

Step 1: Treat with a subcutaneously administered antibody (erenumab, galcanezumab, or fremanezumab) X 2–3 doses.

Step 2: Assess for treatment response and side effects. If improving, and well tolerated, continue. If not improving, but well tolerated, consider increasing dose (if applicable) vs. changing to a different antibody (e.g., if using erenumab [which targets the canonical CGRP receptor] consider changing to one that binds CGRP itself. Alternatively, consider changing the route of administration).

Step 3: Assess for treatment response and side effects. If an effective option has still not been found, consider adjusting dose or changing to another agent vs. changing to another class of preventive treatment.

The table shows dosing, routes of administration, and half-lives for the four CGRP pathway monoclonal antibodies available in the United States (Table 2).

Table 2 Dosing, routes and half-lives of the CGRP pathway monoclonal antibodies.

	Target	FDA-approved for adults	Dosing	Half-life
Erenumab	CGRP receptor	May 2018	70 or 140 mg SC every 28 days, via auto-injector	28 days
Fremanezumab	CGRP	Sept 2018	225 mg SC every 28 days or 675 mg SC quarterly, via auto-injector	31 days
Galcanezumab	CGRP	Sept 2018	240 mg loading dose followed by 120 mg SC every 28 days, via auto-injector	27 days
Eptinezumab	CGRP	Feb 2020	100 mg or 300 mg IV quarterly	27 days

Gepants

Gepants are small-molecule oral medications that antagonize the CGRP receptor. They can be used for either acute or preventive treatment of migraine. In contrast to the CGRP pathway monoclonal antibodies, they have considerably shorter half-lives, and are hepatically metabolized. While issues with liver toxicity occurred with an earlier generation of gepants, hepatotoxicity has not occurred with the newer generation gepants.[18]

For patients and families

Gepants have been studied in adults and shown to be effective for acute treatment of migraine.[19–22] Dosed regularly, at least some gepants are also effective as preventives (i.e., frequency lowering treatment) in adults.[23, 24] Studies in children and adolescents are underway, but results are not yet available as of the time of this writing. If you/your child has not found triptans helpful, or has a contra-indication to triptans (for example, hemiplegic migraine), gepants may be a good alternative option. As they are newer, they tend to be costly and insurance companies may require multiple trials of other acute treatments before covering these. As blocking the CGRP pathway is, if anything, helpful for decreasing migraine frequency, there does not seem to be potential for gepants to cause "medication-overuse headache"—i.e., the phenomenon where frequent use of certain acute headache medications may lead to an increase in headache frequency. In adult trials, gepants appear to have a relatively good side effect profile—fatigue or nausea may occur rarely.

For primary care providers

It is most likely that a headache specialist or neurologist would be the one to prescribe a gepant. Medication interactions to be aware of are that strong inhibitors of CYP3A4 (e.g., ketoconazole, itraconazole, clarithromycin) may lead to increased serum levels of gepants.

For headache specialists

As of early 2021, there are two gepants available in the United States: rimegepant and ubrogepant. Rimegepant is available as a 75 mg oral dissolving tablet (with a light mint flavor) and has a half-life of approximately 11 h. The dissolving formulation means it can be taken without water, which may have practical implications. In addition to its use as an acute treatment, every other day dosing of rimegepant has been shown in adults to be effective for migraine prevention.[23] Ubrogepant is available as a tablet (50 or 100 mg) and has a half-life of 5–7 h. It is packaged in a sachet, which might be practical as a teenager could put one in their pocket or purse without having to take the whole pack. Rimegepant has a maximum of 75 mg (i.e., one dose) in 24 h, whereas ubrogepant has a maximum of 200 mg in 24 h, and therefore the option of redosing 2-h or more after the first dose was given. While not yet available clinically, atogepant has been studied for migraine prevention in adults (dosed once or twice daily) and shown to be effective in a phase 2b/3 trial.[24]

References

1. Hay DL, Walker CS. CGRP and its receptors. *Headache.* 2017;57(4):625–636.
2. Hansen JM, Hauge AW, Olesen J, Ashina M. Calcitonin gene-related peptide triggers migraine-like attacks in patients with migraine with aura. *Cephalalgia.* 2010;30(10): 1179–1186.
3. Szperka CL, VanderPluym J, Orr SL, et al. Recommendations on the use of anti-CGRP monoclonal antibodies in children and adolescents. *Headache.* 2018;58(10):1658–1669.
4. Goadsby PJ, Reuter U, Hallstrom Y, et al. A controlled trial of erenumab for episodic migraine. *N Engl J Med.* 2017;377(22):2123–2132.
5. Ashina M, Goadsby P, Reuter U, et al, eds. *Long-term safety and tolerability of erenumab: three-plus year results from an ongoing open-label extension study in episodic migraine. 2018 American Headache Society Annual Scientific Meeting June 28–July 1, 2018;* 2018. San Francisco, CA.
6. Ashina M, Tepper S, Brandes JL, et al. Efficacy and safety of erenumab (AMG334) in chronic migraine patients with prior preventive treatment failure: a subgroup analysis of a randomized, double-blind, placebo-controlled study. *Cephalalgia.* 2018;38(10): 1611–1621.
7. Dodick DW, Ashina M, Brandes JL, et al. ARISE: a phase 3 randomized trial of erenumab for episodic migraine. *Cephalalgia.* 2018;38(6):1026–1037.
8. Reuter U, Goadsby PJ, Lanteri-Minet M, et al. Efficacy and tolerability of erenumab in patients with episodic migraine in whom two-to-four previous preventive treatments were unsuccessful: a randomised, double-blind, placebo-controlled, phase 3b study. *Lancet.* 2018;392(10161):2280–2287.
9. Aurora SK. Editor efficacy of galcanezumab in patients who failed to respond to preventives previously: results from EVOLVE-1, EVOLVE-2, and REGAIN studies. In: *American Academy of Neurology Annual Scientific Meeting;* 2018. Los Angeles, CA.
10. Skljarevski V, Matharu M, Millen BA, Ossipov MH, Kim BK, Yang JY. Efficacy and safety of galcanezumab for the prevention of episodic migraine: results of the EVOLVE-2 phase 3 randomized controlled clinical trial. *Cephalalgia.* 2018;38:1442–1454.
11. Stauffer VL, Dodick DW, Zhang Q, Carter JN, Ailani J, Conley RR. Evaluation of Galcanezumab for the prevention of episodic migraine: the EVOLVE-1 randomized clinical trial. *JAMA Neurol.* 2018;75:1080–1088.
12. Silberstein SD, Dodick DW, Bigal ME, et al. Fremanezumab for the preventive treatment of chronic migraine. *N Engl J Med.* 2017;377(22):2113–2122.
13. Dodick DW, Silberstein SD, Bigal ME, et al. Effect of Fremanezumab compared with placebo for prevention of episodic migraine: a randomized clinical trial. *JAMA.* 2018;319(19):1999–2008.
14. Dodick DW, Lipton RB, Silberstein S, et al. Eptinezumab for prevention of chronic migraine: a randomized phase 2b clinical trial. *Cephalalgia.* 2019;39(9):1075–1085.
15. Ashina M, Saper J, Cady R, et al. Eptinezumab in episodic migraine: a randomized, double-blind, placebo-controlled study (PROMISE-1). *Cephalalgia.* 2020;40(3):241–254.

16. Saely S, Croteau D, Jawidzik L, Brinker A, Kortepeter C. Hypertension: a new safety risk for patients treated with erenumab. *Headache*. 2021;61(1):202–208.

17. Greene KA, Gentile CP, Szperka CL, et al. Calcitonin gene-related peptide monoclonal antibody use for the preventive treatment of refractory headache disorders in adolescents. *Pediatr Neurol*. 2021;114:62–67.

18. Goadsby PJ, Tepper SJ, Watkins PB, et al. Safety and tolerability of ubrogepant following intermittent, high-frequency dosing: randomized, placebo-controlled trial in healthy adults. *Cephalalgia*. 2019;39(14):1753–1761.

19. Croop R, Goadsby PJ, Stock DA, et al. Efficacy, safety, and tolerability of rimegepant orally disintegrating tablet for the acute treatment of migraine: a randomised, phase 3, double-blind, placebo-controlled trial. *Lancet*. 2019;394(10200):737–745.

20. Lipton RB, Croop R, Stock EG, et al. Rimegepant, an Oral calcitonin gene-related peptide receptor antagonist, for migraine. *N Engl J Med*. 2019;381(2):142–149.

21. Voss T, Lipton RB, Dodick DW, et al. A phase IIb randomized, double-blind, placebo-controlled trial of ubrogepant for the acute treatment of migraine. *Cephalalgia*. 2016;36(9):887–898.

22. Lipton RB, Dodick DW, Ailani J, et al. Effect of ubrogepant vs placebo on pain and the Most bothersome associated symptom in the acute treatment of migraine: the ACHIEVE II randomized clinical trial. *JAMA*. 2019;322(19):1887–1898.

23. Croop R, Lipton RB, Kudrow D, et al. Oral rimegepant for preventive treatment of migraine: a phase 2/3, randomised, double-blind, placebo-controlled trial. *Lancet*. 2020;397:51–60.

24. Goadsby PJ, Dodick DW, Ailani J, et al. Safety, tolerability, and efficacy of orally administered atogepant for the prevention of episodic migraine in adults: a double-blind, randomised phase 2b/3 trial. *Lancet Neurol*. 2020;19(9):727–737.

Nonpharmaceutical options for pediatric headache: Nutraceuticals, manual therapies, and acupuncture ☆

20

Amanda Hall, MSN, FNP-C, Andrea Brand, MAc LAc, and Sita Kedia, MD, MPH

Complementary therapies are commonly sought for treatment of pediatric headache by primary care physicians, specialists, and parents alike. Herein, we describe the use of nutraceuticals, manual therapies, and acupuncture for headache treatment. We specifically address safety and efficacy evidence when available for children and teens.

Nutraceuticals

What patients and families need to know

What are nutraceuticals?

Nutraceutical is a word used for supplements that may help a medical symptom or condition. Dietary supplements contain an ingredient already found in the body. Supplements that may help headaches in children include: Riboflavin (B2), Coenzyme Q10, Magnesium, Omega-3 Polyunsaturated Fatty Acids, Vitamin D, Melatonin, and Folic Acid. These supplements are used as medicine when prescribed to correct a deficiency or as a high-dose treatment. Many of them can also be found in certain foods. Herbal supplements derived from plants that might help headaches include: Feverfew, Butterbur, Capsaicin, Peppermint, and Lavender. You might read about other nutraceuticals being studied to help headaches in children in the future.

☆Editors' note: The authors carefully describe potential benefits and risks of a wide variety of therapies. Complementary therapies are used very commonly by patients, but clinicians don't always know enough to guide. This comprehensive review of the literature is invaluable, and will assist both families and clinicians in shared decision-making.

Pediatric Headache. https://doi.org/10.1016/B978-0-323-83005-8.00025-2

Do nutraceuticals work to stop or prevent headache?

The cause of your child's headache should be diagnosed by a clinician before a supplement is used. Most of the studies looking at supplements for headache are small and in adults with migraine. However, children and teens with different headache types have reported feeling better after trying select supplements. When choosing which treatment, brand, and dose is best for your child, it is important to talk to your child's clinician. She/he may ask about other symptoms, dietary habits, or sleep patterns. Laboratory testing may be done before suggesting a supplement for your child. When reading about supplements on the internet, search trusted sources (e.g., NIH, FDA, USDA) and avoid those selling products.

Are nutraceuticals safe?

Before buying a supplement, ask your child's healthcare provider about safe products. You may see supplements advertised as "natural" remedies with no side effects. Just like medicines, supplements can cause side effects and interactions with other medicines. Just like with medicines, supplements cause both known and unknown chemical reactions in the body to occur. Companies do not have to prove a product works or that it is safe in humans before selling it. There have been reports of variable strengths, unidentified ingredients, and contaminants in supplements on the market. There are even concerns with some of the supplements used for headache treatment, so please continue reading for more information.

What a PCP and headache specialist needs to know

Why prescribe nutraceuticals for pediatric headache?

Poor regulation

Why not just provide patients with a list of supplements and let them decide what to purchase? Nutraceuticals are regulated under The Federal Drug Administration's (FDA's) Dietary Supplement Health and Education Act (DSHEA) of 1994, which restricts the FDA from evaluating supplements for safety or efficacy prior to being sold. This allows the release of supplements in any combination at any concentration without the efficacy or safety studies in humans required of pharmaceuticals. The FDA is authorized to take supplements off market, if they are misrepresented or unsafe but this must be proven. As a result, there may be many unsafe products on the market today which are falsely advertised or not yet proven harmful.[1]

Shared-decision making

Many of our patients are already using nutraceuticals or other forms of Complementary and Alternative Medicine (CAM) and do not tell us.[2–4] By prescribing nutraceuticals, providers can direct patients to certified brands with known adherence to good manufacturing practices, accurate ingredients, and in doses shown to provide benefit without inflicting harm. Patients and families may then be more comfortable discussing their use of other CAM treatments allowing for informed discussions and shared decision making.

Limitations of pharmaceuticals

For headache prevention, the available first line pharmaceutical options in children carry the risk of adverse effects and most do not outcompete placebo.[5] For acute treatment of headache in children, there are effective agents such as triptans, acetaminophen, and ibuprofen, but their use is limited due to concerns for developing Medication Overuse Headache (MOH).[6] This leaves several days without treatment options when nutraceuticals may be useful alternatives.

Efficacy, tolerability, mechanisms of action

While nutraceuticals have not been proven efficacious for headache prevention in children, several hold promise in adults, are well-tolerated, and may leverage an already robust placebo response (up to 66.6%)[7] seen in this population.[8] There are several nutraceuticals of interest in pediatric headache. These can be categorized by endogenous dietary supplements and herbal supplements.

Endogenous dietary supplements

The most studied include: Riboflavin (B2), Co-enzyme Q10, and Magnesium.

Riboflavin (B2)

Riboflavin has been assigned Level B (probably effective) rating by the AAN and AHS for headache prevention in adults with five positive studies, including one Class I trial.[9]

There have been four studies examining riboflavin for prevention of pediatric headache. Of the four studies, two were rated Class I trials by AAN/AHS but produced conflicting results. Despite the inability to outcompete placebo in all trials, riboflavin was extremely well tolerated and improvements in headache were observed in all groups. The most common side effect with riboflavin is urine discoloration.

The first double-blinded RCT revealed greater reductions in headache frequency in the placebo group compared to the riboflavin 200 mg group over twelve weeks.[7] To determine if 400 mg of riboflavin would be more efficacious, a comparison trial (200 mg vs 400 mg) was conducted. Both riboflavin groups reported better responses to abortive medication and 2/3 experienced at least a 50% reduction in headache frequency at 4–6-month follow-up with no significant difference between 200 or 400 mg/day dosing, age, or migraine type.[10] The third trial, a randomized double-blind cross over, then examined the efficacy of riboflavin for pediatric headache prevention at a lower dose, 50 mg, resulting in no significant difference from placebo.[11] The most recent study was a double-blinded RCT using 400 mg of riboflavin or placebo in 98 adolescents with headaches for three months. Headache frequency, duration, and disability were all decreased in the second and third months compared to placebo.[12]

The improvements seen with riboflavin supplementation at higher doses could be attributed to correcting underlying deficiency,[13] its ability to provide mitochondrial support,[14,15] and potential to lower total homocysteine levels.[16] It may also act as a prebiotic promoting the growth of beneficial gut microbes shown to produce antiinflammatory peptides and improve gut barrier function.[17]

Co-enzyme Q10

Co-enzyme Q10 was designated as Level C (possibly effective) for migraine prevention in adults by the AAN and AHS in a 2012 guideline update with one positive Class II study.[9] A 2019 meta-analysis including five studies with 346 patients (226 adult and 120 pediatric) concluded CoQ10 was effective in both decreasing migraine days per month and migraine duration; however, migraine severity and attacks per month was not significantly improved compared to placebo.[18]

There are two studies in children/adolescents with migraine. The first included children with low CoQ10 levels (>30% of 1550 seen in a pediatric headache center) who were then supplemented 1–3 mg/kg/day of liquid gel for more than two months. Subsequent rises in CoQ10 serum levels were documented and significant improvements in headache frequency and disability were seen with CoQ10 supplementation.[19] A second crossover RCT ($n = 76$) supplementing with 100 mg CoQ10 daily reported a placebo response with an early trend towards improvement in the CoQ10 group. All groups improved over time without significant differences at day 224.[20]

Proposed mechanisms of action for Co-enzyme Q10 include correcting deficiency,[19] providing mitochondrial support,[15,16] stabilizing endothelial function by protecting lipoproteins,[16] and modulating inflammatory pathways.[21] Co-enzyme Q10 may increase energy, so can also cause insomnia as well as stomach upset.

Magnesium

The AAN and AHS found Magnesium to be Level B, probably effective for migraine prevention based on two positive Class II studies while considering one negative Class III study.[9] Since these recommendations, a meta-analysis of RCTs in adults was conducted. Eleven studies (789 participants) examined the effects of oral magnesium for headache prevention and thirteen studies (948 participants) examined IV magnesium for acute treatment of migraine. Oral magnesium was found to significantly reduce migraine intensity and severity when used alone or in combination with other treatments (e.g., flunarizine hydrochloride, venlafaxine, ʟ-carnitine, riboflavin plus feverfew) over 4–12 weeks. The use of IV magnesium for acute treatment was found to significantly improve migraines within 15–45 min, at 120 min, and 24 h when used alone or in combination with metoclopramide, Ozagrel, lidocaine, or potassium aspartate.[22]

There have been three studies in pediatric patients. The first study was a double-blinded RCT in 86 pediatric patients with migraine receiving magnesium oxide at 9 mg elemental mg/kg (divided in three doses with food) based on positive adult trials using 600 mg elemental Mg daily. Over 16 weeks, there was a trend towards headache reduction, fewer headache days, and headache severity with magnesium.[23] The second was a replication series (with subsequent 1-year follow-up) examining the effect of magnesium pidolate (2.25 g) dosed twice daily for two months in nine pediatric patients with tension-type headaches (5=episodic, 4=chronic). The authors do not report the dose of elemental magnesium. Eight of the nine patients reported a 50% or more reduction in headache with marked decreases in the use of acute medications sustained at 1-year.[24,25] The third showed the 400 mg of magnesium salt daily increased efficacy of acute medications ibuprofen and acetaminophen in pediatric patients without concerns for adverse effects over 18-months of treatment.[26]

Proposed mechanisms for magnesium in the treatment of headache were reviewed by Taylor[16] to include: (1) correcting and preventing magnesium depletion, (2) maintaining magnesium and calcium homeostasis, (3) calcium channel blocking effect on vascular smooth muscle, (4) antidepressant and anxiolytic effects. Magnesium can cause diarrhea or abdominal discomfort.

Other dietary supplements being investigated in the treatment of migraine include Omega-3 Polyunsaturated Fatty Acids, Vitamin D3, Melatonin, Other B vitamins (Folic Acid, B12), Other antioxidants (Vitamin E, Vitamin C), and probiotics.

Omega-3 polyunsaturated fatty acids

Omega-3 supplementation was rated a Level U by the AAN and AHS, inadequate or conflicting data to support or refute medication use, based on one Class I study in adults. Adults with migraine were given 3 g of omega-3 twice daily for 4 weeks. The omega-3 group experienced a 55% decrease in headaches, the placebo group 45%, suggesting a robust placebo response.[27] A meta-analysis (including four additional small RCTs) reported omega-3 supplementation may reduce headache duration but concluded that there were no significant reductions in frequency or severity given available data.[28]

Of these RCTs, one was a crossover design conducted in adolescents with recurrent migraines. The treatment group (n = 14) were given 2 g of fish oil daily for 2 months while the control received olive oil capsules. More than 75% reported benefit, with nearly all participants (91%) stating they would recommend fish oil or olive oil to a relative or friend with headache.[29]

Omega-3 Polyunsaturated Fatty Acids possess antivasopressor effects,[30] ability to decrease the production of leukotrienes and prostaglandins, and are antiinflammatory.[29]

Vitamin D3

There have been two large reviews both concluding vitamin D supplementation may be helpful for reducing headache frequency, especially in patients with migraine and a documented deficiency.[31,32]

One retrospective pediatric migraine trial compared the effects of vitamin D 2000 iu/day (2 months) then 600–1000 iu/day (6 months) in patients with low baseline 25-OH levels (n = 42) versus those with normal levels (n = 50). Patients with a baseline deficiency in vitamin D experienced significant reductions in migraine frequency, duration, and disability.[33]

Vitamin D holds neuroprotective and antioxidant properties while possessing ability to modulate neuronal calcium and mechanism for detoxification.[34] A meta-analysis confirmed serum 25(OH)D is consistently lower in people with migraine than healthy controls[35] suggesting correction of insufficiency or deficiency as a potential mechanism of action.

Melatonin

A review and meta-analysis found that melatonin was effective and safe for migraine prevention in adults based on 3 positives and 1 negative RCT but data in children was limited (1 RCT). Also reviewed were adult comparison trials revealing melatonin was more effective than pizotifen but did not outcompete amitriptyline, sodium valproate, or propranolol.[36]

The RCT in pediatric patients (80 participants) found improvements in 62% of those treated with melatonin (0.3 mg/kg or max 6 mg) and in 82.5% treated with amitriptyline (1 mg/kg/day or max 50 mg) over three months. Both were determined to be effective and safe. While amitriptyline demonstrated superior efficacy, melatonin was better tolerated.[37] An earlier open-label trial of 22 children with tension-type headache reported improvements in headache frequency and duration in 14/21 participants after 3 months of melatonin 3 mg.[38]

Melatonin has been shown to have an analgesic effect of gamma-aminobutyric acid, protect against glutamate toxicity, modulate dopamine and serotonin,[39] possess antiinflammatory properties,[40] anxiolytic effects,[41] and decreases pain peptides.[42] Supplementation may correct an endogenous dysregulation.[43] Melatonin is also used for delayed sleep phase syndrome and insomnia which may worsen headaches in some pediatric patients.[44,45]

Other B vitamins (folic acid, B6, B12)

There have been a few studies (3) in adults and one in children evaluating supplementation of folic acid, B6, and/or B12 on migraine. The study in children was a small, uncontrolled trial of sixteen patients with documented hyperhomocysteinemia, and a methylenetetrofolate reductase (MTHFR) gene mutation with at least a one-year history of recurrent migraine. After 6 months of supplementation with 5 mg folic acid daily, all sixteen patients had normal plasma homocysteine levels and reported at least a 50% reduction in headache frequency.[46]

The interest in folic acid, vitamin B6, and B12 likely stems from their ability to lower total homocysteine levels.[47] Homocysteine levels have been found to be elevated in people with migraine with aura, particularly those with MTHFR gene mutation.[48,49] These mutations may disrupt the enzymatic activity of MTHFR which interferes with the remethylation of homocysteine resulting in increased plasma levels. Lower folate levels, elevated homocysteine levels, and MTHFR mutations have also been observed as more common amongst pediatric migraineurs.[50]

Other antioxidants (vitamin E, vitamin C, NAC)

There are four studies in adults examining the efficacy of other antioxidants on migraine prevention in adults. The first was an uncontrolled preliminary study in 12 patients with refractory migraines demonstrating significant reductions in headache frequency, severity, and disability with a combination of pine bark extract (flavonoid) 120 mg, vitamin C 60 mg, and vitamin E 30 IU dosed daily over three months.[51] Sustained benefit and ongoing improvement were later observed at 12-months.[52] Vitamin E may be beneficial for menstrual migraine (1 RCT) while combination N-acetylcysteine 300 mg, vitamin E 125 IU, and vitamin C 250 mg (dosed two capsules twice daily) demonstrated promise in episodic migraine (1 randomized sham-controlled pilot).

Exploring potential benefits from CoQ10 and other antioxidants for migraine treatment is appealing given the established role of oxidative stress, generation of free radicals, and neurogenic inflammation on migraine pathophysiology.[53]

Probiotics

Preliminary evidence (1 positive DBRCT, 1 negative RCT, 2 positive open-label trials) exists for daily supplementation with a diverse probiotic in both episodic and chronic adult migraineurs.[54–57]

Migraine may lead to a disruption in microflora composition in the gut affecting the gut-brain axis.[58] In turn, alterations in microflora have been shown to alter tryptophan metabolism, immune, and enteroendocrine cells resulting in an increase in peptides (CGRP) and inflammatory cytokines while decreasing serotonin which may trigger migraine.[59] Connections between dysbiosis and migraine could explain the higher prevalence of GI disorder amongst patients with migraine(IBS, IBD, CD, gastroparesis, and HP infections).[59]

Although unclear, proposed mechanisms for the efficacy of probiotic use in migraine include: increase in gastric emptying rate, improving intestinal integrity, and decreasing inflammatory cytokines via suppression of nuclear factor kappa-B pathway.[58]

Herbal supplements

The most studied include: Feverfew and Butterbur.

Feverfew (*Tanacetum parthenium*)

The AAN and AHS determined MIG-99 (a CO_2 stabilized extract of feverfew) was probably effective (Level B) for migraine prevention in adults based on one positive Class I, one positive Class II, and one negative Class II trial. This recommendation was continued from the earlier recommendation supported by 2 positive Class II and one negative Class III study.[9] The CHS recommends against the use of feverfew based on poor quality evidence (rated by AAN/AHS as Class I).

The initial Cochrane Review concluded feverfew was ineffective for adult migraine prevention based on five trials with conflicting outcomes and heterogeneous interventions, participants and designs. The review was updated to include the larger positive RCT using MIG-99 (a CO_2 stabilized extract of feverfew) finding there is now low quality evidence to support its use without safety concerns.[60] It is theorized that earlier studies were conflicting due to the instability of feverfew extracts, varying as much as 400% in parthenolide content.[61]

While most studies have examined the use of feverfew for prevention, one RCT found a combination of feverfew and ginger given sublingually may also be effective for acute migraine relief.[62]

In children, an observational study of 91 pediatric patients with migraine or tension-type headaches evaluated the effect of a combination supplement containing Magnesium 169 mg, CoQ10 20 mg, Vitamin B2 48 mg, and Feverfew 150 mg (1,2 mg Parthenolides), and *Andrographis paniculata* 100 mg. Improvements in headache frequency were observed without safety concerns reported.[63]

While there were no adverse effects linked to feverfew in adult migraine trials, there was a possible "post-feverfew" syndrome observed following withdrawal. Symptoms included: anxiety, nervousness, sleep problems, and musculoskeletal aches/pains.[60]

Proposed mechanisms reviewed by Taylor[16] for feverfew in the treatment of headache include the inhibitions of prostaglandin biosynthesis, Phospholipase A, Nuclear factor kappa B (NF-0B), NO synthesis, and platelet aggregation. It may also increase serotonin release from WBCs and platelets.

Butterbur (*Petasites hybridus*)

Petasites was granted a Level A classification and determined to be effective for migraine prevention in adults by the AAN and AHS based on two Class I trials.9 These recommendations were later withdrawn in 2017 given concerns for hepatoxicity with petasites/butterbur products in the United Kingdom. While commercially prepared forms, such as Petadolex, are reportedly free of the hepatotoxic pyrrolizidine alkaloids found in petasites prior to purification, there have still been case reports of transaminitis,[64] so petasites are not currently recommended.

There are two small trials examining the effect of Petasites preparations for headache prevention in children. The first was an open-label trial in 108 children with migraine given the brand supplement Petadolex 25–50 mg 2–3 times daily for 4 months. More than 75% of participants experienced at least a 50% reduction in headaches, while nearly all (91%) reported feeling improvements.[65] The second was a 3-armed RCT comparing music therapy to Petadolex (25–50 mg 2–3 times daily). All groups reported a decrease in headaches. At 12-weeks, music therapy outcompeted placebo then at 6-month follow-up both music therapy and Petadolex surpassed placebo.[66]

The benefits from butterbur in migraine prevention is thought to be attributed to its antiinflammatory properties, ability to regulate calcium channels, and inhibit leukotriene biosynthesis.[16]

Other botanicals of interest include: Capsaicin, Peppermint, Lavender, *Boswellia serrata*, Andrographis paniculate, and Marijuana.

Capsaicin

Small studies have shown that capsaicin may be helpful in both the prevention and acute treatment of headache disorders in adults. A series of trials demonstrated potential benefit for cluster headache patients with the nasal administration of capsaicin[67–69] followed by one very small RCT reporting possible benefits with repeated intranasal capsaicin for chronic migraineurs.[70] More recently, a topical formulation capsaicin jelly was shown to reduce scalp tenderness in adult migraineurs.[71]

There are no pediatric studies to date, although one case report exists for migraine relief in an adolescent after ingesting capsaicin containing "chili sauce." She had previously suffered from 6 months of intense headaches before finding relief with "chili sauce."[72]

As an agonist of the transient receptor potential vanilloid type 1, Capsaicin induces the release and subsequent inactivation of CGRP and other pain peptides. Desensitization of sensory neurons may lead to a decrease in headache severity.[71,73]

Peppermint (Mentha × piperita)

There have been small trials supporting the use of topical peppermint preparations for the acute relief of headache. Interest in peppermint for headache relief may have been partly inspired by an early RCT finding a topical peppermint oil preparation (peppermint 10 g plus ethanol 90%) decreased pain sensitivity, improved mood, and promoted relaxation of the temporalis muscle on EMG when applied to the foreheads and temples of thirty-two healthy adult subjects following acute head pain induction.[74] Subsequent trials demonstrated benefit from topical peppermint preparations for the acute treatment of tension-type headache,[75,76] migraine pain, nausea, photophobia, and phonobia.[77] Intranasal administration of peppermint oil may also be efficacious in migraine rescue.[78]

Oral peppermint may be safe and effective in alleviating symptoms of IBS in children,[79] however there are no trials to date evaluating peppermint for headache relief in children.

Peppermint likely improves tension and migraine headaches given its spasmolytic and analgesic properties achieved via stimulation of cation channels.[77]

Lavender

One trial in adults found that inhalation of lavender essential oil for 15 min at the onset of migraine may be an effective rescue treatment,[80] while another supports consideration of oral lavender essential oil for migraine prevention.[81] Topical administration of lavender oil was found to reduce pain prior to dialysis needle insertion in adults suggesting potential benefit with procedural pain associated with injection headache treatments.[82]

There are no studies in children examining the use of lavender for headache prevention or rescue treatment, although, one study found inhaled lavender decreased the use of analgesics in pediatric patients post-tonsillectomy.[83]

Like peppermint, lavender possesses analgesic and spasmolytic properties[81] which may lead to headache relief. Lavender is also an anxiolytic with sedative effects[81] which may be of additional benefit to those identifying sleep problems or anxiety as potential headache triggers.

Marijuana

While a large body of evidence supports consideration of marijuana for chronic pain,[84] evidence in headaches is limited to mostly retrospective case studies, case series, surveys, and reports. There was one controlled trial examining the use of a synthetic formulation, Nabilone. This was a double-blind RCT with crossover design in 26 patients with MOH refractory to treatment. Nabilone 0.5 mg daily compared to 400 mg ibuprofen daily for 8 weeks with one week washout in between significantly decreased headache pain, medication use, and disability.[85]

The most recent survey collected data from a vast number of adult participants (1019 with migraine and 1876 with other headaches) using Stainprint a free medical cannabis app collecting strains and dosing in addition to headache response. Users reported nearly a 50% reduction in both migraine and other headaches with cannabis. The concentrate was reportedly more effective for headache, while there were no differences pertaining to strain or dose in migraine patients. Tolerance was observed but patients appeared to self-titrate with no concerns for MOH detected in either group.[86] Another survey based study of 445 headache patients identified the top 15 preferred strains using data from ID Migraine questionnaire. All preferred strains were hybrid, most being high THC: low CBD.[87]

While young adults using cannabis have reported self-medicating for pain, anxiety, or depression,[88] there is only one pediatric case study reporting the effects of dronabinol on two adolescents with refractory depression and neuropathic pain. Only one of the participants endorsed a decrease in pain severity, but both noted improvements in pain perception, mood, sleep, academic performance, relationship, and activities of daily life with dronabinol.[89]

Marijuana contains a variety of active compounds. While the cannabinoids CBD and THC have been the most studied to date, the plant contains hundreds of phytochemicals including cannabinoids, terpenes, terpenoids, flavonoids, and many other compounds. Mechanisms proposed for headache relief are believed to be complex and dependent on the constitution of the strain since these phytochemicals vary in ratios from strain to strain producing a wide variety of effects. Cannabinoids alone modulate inflammation and pain pathways extensively by binding to cannabinoid receptors located along the pain pathway and in immune cells influencing releases of cytokines, chemokines, glutamate, 5-hydroxytryptamine (5-HT) (serotonin), acetylcholine, gamma-aminobutyric acid (GABA), noradrenaline, dopamine, D-aspartate, and cholecystokinin receptors while also acting at serotonin, opioid, and NMDA receptors (see review by Baron 2018).[90]

While there is the potential for benefit from marijuana, or specifically CBD and THC, there are also potential risks. Marijuana has been associated with prolonged vomiting, psychosis, and cognitive changes amongst other problems. The long-term side effects of marijuana use in children and teens are not known.

Boswellia serrata, Andrographis paniculate, basil essential oil,
Homeopathy

Small adult trials exist for *Boswellia serrata*,[91,92] Andrographis paniculate,[63] Basil essential oil,[93] and homeopathy[62,94] in the prevention of headaches. Since nearly 200 medicinal plants have been documented for use in headaches dating back to the 6th century,[95] it is likely that nutraceuticals will continue to be investigated for headache management in years to come.

When and how to prescribe nutraceuticals for pediatric headache?

Primary headaches

The use of nutraceuticals in pediatric headache assumes that diagnostic work-up is complete and that secondary causes of headache have been excluded (Table 1).

Disability

While pediatric data for pharmaceutical preventive treatments is conflicting, the AAN and AHS 2019 practice guideline update assigned level B recommendations to discuss pharmaceutical options with patients and families when PedMIDAS score is >30 and/or headaches are frequent and to engage in shared decision making.[5]

Nutraceuticals may be more appropriately presented as complementary treatment when disability is moderate to severe and a monotherapy option if disability is low, pharmaceutical agents were not tolerated or ineffective.

Table 1 Considerations prior to prescribing nutraceuticals for pediatric headache.

Nutraceutical	Laboratory Data[96]	Sources[96]	Adverse effects reported in pediatric headache trials	Other possible adverse effects[96]
Magnesium	Magnesium, RBC Ionized magnesium Magnesium, plasma Tolerance test, urine	Almonds, spinach Cashews	Diarrhea or soft stools (58)[23] Unpleasant taste[24, 25] None reported[26]	Nausea, abdominal cramping Toxicity (>5000 mg/d) Avoid in pregnancy (fetal skeletal abnormalities)[97] Avoid in renal failure (inability to remove Mg) Medication Interactions: fluoroquinolones, tetracyclines, bisphosphonates, diuretics, proton pump inhibitors

Continued

Table 1 Considerations prior to prescribing nutraceuticals for pediatric headache—Cont'd

Nutraceutical	Laboratory Data[96]	Sources[96]	Adverse effects reported in pediatric headache trials	Other possible adverse effects[96]
CoQ10 *(Ubiquinol, Ubiquinone)*	CoQ10, plasma CoQ10/ cholesterol ratio[b,98]	Meat, poultry, fish Nuts[99]	None reported[19, 20]	Insomnia, digestive upset May make warfarin less effective May interact with insulin and cancer treatments
Vitamin D	Serum 25(OH) D levels (ng/ mL) Calcium, phosphorus alkaline phosphatase, parathormone	Fatty fish (cod liver, trout, salmon), sun exposed mushrooms Sun exposure	None reported[33]	Hypercalcemia (rare) Long term toxicity may be possible >10,000IU daily or 25(OH)D > 50–60ng/mL Medication interactions: orlistat, statins, steroids, thiazide diuretics
Melatonin	Prolactin	Darkness	Daytime sleepiness (3)[37](1)[38]	Nocturia, headache, dizziness, agitation, nausea Avoid long term use in children Monitor for changes in menstrual cycles or delays in puberty May worsen or improve seizures May increase effects of warfarin
Riboflavin	Erythrocyte glutathione reductase activity coefficient (EGRAC)	Beef liver, oats Cereals, yogurt Milk, clams, beef	Diarrhea (12), Polyuria (18)[12] Vomiting (1), Appetite increase (1)[10] None reported[7, 11] Bright yellow/ orange urine[10]	No known medication interactions No known adverse effects from 400mg/day for 3months

Table 1 Considerations prior to prescribing nutraceuticals for pediatric headache—Cont'd

Nutraceutical	Laboratory Data[96]	Sources[96]	Adverse effects reported in pediatric headache trials	Other possible adverse effects[96]
B6	Pyridoxal 5′ phosphate (PLP) B6, RBC B6, plasma	Chickpeas, beef liver, tuna, salmon, chicken	N/A	Toxicity (1-6g for 1–3 years) may cause neuropathy, skin lesions, photosensitivity, nausea, and heartburn Neuropathy reported in doses <500 mg/d Medication Interactions: antiepileptics, theophylline, cycloserine
B12	B12, plasma Methylmalonic acid	Clams, beef liver, trout, salmon, tuna, nutritional yeast, haddock, beef, milk, yogurt, cheese	N/A	No known adverse effects B-vitamins are Possibly carcinogenic especially with long-term use[100,101] Medication interactions: Chloramphenicol, Proton pump inhibitors, H2 receptor antagonists, and metformin may all interfere with B12 absorption
Folic acid	Folate, RBC Folate, plasma	Beef liver, spinach, black-eyed peas	None reported[46]	May mask B12 deficiency by correcting anemia High doses may accelerate preneoplastic lesions High doses (>1000 µg/d) may impair cognitive development when taken periconception Medication interactions: methotrexate, antiepileptic, sulfasalazine

Continued

Table 1 Considerations prior to prescribing nutraceuticals for pediatric headache—Cont'd

Nutraceutical	Laboratory Data[96]	Sources[96]	Adverse effects reported in pediatric headache trials	Other possible adverse effects[96]
Omega 3	Omega-3 Index (% in RBC)[a] Omega Check[a] Omega-3 and -6, plasma[a]	Salmon, fatty fish	None reported[29]	Unpleasant taste, bad breath, heartburn, nausea, gastrointestinal discomfort, diarrhea, headache, odoriferous sweat May decrease immune response at high doses Antiplatelet effects are possible with high doses Medication interactions: Anticoagulants
Probiotics	None[a]	Yogurt, kimchi, kombucha, sauerkraut, miso, pickles, apple cider vinegar, and other fermented foods	N/A	Flatulence Some strains (unlikely lactobacillus or bifidobacterium) may increase opportunistic infection (review strain/ indication especially immunocompromised individuals)
Vitamin C	Vitamin C, plasma	Citrus fruits, broccoli, strawberries, Brussel sprouts, tomato, melon, cabbage, cauliflower	N/A	GI upset (diarrhea, nausea, abdominal cramps) Conflicting evidence for increasing risk for kidney stones, cardiovascular mortality, cancer under certain conditions, B12/copper deficiency, erosion of enamel, or allergic responses Medication interactions: Chemotherapy, statins

Table 1 Considerations prior to prescribing nutraceuticals for pediatric headache—Cont'd

Nutraceutical	Laboratory Data[96]	Sources[96]	Adverse effects reported in pediatric headache trials	Other possible adverse effects[96]
Vitamin E	Vitamin E (alpha-tocopherol), plasma	Wheat germ oil, sunflower seeds, almonds, sunflower oil, safflower oil, hazelnuts	N/A	Antiplatelet at high doses, hemorrhagic effects Increased risk of prostate cancer unclear Increased morality risk unclear with >150 iu in combination with other supplements Medication Interactions: anticoagulants, antiplatelets, chemotherapy, statins
Feverfew Tenacetum Partheniunim	None	N/A	N/A	Nausea, bloating, digestive problems Withdrawal (pain, anxiety, insomnia) Avoid in pregnancy (uterine contractions) Avoid if tree allergies
Butterbur Petasites (Petadolex)	Liver function tests	N/A	GI upset, bitter taste, dermal/allergic, dizziness, fatigue, pain, asthma flares (similar to placebo)[66] Burping (4), nausea (1), abdominal pain (1)[65]	Transaminitis Belching, headache, itchy eyes, diarrhea, breathing difficulties, fatigue, upset stomach, and drowsiness. Avoid in pregnancy Avoid if plant allergies (ragweed, chrysanthemums, marigolds, and daisies)
Capsaicin	None	Chili peppers (powders, sauces, etc.)	N/A	Burning[67, 69] and rhinorrhea with nasal formulation[67, 68] Heat, ache, itching, dislike of odor[71]

Continued

Table 1 Considerations prior to prescribing nutraceuticals for pediatric headache—Cont'd

Nutraceutical	Laboratory Data[96]	Sources[96]	Adverse effects reported in pediatric headache trials	Other possible adverse effects[96]
Lavender	None	Herb source (used in drinks or cooking), lavender tea or water	N/A	Gynecomastia (dose-dependent) Contact dermatitis
Peppermint	None	Herb source (used in drinks or cooking), peppermint tea or water	N/A	Allergic reactions Heartburn (avoid in patients with reflux) Expected burning sensation (use in small amounts)
Marijuana (THC, CBD, terpenes, flavonoids, other compounds)	Liver function tests	THC, CBD - Hempseeds, hempseed oil Terpenes— wide variety of herbs (cooking and medicinal), spices, fruits, vegetables, hops Flavenoids— many fruits and vegetables[90]	N/A	Avoid in pregnancy (low birth weight) Increased risk for motor vehicle accidents and other injuries Craving, withdrawal, lack of control, negative impact on work/family responsibilities Orthostatic hypotension, worsening psychiatric symptoms Lung injuries when smoked CBD only—diarrhea, fatigue, transaminitis[102]

[a]May only be available through specialty labs.
[b]Obtaining Serum Coq10/cholesterol ratio may be preferred because coq10 levels may be artificially increased due to cholesterol (19,20).

Offer an individualized approach

Coexisting symptoms, medications, diet, and lifestyle should be assessed and considered. Like pharmaceutical agents, there are secondary benefits with select nutraceuticals. Certain medications, dietary habits, lifestyle, or genetic mutations may predispose one to a deficiency. While laboratory data exists for many of these endogenous therapies, they should be ordered and interpreted with caution given the variabilities (biologic and analytic), potential for recent dietary influences and costs associated with serial testing. Patients should be directed to avoid taking supplements or making changes in diet for one week prior to lab testing. If labs are inconsistent or unavailable, it is reasonable to rely on clinical responsiveness.

Quality

If prescription grade supplements are unavailable, nutraceuticals labels should be assessed for disclosure statements in addition to seals or notations representing degrees of voluntary paid regulation by third parties (e.g., National Nutritional Foods Association (NNFA)) GMP confirms the facility complies with manufacturing procedures. NNFA TruLabel certifies product quantity and freedom from contaminants. NSF International and U.S. Pharmacopeia (USP) seals verify good manufacturing practices in addition to accuracy of contents, quantity, and freedom of contaminants. Consumer Labs (CL) further assesses products for bioavailability. Labdoor adds a quality score considering safety and efficacy data. Some companies attest to internal product testing.

Dose and duration

Dosing should be guided by age, weight, patient history, safety, and efficacy data (see Table 2). Weekly titrations may prevent adverse effects. As with pharmaceuticals, benefits from nutraceuticals may not be achieved for three months or longer. The long-term use of nutraceuticals should be avoided due to lack of long-term safety data. Consider switching to dietary sources when available by encouraging a diverse diet in whole foods.

Medication interactions

Studies identifying supplements-drug interactions are limited, although several interactions (inhibitory and synergistic) have been identified.[112] To assess supplement-drug interactions or pre-operative risks, consider using a drug interaction checker tool. If the supplement is not found, interaction information may be found using a Pubmed database searches (herb-drug or herb-herb).

Surgical clearance

Consider advising patients to withhold supplements one week prior to any surgical procedure given unknown risks and potential for hematologic interactions.

Provider references and patient education

Other sources of information on supplements for providers and patients include: The National Institutes of Health, Dietary Supplement Fact Sheets, herbal monographs (The American Herbal Pharmacopeia, The American Botanical Counsel German Commission E Monographs, The European Union's European Medicines Agency, Health Canada), or institutional fact sheets: Mayo Clinic, Memorial Sloan Kettering Cancer Center.

Table 2 How to prescribe nutraceuticals for pediatric headache.

Nutraceutical	Formulations/sources	Dosing (Children <12yo)	Adult dosing	Prescribing notes
Magnesium (Mg) Salt	Tablets, capsule, or powder Oxide,[23] pidolate,[24, 25] Citrate, Trimagnesium dicitrate, 2-propylvalerate, aspartate, sulfate[22] Others: Malate, Gluconate, Taurate, Glycinate, etc.	9mg/kg/day (bid)[23]	102–800mg (divided 1–3 times daily)[22]	Titrate as tolerated Oxide used to treat constipation, inexpensive Citrate is better absorbed, inexpensive Glycinate if diarrhea Chelated forms better tolerated Adults may tolerate up to 400mg tid
CoQ10 (Ubiquinol, Ubiquinone)	Liquid gel capsules 100mg chewable tablets 100mg liquid melt, liquid	1–3mg/kg/day[19] 100mg/day[20]	100–400mg/day[18]	Liquid best absorbed Frequent dosing may be more effective
Vitamin D	Ergocalciferol (vitamin D2) or Cholecalciferol (vitamin D3) 50,000IU capsule (prescription) Tablet, capsule, liquid, or dissolvable (400, 1000, 2000, 5000 and 10,000)	400–5000IU/day[34]	50,000IU weekly for 12weeks or 800–5000IU daily[32]	Consider maintenance dosing once deficiency corrected vitamin D3 may be better absorbed
Melatonin	Tablet, capsules, liquid, or dissolvable (0.3, 0.5, 1, 3, 5mg), immediate or extended release	0.3mg/kg, (up to 6mg)[103]	3–10mg HS[104]	Lower doses may be more effective for insomnia Higher doses may be more effective for anxiety Take 1–2h HS

Riboflavin (B2)	Tablet or capsule (25, 50, 100, 200, or 400mg)	200–400mg/day[7,10]	400mg daily[105]	Water soluble, split dose Take with food
B6	Tablet (sublingual, chewable), capsule, liquid dissolvable	N/A	80mg daily[106]	Water soluble, split dose Take with food
B12 plus B6 plus folic acid	Tablet or capsule	N/A 5mg/day[46]	400 μg (B12), 25mg (B6), 2mg/day (folic acid)[47]	Take with food
Folic acid	Tablet or capsule		2mg/day[47]	
Omega 3	Capsules, liquid	1–2g/day[29]	1–6g/day[28]	Confirm Omega 3 contains both eicosapentaenoic acid (EPA) +docosahexaenoic acid (DHA)
Probiotics	Capsules, powders, liquids	N/A	2×10^9 CFU/day[54]	CFU count should be listed as by expiration date vs time of packaging Contains prebiotics (inulin and other fructo-oligosaccharides)
Vitamin E	Tablets, capsules	N/A	400–500 iu/day[53,107]	Take with food
N-acetylcysteine +Vitamin E +Vitamin C	Capsules	N/A	NEC (NAc 600mg) bid Vitamin E 250 iu bid Vitamin C 500mg bid[53]	Take with food
Feverfew *Tenacetum Partheniunim*	Capsules, liquid extract	N/A	6.25mg tid[108]	CO2 stabilized formula Monitor for allergic reaction
Butterbur *Petasites*	Petadolex 25mg capsules	25–75mg bid[65,66]	50–75mg bid[109,110]	Needs to be PA free Monitor for allergic reaction

Continued

Table 2 How to prescribe nutraceuticals for pediatric headache—Cont'd

Nutraceutical	Formulations/sources	Dosing (Children <12yo)	Adult dosing	Prescribing notes
Capcaisin	Intranasal, topical	N/A	Intranasal 300µL/100µL suspension daily via pipette in one or both nostrils for 5–7 days or as tolerated[67, 68, 70] or 100µL of a 10^{-2}M solution 3% camphor in 0.025% applied via cotton tip one-half inch up the nostril ipsilateral to headache bid for 7 days[69] Topical 1 g tid (0.05%)[111] or 0.05–0.10mL 0.1% to each temporal artery for 30min[71]	N/A
Lavender	Liquid, capsules, aromatherapy, topical	N/A	PO 10 drops of extract into water (1 mL from 100 g dried plant in ethanol/water 80/20) nightly[81] Aromatherapy 15min at onset of headache[80]	If PO, use ingestible grade essential oil Monitor for allergic reaction Oral was standardized linalyl acetate (0.6%) and linalool (0.4%)[81]
Peppermint Menthol (33%–60% peppermint)	Liquid, capsules, aromatherapy, topical	N/A	Apply 1 mL of topical solution (peppermint or menthol 10% in ethanol preparation) to forehead/temples for 3min at onset, 15min, 30min[74, 77]	If PO, use ingestible grade essential oil Monitor for allergic reaction

bid, twice daily; tid, three times daily; PO, by mouth; HS, before bedtime; N/A, not available.

Manual therapies
What patients and families need to know?

As a patient or caregiver, nonpharmacological treatment options are appealing given the side-effects that are associated with pharmaceuticals. When choosing a manual therapy, it is recommended to consider the type of the practitioner and the cost. If working with chiropractors, it is important to request to avoid any high-velocity manipulations of the cervical spine until more evidence for safety in pediatric populations is available. Chiropractors, physical therapists, and osteopaths use a variety of techniques that are not cervical manipulations such as cervical mobilizations, massage, and stretching techniques that may be useful for headache. These techniques are safe and may be helpful for treating neck pain tension, and headaches. It is best to work with your primary care provider or headache specialist for a recommendation and referral to a trusted practitioner. Insurance companies may cover the cost of these treatments, but is entirely dependent on your coverage with your insurance carrier.

What a PCP and headache specialist needs to know
What are manual therapies?

Manual therapies include five distinct techniques that are used in combination or isolation. These include (1) manipulation, (2) mobilization, (3) massage, (4) stretching, and (5) muscle energy techniques. While professionals and the literature may use manipulation and mobilization interchangeably, here forth, manipulation will refer to methods using high-velocity low-amplitude thrust and mobilization to techniques without thrust that are low-velocity and low-amplitude. Stretching includes static and dynamic stretching, the former is holding a joint position at maximal range of motion for no longer than 60 s in general, and the latter is moving a joint in its full range of motion repetitively but not holding longer than a few seconds. Muscle energy techniques, although a form of stretching, is generally considered separately, as stretching can be taught to the individual and self-performed, in contrast to muscle energy technique needs a practitioner coaching and manually helping the individual stretch using contraction/relaxation method. These five techniques are used by a variety of health care professionals, including doctors of medicine and osteopathy, chiropractors, massage therapists, and physical therapists.

Manual therapies are commonly sought out by individuals who have recurrent headaches.[3,113-115] The body of literature for manual therapies is heterogeneous (for both modality and diagnosis), sparse, and observational in nature. Furthermore, it is difficult to correlate studies where a single technique is used in isolation to how individuals are treated in practice where multiple techniques may be used in a single session. Despite the growing number of children and adolescents accessing these therapies,[116] it is clear that the evidence for evaluating the effectiveness of treatment for pediatric headache is trailing behind.

Most manual therapies center on treatment of the neck and the associated musculoskeletal dysfunctions seen in individuals with headaches. Patients with migraine and tension-type headache commonly experience neck pain[117] and seek treatment for this neck pain.[118] More importantly, neck pain plays a role in the pathophysiology of migraine and tension-type headache.[119] Specifically, the convergence of C1–3 nerve roots and the first division of the trigeminal nerve onto the trigeminal cervical complex may give rise to the connection between neck pain and migraine[119] (Fig. 1). Patients with recurrent headaches also exhibit decreased range of motion in their neck, myofascial tenderness, cervical, and trapezius tension, as well as a forward head posture.[120–125] Commonly we see a forward head posture that can be quantified by the angle at C7 with a line horizontal from C7 and the other line through the tragus of the ear (Fig. 2) using a goniometer to help follow this angle overtime. Manual therapies work on these symptoms to try to relieve neck pain, improve posture, or alleviate headaches themselves.

This section will discuss what each of the manual methods, the potential side-effects or adverse events associated with these therapies, and the evidence, if any is available for its effectiveness in pediatrics.

Manipulation

Manipulation is a high-velocity low-amplitude thrust[126] most commonly provided by chiropractors, but also by physical therapists and osteopaths. Manipulations can be for any region along the spine, but also for other joints in the body. Individuals may have reoccurring headaches because of malalignment of their cervical spine, posture, or muscular tension in their cervical and upper thoracic regions.[120–125] Manipulations for headache are focused on malalignment of the cervical spine and improved range of motion.

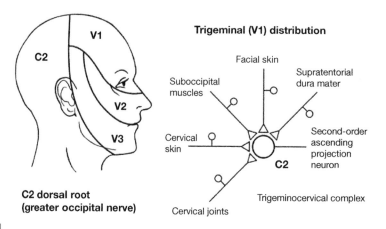

FIG. 1

Confluence of cervical nerve roots, trigeminal nerve (V1) onto the Trigeminocervical complex.
Adapted from Bartsch T, Goadsby PJ. The trigeminocervical complex and migraine: Current concepts and synthesis. Curr Pain Headache Rep. 2003;7(5):371-376. doi:https:/doi.org/10.1007/s11916-003-0036-y.

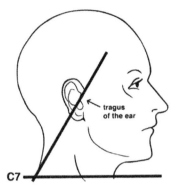

FIG. 2

Assessment of a forward head posture quantified by the angle created at C7 with one line horizontal from C7 and the other line through the tragus of the ear.

There are no pediatric RCTs using manipulations as a treatment for pediatric migraine. In a single pediatric study, 52 children with suspected cervicogenic headache were randomized to either spinal manipulation or an active control where children received light touch with a manipulation to a different region thought not to be contributing to the child's pain. Both groups showed improved headache days and no significant differences between groups.[127] There are a few more studies evaluating the role of manipulation for adults with recurrent headaches. In one adult based study, spinal manipulation led to reduced migraine days and pain/intensity.[128] In another study, spinal manipulation was as effective as amitriptyline for the treatment of adults with migraines.[129] Spinal manipulation has been effective in reducing pain in cervicogenic and tension type headaches in adults as well.[130–134]

Of all the manual based treatments, manipulations may have the highest risk of serious adverse events resulting it to be rarely recommended by pediatricians, neurologists, and headache specialists alike. In a systematic review of adverse events associated with pediatric spinal manipulation, nine serious adverse events were reported in observational studies and case reports including permanent disability or death.[135] In a clinical trial with 171 children receiving spinal manipulation for treatment of enuresis, authors reported two moderate adverse events: severe headache and stiff neck which improved over two weeks, and a second case of transient acute lumbar pain.[136] In a feasibility study, nine children received spinal manipulation for treatment of chronic otitis with effusion, with two minor adverse events reported: transient mid back soreness and transient irritability.[137] A randomized clinical trial of 9–15 years old children receiving spinal manipulation for back or neck pain reported no adverse events after spinal manipulation in 123 children.[138]

At this time, given the limited evidence of cervical spinal manipulation for treatment of pediatric headache, it is recommended that cervical spinal manipulation be avoided in pediatric populations until safety can be determined in large prospective pediatric cohorts.

Mobilization

Mobilization is a gentle low-velocity and low-amplitude adjustments that are used by chiropractors, physical therapists, and osteopaths. The theory for use in headache is similar to manipulations. Mobilizations are generally safe in children and adolescents and no studies have reported harm from cervical or full spinal mobilization.[139] There are no current studies published on the effects of mobilization technique used in isolation in either adult or pediatric headache cohorts.

Typically in practice manual therapists such as chiropractors, physical therapists, and osteopaths, combine other manual therapies, especially manipulations, with mobilizations. There are a few low quality RCTs that evaluate this combination of manipulations with mobilizations in the treatment adult headache. A study in cervicogenic headaches, showed no differences between spinal manual therapies (manipulation and mobilization) compared to an exercise group, and a control group with no treatment at all.[140] In another study, patients with tension type headache received massage and then randomly assigned to either manipulation or mobilization. Both groups showed improvement from baseline.[141] Lastly, a small RCT with 10 individuals with post-traumatic headache receiving a combination of manipulation, muscle energy technique, and mobilization and 9 control subjects receiving cold pack treatment, showed both groups improving but no differences between groups at follow up.[142]

In summary, spinal mobilizations are gentle and safe,[139] however the efficacy of them for treatment of pediatric headache is not established.

Massage

Massage includes a variety of techniques including deep tissue, Swedish, and myofascial trigger points or release. Each provides a manual pressure or manipulation of the soft tissue to improve aches and pains. The mechanism of action for massage is multilevel including physical relaxation, stress relief, and mental relaxation, and increasing circulating endorphins.[143] Other mechanisms may include gate-control theory and balance towards parasympathetic state.[144] Massage generally has minimal side-effects and is tolerated well.[145,146] Despite its wide use for headache,[4,147] no randomized controlled studies exist for pediatric headache. One pilot study of 9 girls with tension type headache receiving myofascial trigger showed improvement in headache frequency, intensity, and duration.[145] Massage in adults suffering from headaches may be effective,[148] with small studies with favorable results in migraine[149] and tension type headache.[150,151]

In summary, massage is safe and tolerated well, however there are virtually no studies evaluating the efficacy of massage for pediatric headache, but its use in adults with headaches is promising.

Static and dynamic stretching

Static stretching is taking the joint to the maximal point in its range of motion and holding for a period of time usually less than 1 min. Dynamic stretching which involves controlled movement through the active range of motion of a joint.

Individuals with reoccurring headaches and specifically cervicogenic headache may suffer from significant cervical and trapezius tension and decreased range of motion and cervical tension.[121,152] Cervical and upper body stretches can easily be taught to most children and adolescents to be implemented at home. These stretches are generally safe without adverse effects.[153] There are no pediatric studies showing effectiveness of stretching for treatment of headache. In adults with recurrent headache, stretching has favorable studies in the treatment of migraines, tension type headache, and cervicogenic headaches.[154–156]

In summary, stretching is safe and well tolerated in pediatric populations, it lends itself for a cost-effective treatment that can be taught to the child. Efficacy of stretching in pediatrics is unknown for headaches, however favorable in adults.

Muscle energy technique (MET)

MET a technique where the patient is an active participant with the therapist to stretch the muscle by using series of isometric contraction and then relaxation exercises to stretch the muscle. In this technique the muscle is using its own energy and golgi tendon organ. These can be applied carefully by the provider on the levator scapula and trapezius muscles to assist individuals with cervical range of motion and pain.[157,158] Muscle energy technique is generally safe.[159] There are no pediatric or adults studies evaluating the effectiveness of MET for treatment of headache.

Acupuncture

What patients and families need to know

What is traditional Chinese medicine and how is it related to acupuncture?
Traditional Chinese Medicine (CM) is an ancient healing art, which takes into consideration the whole individual (mind, body, and spirit) when looking at a disease process and the symptoms. Chinese Medicine is based entirely on the laws of nature and principles of creating balance in the body, mind, and spirit (which in CM are interconnected and mutually inform one another. Therefore, the health of the body impacts the health of the mind, and vice versa).

CM works directly with the "qi" of an individual to assess and treat symptoms. Qi is most easily translated as "life force" or "energy." The dictionary gives many meanings, including "air," "gas," and "vapor." To the early Chinese naturalists, this term seemed to bear some resemblance to what we now call "matter-energy," corresponding to the pneuma of the ancient Greeks and the prana of the ancient Hindus." (Peng Yoke Ho, *Li, Qi and Shu*, 2002, p. 3).

> "There must be some primal force, but it is impossible to locate. I believe it exists, but cannot see it. I see its results, I can even feel it, but it has no form." (Zhuang Zi, Inner Chapters, Fourth Century B.C.E.)

Qi flows through the body via the meridians. Through a Chinese Medicine lens, we assess the health of the qi to determine the state of the meridian systems, to identify pathology, and ultimately support qi by using acupuncture points that fall along the meridian systems.

When acupuncturists are assessing an individual's symptoms, they are looking for patterns of dis-harmony in the mind/body/spirit and using the points on the meridians to rectify the imbalance(s). Each meridian system relates to the metaphysical function of the organ systems. There are 12 primary meridians: heart, small intestine, bladder, kidney, pericardium, Triple heater (not recognized as an actual organ or system in western medicine), gall bladder, liver, lung, large intestine, spleen, and stomach. Each system has acupoints that lie along the meridians, where the energy of that system can be accessed using acupuncture needles or body work.

Each acupuncture point also has a *geographical region of influence* based on where it is located on the body (qi follows structure), as well as a *point function* in terms of what a particular acupuncture point's job is. For example, Spleen 10 (SP 10) is a great point to use to support medial knee pain because of where its located *(geographical influence),* as well as a great point to invigorate blood and qi, which can help with digestive issues, head pain, sleep problems, or feelings of sluggishness *(point function).*

In addition to acupuncture, CM practitioners use a variety of modalities to help move or sedate excess qi, tonify deficient qi, and warm stuck qi to assist the body/mind/spirit in finding a more homeostatic place and reduce symptoms. A short list of modalities under the Chinese Medicine umbrella include: tuina (a form of body work which uses massage techniques along the primary meridian systems and muscle bodies),[160] moxibustion (burning of the dried herb mugwort, directly with removal or indirectly on a needle on an acupuncture point or region of the body), cupping and guasha, Chinese Herbal medicine, and dietetic/nutrition therapies, and lifestyle coaching (integration of intentional movement and shifting unhealthy habits).

How to find an acupuncture practitioner?

Most states regulate the practice of acupuncture. Acupuncturists should have no less than a Master's Degree in Chinese Medicine (3 year program) from an accredited school or university. Some states require completion of the national board exam along with a master's degree to practice acupuncture. With this training, practitioners should have a solid understanding of anatomy and physiology, point location, Chinese Medical theory (which is considered a whole system of science), as well as the energetics of each meridian system. Medical Doctors can take a certificate course, however there is little emphasis on CM theory in these courses and they are more prescriptive and standardized in nature.

Working with a medical provider for a referral to an acupuncturist is likely the best place to start. If your physician does not have a recommendation, a simple internet search can be performed, keeping in mind that anyone to be considered should meet the minimum education requirements. If there is an accredited complementary medicine institution or university nearby, you may also contact the school for a list of graduates.

What to expect from an acupuncture treatment?

Receiving acupuncture is a very individualized experience. People tend to report a wide range of feelings or observations while receiving treatment, and most commonly report a feeling of deep relaxation or a "tired" feeling. As a way to empower the patient to build body awareness, practitioners work with the patient and their families to identify primary concerns prior to treatment. Assessments will include pain scale and range of motion, especially if the neck is stiff or a back or shoulders are tight or tender. Actively working with the child and integrating them in the treatment experience, will help young people notice changes in their head pain, and improvements, even if subtle.

Often patients will report noticing a positive impact on their symptoms after one session, however, it is more common for the reduction or resolution of pain to take place over a number of treatments. We recommend patients come more frequently when treatment first starts at no less than $1 \times$ a week for about 4–6 weeks. Then individuals can space out treatment over time and eventually reach a maintenance phase, where their visits are more frequent during periods of recurrence and less frequent when symptoms are stable or improved. Patience is key here because often families are desperate and anxious to help their child feel better so setting realistic expectations at the outset is crucial.

Sometimes people are surprised by the placement of pins. In conventional medicine we target the symptoms with a linear intervention (for example, "my head hurts, I will take medicine to stop the head from hurting"). Here acupuncturists not only insert pins "where it hurts" but insert pins in other areas. Many of the points which help reduce head pain happen to lie on the bottom half of the body. By using these points with some frequency, acupuncturists see a positive impact on headache symptoms. It should also be noted that since Chinese Medicine is a whole system modality, a youngster may observe the resolution or reduction of symptoms other than the headache for which they are seeking treatment.

Often children and adolescents with headaches also have sleep pathology, anxiety, and digestive issues. With the use of acupuncture, as well as some nutritional counseling and lifestyle coaching, acupuncturist can shift the overall symptoms, and sometimes even the resolution of a secondary or tertiary concern before the headaches resolve. Practically, when using CM to treat an individual, practitioners, and families need to understand the interconnectedness of the mind/body/spirit. Practitioners will evaluate for these comorbidities, evaluate activity level (distinguishing between being incredibly active and engaged with little downtime from academics or sport, or being very sedentary, lacking intentional movement, and drive in their life), hydration, and sleep. With CM, practitioners are looking at patterns of excess and deficiency to help maintain a level of balance. Practitioners will commonly include lifestyle coaching and nutrition, including a try elimination of refined sugars, dairy, or gluten.

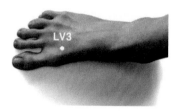

FIG. 3

Liver point 3.

Are there any acupressure points I can try at home?
Liver 3 (LV3): Supreme rushing

This point is frequently used by practitioners because it is multifaceted, easy to access (dorsal side of the foot, in the depression between first and second metatarsal, just distal the junction of the two bones) (Fig. 3), and can have a powerful impact. LV3 has a profoundly calming effect on the mind and regulates the smooth flow of qi (headaches are often a result of stuck qi, or stasis, rebellions qi- qi moving too fast in the correct direction or moving entirely in the wrong direction—for a headache the qi rises and cannot descend). Young women with headaches will often observe their headaches may have something to do with their menstrual cycle, and this point also has a powerful effect on gynecological health and the reproductive system. With this point, one can support smoother flow of qi, invigorate, and move stagnant blood and qi (as well as offer support for a painful period for young girls), and promote a sense of calm in the mind/body/spirit. Acupuncturists will affectionately call LV3 "Happy Calm" because of its relaxant affect, and we know living with pain causes a level of agitation that could be greatly benefited by easing the body/ mind/spirit.

GV20, Governor Vessel 20: Assembly of ancestors

This point is actually on the head. It lies on the midline of the scalp, several inches posterior to the hairline, in a depression that can be found by drawing an invisible line from the apex of each ear and meeting at the top of the head (Fig. 4). This point is a great one to show patients how to self-administer acupressure because it is so easy to find. GV 20 is particularly helpful for headaches that tend to reside at the top of the head as well as headaches that lie behind the eyes. This point is often selected for the person that carries a lot of stress in the top region of their body, presents with head pain and also may present with a level of lack of "get up and go", as this point can release excess qi to the exterior but it also helps invigorate sinking or prolapsed qi.

In summary, acupuncture has been used for treating headaches for many centuries. In the hands of a skilled practitioner it can be an excellent treatment either alone or in conjunction with traditional medicine. Developing a treatment plan that involves the patient, family and other practitioners produces the best outcome.

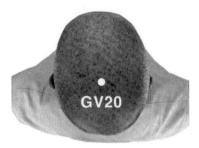

FIG. 4

Governing Vessel 3.

What a PCP and headache specialist needs to know

What is acupuncture?

Acupuncture is a practice originally from China (dating to 1800 BCE) where specific meridian points are stimulated with the placement of fine hypodermic needles. Electric currents, point pressure, and heat may also be applied to these points for similar effects.

Acupuncture relies on the knowledge of several Chinese medicine principles of Yin and Yang, Qi (Life Force or Energy), 5 elements (fire, water, earth, wood, and metal) and their phases, meridian channels, and specific acupoints. In general, according to Chinese medicine, disease arises from imbalances in these systems and blockages present in meridian channels. Acupuncture alleviates these blockages and works to restore balance in these systems.

Is acupuncture safe?

Acupuncture delivered to children and adolescents is safe and well-tolerated, as long as it is performed with sterile needles.[161–165] A systematic review in 2011 found a majority of adverse events associated with acupuncture were mild and found acupuncture safe when performed by appropriately trained practitioners.[164] Individuals may experience pain, bruising, bleeding, and worsening of symptoms.[164] This systematic review also reported rare serious adverse events including five cases of infections and single cases of each of the following: cardiac rupture, pneumothorax, nerve impairment, subarachnoid hemorrhage, intestinal obstruction, hemoptysis, reversible coma, and overnight hospitalization.[164] Children and adolescents tolerate the use of acupuncture needles,[166] however if they have a needle phobia, other forms of acustimulation can occur with the use of electrical or laser stimulation, as well as acupressure.

Certified practitioners of acupuncture hold a minimum of a Master's Degree with some variability in training. Practitioners of Traditional Chinese Medicine (TCM) often use a variety of other treatments in addition to acupuncture which may include: herbal remedies, moxibustion (dried herbs burned above skin), or cupping (heated cups creating suction on skin), dietary changes. It is important to encourage patients to disclose their treatment plan or develop a relationship with a trusted practitioner with whom care can be coordinated. While most TCM practices are likely safe, combination herbal remedies are commonly used with side effect and interaction potentials. It is also important to consider the impact treatment with complementary practitioners have on the patient and family's perception of the condition, psychological wellness, financial stressors, time constraints interfering with school work or social events, and relationships with conventional providers (e.g., trust in allopathic medicine if an emergency arises). These factors further support the need for integrative approaches and open communication between providers and between providers, patients, and their families.

Is acupuncture helpful for headaches?

The majority of studies evaluating the efficacy of acupuncture treatment for headache are in adult populations. Gottschling and colleagues showed in 43 children receiving either placebo or laser acupuncture with headache with decreased frequency, duration, and severity of headaches.[167]

A multicenter single-blinded RCT conducted by Wang et al. (2012) examined the use of acupuncture for acute treatment of migraines in adults. The trial included 140 subjects, 72 in the "true" acupuncture group and 68 in the sham acupuncture group. Treatments were administered for 30 min during acute migraine. Response was then assessed at 24, 48, and 72 h post treatment. Pain and migraine related symptoms improved in both groups. Treatment using "true" acupuncture resulted in less acute medication usage and slightly better pain relief.[168]

Efficiency for acupuncture as episodic migraine prophylaxis in adults was examined in an updated Cochrane Review by Linde and colleagues[169] including 22 trials (4985 participants). Comparator groups included no-treatment group (5 trials), sham acupuncture (15 trials), and prophylactic pharmaceutical controls (5 trials). In all analyses, acupuncture was superior to controls. When compared to sham acupuncture, there was a statistically significant, albeit small, reduction in headache frequency.[169]

Another updated Cochrane Review conducted by Linde and colleagues[170] examined the use of acupuncture for both episodic and chronic tension type headache (TTH) with twelve trials (2349 participants). There were two trials reporting short-term benefits (decreased pain intensity, number headache days) from acupuncture compared to routine care without examining long term effects. Five trials found small improvements in true acupuncture versus sham acupuncture. Altogether, the meta-analysis suggest that acupuncture is an effective treatment for episodic and chronic tension headaches.[170]

While benefits from acupuncture in headache management appear promising, authors caution effect size estimates are crude given heterogeneity.[171,172] Colquhoun and Novella[173] provided broader interpretations of the acupuncture literature identifying significant limitations due to heterogeneity of design and treatment (electroacupuncture, laser), inability to blind, publication bias, and minimal effect sizes with large placebo effect.

One of the challenges researchers face is that the treatment provided in nonresearch setting by an acupuncturist is typically highly individualized. Treatments are often adapted during a session to meet the needs or symptoms of the individual (e.g., insomnia is identified in addition to headache). Depending on the acupuncturist's training and practice style, the sites selected and complementary modalities used will vary unlike in a research setting where they remain consistent.

How does Acupuncture work to help headache?

The mechanism of action for true acupuncture, sham acupuncture, acupressure, electroacupuncture, and laser acupuncture is largely unknown. Some forms of acupuncture may produce analgesia using the following: (1) the HPA axis and endogenous opioid system, (2) the gate control theory (hyperstimulation analgesia via myofascial trigger points), (3) noxious inhibitory control.[168]

Acupuncture may provide a session of relaxation similar to those used in biofeedback (e.g., progressive muscle relaxation, deep breathing, mindfulness, etc.) and is typically conducted in a relaxing environment with music. It also provides patients a sense of control of their self-care with less concern for adverse effects and creates space for processing thoughts, fostering gratitude, self-compassion, etc. These variables may account for insufficient findings when comparing acupuncture to relaxation practices for headache.[171,172]

A meta-analysis of studies using fMRI to study brain activity during an acupuncture session identified activity present in following regions: "sensorimotor cortical network, including the insula, thalamus, anterior cingulate cortex, and primary and secondary somatosensory cortices, and deactivation in the limbic-paralimbic neocortical network, including the medial prefrontal cortex, caudate, amygdala, posterior cingulate cortex, and parahippocampus."[174] Studies examining fMRI results using a phantom limb (e.g., rubber) to administer acupuncture found similar brain activity[175,176] suggesting a mind–body placebo effect accounts for the activity observed in the brain during acupuncture treatment.

Placebo

Placebo, a complex response involving neurobiological and neuropsychological mechanisms,[177] is thought to be higher amongst pediatric patients with headaches.[8] Prescribing placebo is a long standing ethical controversy largely due to the misconception that patients need to be deceived for the treatment to work. Some studies suggest placebo may still be elicited in both pediatric patients and patients with migraine when the placebo mechanism is disclosed, negating the need for deception.[178,179] Since prophylactic medications carry the risk of adverse effects and do not outcompete placebo in pediatric headache,[5] acupuncture may be seen as a more benign placebo prescription for some individuals.

Eliciting placebo via "true" or "sham" points via needles, electrical stimulation, laser stimulation, or acupressure may be most effective when patients report benefits from acupuncture in the past or enthusiastically express interest in the modality. If

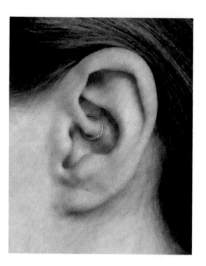

FIG. 5

Daith piercing involving the inner most cartilage fold in the ear, located at the crus of the helix.

prescribing acupuncture, consider also presenting placebo as a validated approach comprised of complicated neurobiological and neuropsychological effects, with efficacy comparable to medications and fewer adverse effects reported. Behavioral therapies, manual therapies, devices, and nutraceuticals could be considered first when reviewing nonmedication treatments since they are arguably less invasive.

Daith piercing

It is pertinent to mention daith piercing, which has gained popularity over the last decade for treatment of recurrent headaches and migraines. Daith piercing involves the bilateral ear piercing, at the crus of the helix (Fig. 5). Although mechanism or efficacy has not been studied, daith piercing involves similar areas used for auricular acupuncture and may have overlapping mechanism. Additionally, of note, the sensory innervation of the helix is supplied both the trigeminal and vagal nerves and may activate the vagal pathways.[180] At this time, more research is needed to make conclusions on the benefits or mechanism for daith piercing.

References

1. U.S. Food and Drug Adminstration. What you Need to Know About Dietary Supplements, (n.d.).
2. Kristoffersen ES, Aaseth K, Grande RB, Lundqvist C, Russell MB. Self-reported efficacy of complementary and alternative medicine: the Akershus study of chronic headache. *J Headache Pain.* 2013;14(1):1–5. https://doi.org/10.1186/1129-2377-14-36.
3. Gaul C, Eismann R, Schmidt T, et al. Use of complementary and alternative medicine in patients suffering from primary headache disorders. *Cephalalgia.* 2009;29(10):1069–1078. https://doi.org/10.1111/j.1468-2982.2009.01841.x.

4. Dalla Libera D, Colombo B, Pavan G, Comi G. Complementary and alternative medicine (CAM) use in an Italian cohort of pediatric headache patients: the tip of the iceberg. *Neurol Sci.* 2014;35(Suppl 1):145–148. https://doi.org/10.1007/s10072-014-1756-y.

5. Oskoui M, Pringsheim T, Billinghurst L, et al. Practice guideline update summary: pharmacologic treatment for pediatric migraine prevention: report of the guideline development, dissemination, and implementation Subcommittee of the American Academy of neurology and the American headache society. *Neurology.* 2019;93(11):500–509. https://doi.org/10.1212/WNL.0000000000008105.

6. Oskoui M, Pringsheim T, Holler-Managan Y, et al. Practice guideline update summary: acute treatment of migraine in children and adolescents: report of the guideline development, dissemination, and implementation Subcommittee of the American Academy of neurology and the American headache society. *Neurology.* 2019;93(11):487–499. https://doi.org/10.1212/WNL.0000000000008095.

7. MacLennan SC, Wade FM, Forrest KML, Ratanayake PD, Fagan E, Antony J. High-dose riboflavin for migraine prophylaxis in children: a double-blind, randomized, Placebo-Controlled Trial. *J Child Neurol.* 2008;23(11):1300–1304. https://doi.org/10.1177/0883073808318053.

8. Evers S, Marziniak M, Frese A, Gralow I. Placebo efficacy in childhood and adolescence migraine: an analysis of double-blind and placebo-controlled studies. *Cephalalgia.* 2009;29(4):436–444. https://doi.org/10.1111/j.1468-2982.2008.01752.x.

9. Holland S, Silberstein SD, Freitag F, Dodick DW, Argoff C, Ashman E. Evidence-based guideline update: NSAIDs and other complementary treatments for episodic migraine prevention in adults: report of the quality standards Subcommittee of the American Academy of neurology and the American headache society. *Neurology.* 2012;78(17):1346–1353. https://doi.org/10.1212/WNL.0b013e3182535d0c.

10. Condò M, Posar A, Arbizzani A, Parmeggiani A. Riboflavin prophylaxis in pediatric and adolescent migraine. *J Headache Pain.* 2009;10(5):361–365. https://doi.org/10.1007/s10194-009-0142-2.

11. Bruijn J, Duivenvoorden H, Passchier J, Locher H, Dijkstra N, Arts WF. Medium-dose riboflavin as a prophylactic agent in children with migraine: a preliminary placebo-controlled, randomised, double-blind, cross-over trial. *Cephalalgia Int J Headache.* 2010;30(12):1426–1434. https://doi.org/10.1177/0333102410365106.

12. Athaillah A, Dimyati Y, Saing JH, Saing B, Hakimi H, Lelo A. Riboflavin as migraine prophylaxis in adolescents. *Paediatr Indones.* 2012;52(3):132–137. https://doi.org/10.14238/pi52.3.2012.132-7.

13. Smithers G, Gregory JR, Bates CJ, Prentice A, Jackson LV, Wenlock R. The national diet and nutrition survey: young people aged 4–18 years. *Nutr Bull.* 2000;25(2):105–111. https://doi.org/10.1046/j.1467-3010.2000.00027.x.

14. Colombo B, Saraceno L, Comi G. Riboflavin and migraine: the bridge over troubled mitochondria. *Neurol Sci.* 2014;35(S1):141–144. https://doi.org/10.1007/s10072-014-1755-z.

15. Markley HG. CoEnzyme Q10 and riboflavin: the mitochondrial connection. *Headache.* 2012;52:81–87. https://doi.org/10.1111/j.1526-4610.2012.02233.x.

16. Taylor FR. Nutraceuticals and headache: the biological basis. *Headache J Head Face Pain.* 2011;51(3):484–501. https://doi.org/10.1111/j.1526-4610.2011.01847.x.

17. Steinert RE, Sadaghian Sadabad M, Harmsen HJM, Weber P. The prebiotic concept and human health: a changing landscape with riboflavin as a novel prebiotic candidate? *Eur J Clin Nutr.* 2016;70(12):1348–1353. https://doi.org/10.1038/ejcn.2016.119.

18. Zeng Z, Li Y, Lu S, Huang W, Di W. Efficacy of CoQ10 as supplementation for migraine: a meta-analysis. *Acta Neurol Scand.* 2019;139(3):284–293. https://doi.org/10.1111/ane.13051.

19. Hershey AD, Powers SW, Vockell AB, et al. Coenzyme Q10 deficiency and response to supplementation in pediatric and adolescent migraine. *Headache J Head Face Pain.* 2007;47(1):73–80. https://doi.org/10.1111/j.1526-4610.2007.00652.x.

20. Slater SK, Nelson TD, Kabbouche MA, et al. A randomized, double-blinded, placebo-controlled, crossover, add-on study of CoEnzyme Q10 in the prevention of pediatric and adolescent migraine. *Cephalalgia.* 2011;31(8):897–905. https://doi.org/10.1177/0333102411406755.

21. Doring F, Schmelzer C, Lindner I, Vock C, Fujii K. Functional connections and pathways of coenzyme Q10-inducible genes: an in-silico study. *IUBMB Life.* 2007;59(10):628–633. https://doi.org/10.1080/15216540701545991.

22. Chiu H-Y, Yeh T-H, Huang Y-C, Chen P-Y. Effects of intravenous and oral magnesium on reducing migraine: a meta-analysis of randomized controlled trials. *Pain Physician.* 2016;19(1):E97.

23. Wang F, Van Den Eeden SK, Ackerson LM, Salk SE, Reince RH, Elin RJ. Oral magnesium oxide prophylaxis of frequent migrainous headache in children: a randomized, double-blind, placebo-controlled trial. *Headache.* 2003;43(6):601–610. https://doi.org/10.1046/j.1526-4610.2003.03102.x.

24. Grazzi L, Andrasik F, Usai S, Bussone G. Magnesium as a treatment for paediatric tension-type headache: a clinical replication series. *Neurol Sci.* 2005;25(6):338–341. https://doi.org/10.1007/s10072-004-0367-4.

25. Grazzi L, Andrasik F, Usai S, Bussone G. Magnesium as a preventive treatment for paediatric episodic tension-type headache: results at 1-year follow-up. *Neurol Sci.* 2007;28(3):148–150. https://doi.org/10.1007/s10072-007-0808-y.

26. Gallelli L, Avenoso T, Falcone D, et al. Effects of acetaminophen and ibuprofen in children with migraine receiving preventive treatment with magnesium. *Headache J Head Face Pain.* 2014;54(2):313–324. https://doi.org/10.1111/head.12162.

27. Pradalier A, Bakouche P, Baudesson G, et al. Failure of omega-3 polyunsaturated fatty acids in prevention of migraine: a double-blind study versus placebo. *Cephalalgia.* 2001;21(8):818–822. https://doi.org/10.1046/j.1468-2982.2001.218240.x.

28. Maghsoumi-Norouzabad L, Mansoori A, Abed R, Shishehbor F. Effects of omega-3 fatty acids on the frequency, severity, and duration of migraine attacks: a systematic review and meta-analysis of randomized controlled trials. *Nutr Neurosci.* 2018;21(9):614–623. https://doi.org/10.1080/1028415X.2017.1344371.

29. Harel Z, Gascon G, Riggs S, Vaz R, Brown W, Exil G. Supplementation with omega-3 polyunsaturated fatty acids in the management of recurrent migraines in adolescents. *J Adolesc Health.* 2002;31(2):154–161. https://doi.org/10.1016/S1054-139X(02)00349-X.

30. Orr SL, Venkateswaran S. Nutraceuticals in the prophylaxis of pediatric migraine: evidence-based review and recommendations. *Cephalalgia.* 2014;34(8):568–583. https://doi.org/10.1177/0333102413519512.

31. Nowaczewska M, Wiciński M, Osiński S, Kázmierczak H. The role of vitamin D in primary headache–from potential mechanism to treatment. *Nutrients.* 2020;12(1):1–17. https://doi.org/10.3390/nu12010243.

32. Ghorbani Z, Togha M, Rafiee P, et al. Vitamin D in migraine headache: a comprehensive review on literature. *Neurol Sci*. 2019;40(12):2459–2477. https://doi.org/10.1007/s10072-019-04021-z.

33. Kılıç B, Kılıç M. Evaluation of vitamin D levels and response to therapy of childhood migraine. *Medicina*. 2019;55(7):1–9. https://doi.org/10.3390/medicina55070321.

34. Cayir A, Turan MI, Tan H. Effect of vitamin D therapy in addition to amitriptyline on migraine attacks in pediatric patients. *Braz J Med Biol Res*. 2014;47(4):349–354. https://doi.org/10.1590/1414-431x20143606.

35. Liampas I, Siokas V, Brotis A, Dardiotis E. Vitamin D serum levels in patients with migraine: a meta-analysis. *Rev Neurol (Paris)*. 2020. https://doi.org/10.1016/j.neurol.2019.12.008.

36. Liampas I, Siokas V, Brotis A, Vikelis M, Dardiotis E. Endogenous melatonin levels and therapeutic use of exogenous melatonin in migraine: systematic review and meta-analysis. *Headache*. 2020. https://doi.org/10.1111/head.13828.

37. Fallah R, Fazelishoroki F, Sekhavat L. A randomized clinical trial comparing the efficacy of melatonin and amitriptyline in migraine prophylaxis of children. *Iran J Child Neurol*. 2018;12(1):47–54.

38. Miano S, Parisi P, Pelliccia A, Luchetti A, Paolino MC, Villa MP. Melatonin to prevent migraine or tension-type headache in children. *Neurol Sci*. 2008;29(4):285–287. https://doi.org/10.1007/s10072-008-0983-5.

39. Peres MFP. Melatonin, the pineal gland and their implications for headache disorders. *Cephalalgia*. 2005;25(6):403–411. https://doi.org/10.1111/j.1468-2982.2005.00889.x.

40. El-Shenawy SM, OME A-S, Baiuomy AR, El-Batran S, MS A. Studies on the anti-inflammatory and anti-nociceptive effects of melatonin in the rat. *Pharmacol Res*. 2002;46(3):235–243. https://doi.org/10.1016/S1043-6618(02)00094-4.

41. Marseglia L, Manti S, D'Angelo G, et al. Potential use of melatonin in procedural anxiety and pain in children undergoing blood withdrawal. *J Biol Regul Homeost Agents*. 2015;29(2):509.

42. Gitto E, Aversa S, Salpietro CD, et al. Pain in neonatal intensive care: role of melatonin as an analgesic antioxidant: melatonin and neonatal pain. *J Pineal Res*. 2012;52(3):291–295. https://doi.org/10.1111/j.1600-079X.2011.00941.x.

43. Ong JC, Taylor HL, Park M, et al. Can circadian dysregulation exacerbate migraines? *Headache J Head Face Pain*. 2018;58(7):1040–1051. https://doi.org/10.1111/head.13310.

44. Guidetti V, Dosi C, Bruni O. The relationship between sleep and headache in children: implications for treatment. *Cephalalgia*. 2014;34(10):767–776. https://doi.org/10.1177/0333102414541817.

45. Lateef T, Witonsky K, He J, Ries MK. Headaches and sleep problems in US adolescents: findings from the National Comorbidity Survey—adolescent supplement (NCS-A). *Cephalalgia*. 2019;39(10):1226–1235. https://doi.org/10.1177/0333102419835466.

46. Rosa GD, Attinà S, Spanò M, et al. Efficacy of folic acid in children with migraine, Hyperhomocysteinemia and MTHFR polymorphisms. *Headache*. 2007;47:1342–1351.

47. Lea R, Colson N, Quinlan S, MacMillan J, Griffiths L. The effects of vitamin supplementation and MTHFR (C677T) genotype on homocysteine-lowering and migraine disability. *Pharmacogenet Genomics*. 2009;19(6):422–428. https://doi.org/10.1097/FPC.0b013e32832af5a3.

48. Moschiano F, D'Amico D, Usai S, et al. Homocysteine plasma levels in patients with migraine with aura. *Neurol Sci.* 2008;29(SUPPL. 1):2006–2008. https://doi.org/10.1007/s10072-008-0917-2.

49. Liu L, Yu Y, He J, Guo L, Li H, Teng J. Effects of MTHFR C677T and A1298C polymorphisms on migraine susceptibility: a meta-analysis of 26 studies. *Headache.* 2019;59(6): 891–905. https://doi.org/10.1111/head.13540.

50. Bottini F, Celle ME, Calevo MG, et al. Metabolic and genetic risk factors for migraine in children. *Cephalalgia.* 2006;26(6):731–737. https://doi.org/10.1111/j.1468-2982.2006.01107.x.

51. Chayasirisobhon S. Use of a pine bark extract and antioxidant vitamin combination product as therapy for migraine in patients refractory to pharmacologic medication. *Headache.* 2006;46(5):788–793. https://doi.org/10.1111/j.1526-4610.2006.00454.x.

52. Chayasirisobhon S. Efficacy of Pinus radiata bark extract and vitamin C combination product as a prophylactic therapy for recalcitrant migraine and long-term results. *Acta Neurol Taiwan.* 2013;22(1):13.

53. Visser EJ, Drummond PD, Lee-Visser JLA. Reduction in migraine and headache frequency and intensity with combined antioxidant prophylaxis (N-acetylcysteine, vitamin E and vitamin C: NEC): a randomized sham-controlled pilot study. *Pain Pract.* 2020;1–11. https://doi.org/10.1111/papr.12902.

54. Martami F, Togha M, Seifishahpar M, et al. The effects of a multispecies probiotic supplement on inflammatory markers and episodic and chronic migraine characteristics: a randomized double-blind controlled trial. *Cephalalgia.* 2019;39(7):841–853. https://doi.org/10.1177/0333102418820102.

55. de Roos NM, Giezenaar CGT, Rovers JMP, Witteman BJM, Smits M, van Hemert S. The effects of the multispecies probiotic mixture ecologic barrier on migraine: results of an open-label pilot study. *Benef Microbes.* 2015;6(5):641–646. https://doi.org/10.3920/BM2015.0003.

56. Sensenig J, Marrongelle J, Johnson M, Staverosky T. Treatment_of_migraine_with_tar. PDF. *Altern Med Rev.* 2001;6(5):488–494.

57. De Roos NM, Van Hemert S, Rovers JMP, Smits MG, Witteman BJM. The effects of a multispecies probiotic on migraine and markers of intestinal permeability-results of a randomized placebo-controlled study. *Eur J Clin Nutr.* 2017;71(12):1455–1462. https://doi.org/10.1038/ejcn.2017.57.

58. Arzani M, Jahromi SR, Ghorbani Z, et al. Gut-brain Axis and migraine headache: a comprehensive review. *J Headache Pain.* 2020;21(1). https://doi.org/10.1186/s10194-020-1078-9.

59. Cámara-Lemarroy CR, Rodriguez-Gutierrez R, Monreal-Robles R, Marfil-Rivera A. Gastrointestinal disorders associated with migraine: a comprehensive review. *World J Gastroenterol.* 2016;22(36):8149–8160. https://doi.org/10.3748/wjg.v22.i36.8149.

60. Wider B, Pittler MH, Ernst E. Feverfew for preventing migraine. *Cochrane Database Syst Rev.* 2015;2015(4). https://doi.org/10.1002/14651858.CD002286.pub3.

61. Schiapparelli P, Allais G, Castagnoli Gabellari I, Rolando S, Terzi M, Benedetto C. Non-pharmacological approach to migraine prophylaxis: part II. *Neurol Sci.* 2010;31:137–139. https://doi.org/10.1007/s10072-010-0307-4.

62. Cady RK, Goldstein J, Nett R, Mitchell R, Beach ME, Browning R. A double-blind placebo-controlled pilot study of sublingual feverfew and ginger (LipiGesic™M) in the treatment of migraine. *Headache.* 2011;51(7):1078–1086. https://doi.org/10.1111/j.1526-4610.2011.01910.x.

63. Moscano F, Guiducci M, Maltoni L, et al. An observational study of fixed-dose Tanacetum parthenium nutraceutical preparation for prophylaxis of pediatric headache. *Ital J Pediatr.* 2019;45(1):36. https://doi.org/10.1186/s13052-019-0624-z.

64. Diener H, Freitag F, Danesch U. Safety profile of a special butterbur extract from Petasites hybridus in migraine prevention with emphasis on the liver. *Cephalalgia Rep.* 2018;1. https://doi.org/10.1177/2515816318759304, 251581631875930.

65. Pothmann R, Danesch U. Migraine prevention in children and adolescents: results of an open study with a special butterbur root extract. *Headache.* 2005;45(3):196–203. https://doi.org/10.1111/j.1526-4610.2005.05044.x.

66. Oelkers-Ax R, Leins A, Parzer P, et al. Butterbur root extract and music therapy in the prevention of childhood migraine: an explorative study. *Eur J Pain.* 2008;12(3):301–313. https://doi.org/10.1016/j.ejpain.2007.06.003.

67. Fusco BM, Marabini S, Maggi CA, Fiore G, Geppetti P. Preventative effect of repeated nasal applications of capsaicin in cluster headache. *Pain.* 1994;59(3):321–325. https://doi.org/10.1016/0304-3959(94)90017-5.

68. Sicuteri F, Fusco BM, Marabini S, et al. Beneficial effect of capsaicin application to the nasal mucosa in cluster headache. *Clin J Pain.* 1989;5(1):49–53. https://doi.org/10.1097/00002508-198903000-00010.

69. Marks DR, Rapoport A, Padla D, et al. A double-blind placebo-controlled trial of intranasal capsaicin for cluster headache. *Cephalalgia.* 1993;13(2):114–116. https://doi.org/10.1046/j.1468-2982.1993.1302114.x.

70. Fusco BM, Barzoi G, Agrò F. Repeated intranasal capsaicin applications to treat chronic migraine [5]. *Br J Anaesth.* 2003;90(6):812. https://doi.org/10.1093/bja/aeg572.

71. Cianchetti C. Capsaicin jelly against migraine pain. *Int J Clin Pract.* 2010;64(4):457–459. https://doi.org/10.1111/j.1742-1241.2009.02294.x.

72. Anand KS, Dhikav V. Migraine relieved by chilis. *Headache.* 2012;52:1041-1041. https://doi.org/10.1111/j.1526-4610.2012.02180.x.

73. Fattori V, Hohmann M, Rossaneis A, Pinho-Ribeiro F, Verri W. Capsaicin: current understanding of its mechanisms and therapy of pain and other pre-clinical and clinical uses. *Molecules.* 2016;21(7):844. https://doi.org/10.3390/molecules21070844.

74. Göbel H, Schmidt G, Soyka D. Effect of peppermint and eucalyptus oil preparations on neurophysiological and experimental algesimetric headache parameters. *Cephalalgia.* 1994;14(3):228–234. https://doi.org/10.1046/j.1468-2982.1994.014003228.x.

75. Göbel H, Fresenius J, Heinze A, Dworschak M, Soyka D. Effectiveness of oleum menthae piperitae and paracetamol in therapy of headache of the tension type. *Nervenarzt.* 1996;67(8):672.

76. Shah Y, Spoo M, Jeitler M, et al. Efficacy and safety of an ethanolic solution of peppermint oil for patients with episodic tension type headache: EUMINZ a randomized controlled trial. *Zeitschrift für Phyther.* 2017;38(S 01):V04. https://doi.org/10.1055/s-0037-1607119.

77. Borhani Haghighi A, Motazedian S, Rezaii R, et al. Cutaneous application of menthol 10% solution as an abortive treatment of migraine without aura: a randomised, double-blind, placebo-controlled, crossed-over study. *Int J Clin Pract.* 2010;64(4):451–456. https://doi.org/10.1111/j.1742-1241.2009.02215.x.

78. Rafieian-Kopaei M, Hasanpour-Dehkordi A, Lorigooini Z, Deris F, Solati K, Mahdiyeh F. Comparing the effect of intranasal lidocaine 4% with peppermint essential oil drop 1.5% on migraine attacks: a double-blind clinical trial. *Int J Prev Med.* 2019;10(1):14–18. https://doi.org/10.4103/ijpvm.IJPVM-530-17.

79. Kline RM, Kline JJ, Di Palma J, Barbero GJ. Enteric-coated, pH-dependent peppermint oil capsules for the treatment of irritable bowel syndrome in children. *J Pediatr.* 2001;138(1):125–128. https://doi.org/10.1067/mpd.2001.109606.

80. Sasannejad P, Saeedi M, Shoeibi A, Gorji A, Abbasi M, Foroughipour M. Lavender essential oil in the treatment of migraine headache: a placebo-controlled clinical trial. *Eur Neurol.* 2012;67(5):288–291. https://doi.org/10.1159/000335249.

81. Rafie S, Namjoyan F, Golfakhrabadi F, Yousefbeyk F, Hassanzadeh A. Effect of lavender essential oil as a prophylactic therapy for migraine: a randomized controlled clinical trial. *J Herb Med.* 2016;6(1):18–23. https://doi.org/10.1016/j.hermed.2016.01.003.

82. Ghods AA, Abforosh NH, Ghorbani R, Asgari MR. The effect of topical application of lavender essential oil on the intensity of pain caused by the insertion of dialysis needles in hemodialysis patients: a randomized clinical trial. *Complement Ther Med.* 2015;23(3):325–330. https://doi.org/10.1016/j.ctim.2015.03.001.

83. Soltani R, Soheilipour S, Hajhashemi V, Asghari G, Bagheri M, Molavi M. Evaluation of the effect of aromatherapy with lavender essential oil on post-tonsillectomy pain in pediatric patients: a randomized controlled trial. *Int J Pediatr Otorhinolaryngol.* 2013;77(9):1579–1581. https://doi.org/10.1016/j.ijporl.2013.07.014.

84. National Academies of Sciences and Medicine E. *The Health Effects of Cannabis and Cannabinoids: The Current State of Evidence and Recommendations for Research.* Washington, DC: The National Academies Press; 2017. https://doi.org/10.17226/24625.

85. Pini LA, Guerzoni S, Cainazzo MM, et al. Nabilone for the treatment of medication overuse headache: results of a preliminary double-blind, active-controlled, randomized trial. *J Headache Pain.* 2012;13(8):677–684. https://doi.org/10.1007/s10194-012-0490-1.

86. Cuttler C, Spradlin A, Cleveland MJ, Craft RM. Short- and long-term effects of Cannabis on headache and migraine. *J Pain.* 2019. https://doi.org/10.1016/j.jpain.2019.11.001.

87. Baron EP, Lucas P, Eades J, Hogue O. Patterns of medicinal cannabis use, strain analysis, and substitution effect among patients with migraine, headache, arthritis, and chronic pain in a medicinal cannabis cohort. *J Headache Pain.* 2018;19(1). https://doi.org/10.1186/s10194-018-0862-2.

88. Osborn LA, Lauritsen KJ, Cross N, et al. Self-medication of somatic and psychiatric conditions using botanical marijuana. *J Psychoactive Drugs.* 2015;47(5):345–350. https://doi.org/10.1080/02791072.2015.1096433.

89. Rudich Z, Stinson J, Jeavons M, Brown SC. Treatment of chronic intractable neuropathic pain with dronabinol: case report of two adolescents. *Pain Res Manag.* 2003;8(4):221–224. https://doi.org/10.1155/2003/675976.

90. Baron EP. Medicinal properties of cannabinoids, terpenes, and flavonoids in Cannabis, and benefits in migraine, headache, and pain: an update on current evidence and Cannabis science. *Headache.* 2018;58(7):1139–1186. https://doi.org/10.1111/head.13345.

91. Abdel-Tawab M, Werz O, Schubert-Zsilavecz M. *Boswellia serrata*: an overall assessment of in vitro, preclinical, pharmacokinetic and clinical data. *Clin Pharmacokinet.* 2011;50:349.

92. Lampl C, Haider B, Schweiger C. Long-term efficacy of Boswellia serrata in 4 patients with chronic cluster headache. *J Headache Pain.* 2013;14(S1):P37. https://doi.org/10.1186/1129-2377-14-s1-p37.

93. Ahmadifard M, Yarahmadi S, Ardalan A, Ebrahimzadeh F, Bahrami P, Sheikhi E. The efficacy of topical basil essential oil on relieving migraine headaches: a randomized triple-blind study. *Complement Med Res.* 2020. https://doi.org/10.1159/000506349, 6816885916.

94. Piraneo S. Unicist homeopathy and primary headache. *Homœopathic Links*. 2014; 27(4):252–255. https://doi.org/10.1055/s-0034-1383200.

95. Zarshenas MM, Petramfar P, Firoozabadi A, Moein MR, Mohagheghzadeh A. Types of headache and those remedies in traditional persian medicine. *Pharmacogn Rev*. 2013; 7(13):17–26. https://doi.org/10.4103/0973-7847.112835.

96. National Institutes of Health: Office of Dietary Supplements. Dietary Supplement Fact Sheets, (n.d.).

97. U.S. Food and Drug Adminstration. *FDA Recommends Against Prolonged Use of Magnesium Sulfate to Stop Pre-Term Labor Due to Bone Changes in Exposed Babies: Safety Announcement*; 2013.

98. Tang PH, Miles MV, DeGrauw A, Hershey A, Pesce A. HPLC analysis of reduced and oxidized coenzyme Q(10) in human plasma. *Clin Chem*. 2001;47(2):256–265.

99. Pravst I, Zmitek K, Zmitek J. Coenzyme Q10 contents in foods and fortification strategies. *Crit Rev food Sci Nutr*. 2010;50(4):269.

100. Kok DEG, Dhonukshe-Rutten RAM, Lute C, et al. The effects of long-term daily folic acid and vitamin B12 supplementation on genomewide DNA methylation in elderly subjects. *Clin Epigenetics*. 2015;7(1):1–14. https://doi.org/10.1186/s13148-015-0154-5.

101. Mahmoud AM, Ali MM. Methyl donor micronutrients that modify DNA methylation and cancer outcome. *Nutrients*. 2019;11(3):1–30. https://doi.org/10.3390/nu11030608.

102. Natiional Center for Complementary and Integrative Health. *Cannabis (marijuana) and cannabinoids: what you need to know*. Natiional Center for Complementary and Integrative Health; 2020. https://www.nccih.nih.gov/health/cannabis-marijuana-and-cannabinoids-what-you-need-to-know.

103. Fallah R, Shoroki FF, Ferdosian F. Safety and efficacy of melatonin in pediatric migraine prophylaxis. *Curr Drug Saf*. 2015;10(2):132.

104. Leite Pacheco R, de Oliveira Cruz Latorraca C, Adriano Leal Freitas da Costa A, Luiza Cabrera Martimbianco A, Vianna Pachito D, Riera R. Melatonin for preventing primary headache: a systematic review. *Int J Clin Pract*. 2018;72(7):1–10. https://doi.org/10.1111/ijcp.13203.

105. Thompson DF, Saluja HS. Prophylaxis of migraine headaches with riboflavin: a systematic review. *J Clin Pharm Ther*. 2017;42(4):394–403. https://doi.org/10.1111/jcpt.12548.

106. Sadeghi O, Nasiri M, Maghsoudi Z, Pahlavani N, Rezaie M, Askari G. Effects of pyridoxine supplementation on severity, frequency and duration of migraine attacks in migraine patients with aura: a double-blind randomized clinical trial study in Iran. *Iran J Neurol*. 2015;14(2):74–80.

107. Ziaei S, Kazemnejad A, Sedighi A. The effect of vitamin E on the treatment of menstrual migraine. *Med Sci Monit*. 2009;15(1):2007–2010.

108. Diener HC, Pfaffenrath V, Schnitker J, Friede M, Henneicke-Von Zepelin HH. Efficacy and safety of 6.25 mg t.i.d. feverfew CO2-extract (MIG-99) in migraine prevention - a randomized, double-blind, multicentre, placebo-controlled study. *Cephalalgia*. 2005;25 (11):1031–1041. https://doi.org/10.1111/j.1468-2982.2005.00950.x.

109. Lipton RB, Göbel H, Einhäupl KM, Wilks K, Mauskop A. Petasites hybridus root (butterbur) is an effective preventive treatment for migraine. *Neurology*. 2004;63(12): 2240–2244. https://doi.org/10.1212/01.WNL.0000147290.68260.11.

110. Grossmann W, Schmidramsl H. An Extract of *Petasites hybridus* is Effective in the Prophylaxis of Migraine. *Altern Med Rev*. 2001;6(3).

111. Fusco BM, Geppetti P, Fanciullacci M, Sicuteri F. Local application of capsaicin for the treatment of cluster headache and idiopathic trigeminal neuralgia. *Cephalalgia.* 1991;11:234–235.

112. Posadzki P, Watson L, Ernst E. Herb-drug interactions: an overview of systematic reviews. *Br J Clin Pharmacol.* 2013;75(3):603–618. https://doi.org/10.1111/j.1365-2125.2012.04350.x.

113. Wells RE, Phillips RS, Schachter SC, McCarthy EP. Complementary and alternative medicine use among US adults with common neurological conditions. *J Neurol.* 2010;257(11):1822–1831. https://doi.org/10.1007/s00415-010-5616-2.

114. Bigal ME, Serrano D, Reed M, Lipton RB. Chronic migraine in the population: burden, diagnosis, and satisfaction with treatment. *Neurology.* 2008;71(8):559–566. https://doi.org/10.1212/01.wnl.0000323925.29520.e7.

115. Sanderson JC, Devine EB, Lipton RB, et al. Headache-related health resource utilisation in chronic and episodic migraine across six countries. *J Neurol Neurosurg Psychiatry.* 2013;84(12):1309–1317. https://doi.org/10.1136/jnnp-2013-305197.

116. Snyder J, Brown P. Complementary and alternative medicine in children: an analysis of the recent literature. *Curr Opin Pediatr.* 2012;24(4):539–546. https://doi.org/10.1097/MOP.0b013e328355a214.

117. Ashina S, Bendtsen L, Lyngberg AC, Lipton RB, Hajiyeva N, Jensen R. Prevalence of neck pain in migraine and tension-type headache: a population study. *Cephalalgia.* 2015;35(3):211–219. https://doi.org/10.1177/0333102414535110.

118. Moore CS, Sibbritt DW, Adams J. A critical review of manual therapy use for headache disorders: prevalence, profiles, motivations, communication and self-reported effectiveness. *BMC Neurol.* 2017;17(1):61. https://doi.org/10.1186/s12883-017-0835-0.

119. Bartsch T, Goadsby PJ. The trigeminocervical complex and migraine: current concepts and synthesis. *Curr Pain Headache Rep.* 2003;7(5):371–376. https://doi.org/10.1007/s11916-003-0036-y.

120. Fernández-De-Las-Peñas C, Cuadrado ML, Pareja JA. Myofascial trigger points, neck mobility and forward head posture in unilateral migraine. *Cephalalgia.* 2006;26(9):1061–1070. https://doi.org/10.1111/j.1468-2982.2006.01162.x.

121. Bevilaqua-Grossi D, Pegoretti KS, Goncalves MC, Speciali JG, Bordini CA, Bigal ME. Cervical mobility in women with migraine. *Headache.* 2009;49(5):726–731. https://doi.org/10.1111/j.1526-4610.2008.01233.x.

122. Griegel-Morris P, Larson K, Mueller-Klaus K, Oatis CA. Incidence of common postural abnormalities in the cervical, shoulder, and thoracic regions and their association with pain in two age groups of healthy subjects. *Phys Ther.* 1992;72(6):425–431. https://doi.org/10.1093/ptj/72.6.425.

123. Watson DH, Trott PH. Cervical headache: an investigation of natural head posture and upper cervical flexor muscle performance. *Cephalalgia.* 1993;13(4):272–284. https://doi.org/10.1046/j.1468-2982.1993.1304272.x.

124. Fernández-De-Las-Peñas C, Alonso-Blanco C, Cuadrado ML, Pareja JA. Forward head posture and neck mobility in chronic tension-type headache: a blinded, controlled study. *Cephalalgia.* 2006;26(3):314–319. https://doi.org/10.1111/j.1468-2982.2005.01042.x.

125. Sjaastad O, Fredriksen TA, Pfaffenrath V. Cervicogenic headache: diagnostic criteria. *Headache.* 1998;38(6):442–445. https://doi.org/10.1046/j.1526-4610.1998.3806442.x.

126. Gross A, Miller J, D'Sylva J, et al. Manipulation or mobilisation for neck pain: a Cochrane review. *Man Ther.* 2010;15(4):315–333. https://doi.org/10.1016/j.math.2010.04.002.

127. Borusiak P, Biedermann H, Boßerhoff S, Opp J. Lack of efficacy of manual therapy in children and adolescents with suspected cervicogenic headache: results of a prospective, randomized, placebo-controlled, and blinded trial: research submission. *Headache*. 2010;50(2):224–230. https://doi.org/10.1111/j.1526-4610.2009.01550.x.

128. Rist PM, Hernandez A, Bernstein C, et al. The impact of spinal manipulation on migraine pain and disability: a systematic review and meta-analysis. *Headache*. 2019;59(4): 532–542. https://doi.org/10.1111/head.13501.

129. Nelson CF, Bronfort G, Evans R, Boline P, Goldsmith C, Anderson AV. The efficacy of spinal manipulation, amitriptyline and the combination of both therapies for the prophylaxis of migraine headache. *J Manipulative Physiol Ther*. 1998;21(8):511–519.

130. Haas M, Bronfort G, Evans R, et al. Dose-response and efficacy of spinal manipulation for care of cervicogenic headache: a dual-center randomized controlled trial. *Spine J*. 2018;18(10):1741–1754. https://doi.org/10.1016/j.spinee.2018.02.019.

131. Dunning JR, Butts R, Mourad F, et al. Upper cervical and upper thoracic manipulation versus mobilization and exercise in patients with cervicogenic headache: a multi-center randomized clinical trial. *BMC Musculoskelet Disord*. 2016;17(1):1–12. https://doi.org/ 10.1186/s12891-016-0912-3.

132. Fernandez M, Moore C, Tan J, et al. Spinal manipulation for the management of cervicogenic headache: a systematic review and meta-analysis. *Eur J Pain*. 2020;1–16. https://doi.org/10.1002/ejp.1632 [June].

133. Morin CM, Hauri PJ, Espie CA, Spielman AJ, Buysse DJ, Bootzin RR. Nonpharmacologic treatment of chronic insomnia. an American Academy of sleep medicine review. *Sleep*. 1999;22(8):1134–1156.

134. Espí-López GV, Rodríguez-Blanco C, Oliva-Pascual-Vaca A, Molina-Martínez F, Falla D. Do manual therapy techniques have a positive effect on quality of life in people with tension-type headache? A randomized controlled trial. *Eur J Phys Rehabil Med*. 2016;52(4):447–456.

135. Vohra S, Johnston BC, Cramer K, Humphreys K. Adverse events associated with pediatric spinal manipulation : a systematic review. *Pediatrics*. 2019;119(1). https://doi.org/ 10.1542/peds.2006-1392.

136. Leboeuf C, Brown P, Herman A, Leembruggen K, Walton D, Crisp TC. Chiropractic care of children with nocturnal enuresis: a prospective outcome study. *J Manipulative Physiol Ther*. 1991;14(2):110–115.

137. Sawyer CE, Evans RL, Boline PD, Branson R, Spicer A. A feasibility study of chiropractic spinal manipulation versus sham spinal manipulation for chronic otitis media with effusion in children. *J Manipulative Physiol Ther*. 1999;22(5):292–298. https://doi.org/10.1016/S0161-4754(99)70061-8.

138. Dissing KB, Hartvigsen J, Wedderkopp N, Hestbæk L. Conservative care with or without manipulative therapy in the management of back and/or neck pain in Danish children aged 9-15: a randomised controlled trial nested in a school-based cohort. *BMJ Open*. 2018;8(9):e021358. https://doi.org/10.1136/bmjopen-2017-021358.

139. Driehuis F, Hoogeboom TJ, der Sanden MWG N-V, de Bie RA, Bart Staal J. Spinal manual therapy in infants, children and adolescents: a systematic review and meta-analysis on treatment indication, technique and outcomes. *PLoS One*. 2018;14(6):1–22. https://doi.org/10.1371/journal.pone.0218940.

140. Jull G, Trott P, Potter H, et al. A randomized controlled trial of exercise and manipulative therapy for cervicogenic headache. *Spine (Phila Pa 1976)*. 2002;27(17):1835–1843. discussion 1843 https://doi.org/10.1097/00007632-200209010-00004.

141. Demirturk F, Akarcali I, Akbayrak T, Citak I, Inan L. Results of two different manual therapy techniques in chronic tension-type headache. *Pain Clin.* 2002;14(2): 121–128. https://doi.org/10.1163/156856902760196333.

142. Jensen OK, Nielsen FF, Vosmar L. An open study comparing manual therapy with the use of cold packs in the treatment of post-traumatic headache. *Cephalalgia.* 1990;10(5): 241–250. https://doi.org/10.1046/j.1468-2982.1990.1005241.x.

143. Ernst E. Massage therapy for low back pain: a systematic review. *J Pain Symptom Manage.* 1999;17(1):65–69. https://doi.org/10.1016/s0885-3924(98)00129-8.

144. Moyer CA, Rounds J, Hannum JW. A meta-analysis of massage therapy research. *Psychol Bull.* 2004;130(1):3–18. https://doi.org/10.1037/0033-2909.130.1.3.

145. von Stulpnagel C, Reilich P, Straube A, et al. Myofascial trigger points in children with tension-type headache: a new diagnostic and therapeutic option. *J Child Neurol.* 2009; 24(4):406–409. https://doi.org/10.1177/0883073808324540.

146. Kemper KJ, Breuner CC. Complementary, holistic, and integrative medicine: headaches. *Pediatr Rev.* 2020;31(2):e17–e23.

147. Groenewald CB, Beals-Erickson SE, Ralston-Wilson J, Rabbitts JA, Palermo TM. Complementary and alternative medicine use by children with pain in the United States. *Acad Pediatr.* 2017;17(7):785–793. https://doi.org/10.1016/j.acap.2017.02.008.

148. Kuruvilla D, Wells RE. Evidence-based integrative treatments for headache. *Headache.* 2019;59(6):971–972. https://doi.org/10.1111/head.13555.

149. Lawler SP, Cameron LD. A randomized, controlled trial of massage therapy as a treatment for migraine. *Ann Behav Med.* 2006;32(1):50–59. https://doi.org/10.1207/s15324796abm3201_6.

150. Kamali F, Mohamadi M, Fakheri L, Mohammadnejad F. Dry needling versus friction massage to treat tension type headache: a randomized clinical trial. *J Bodyw Mov Ther.* 2019;23(1):89–93. https://doi.org/10.1016/j.jbmt.2018.01.009.

151. Espí-López GV, Zurriaga-Llorens R, Monzani L, Falla D. The effect of manipulation plus massage therapy versus massage therapy alone in people with tension-type headache. A randomized controlled clinical trial. *Eur J Phys Rehabil Med.* 2016; 52(5):606–617.

152. Ferracini GN, Florencio LL, Dach F, et al. Musculoskeletal disorders of the upper cervical spine in women with episodic or chronic migraine. *Eur J Phys Rehabil Med.* 2017;53(3):342–350. https://doi.org/10.23736/S1973-9087.17.04393-3.

153. Gross A, Kay TM, Paquin JP, et al. Exercises for mechanical neck disorders. *Cochrane Database Syst Rev.* 2015;2017(6). https://doi.org/10.1002/14651858.CD004250.pub5.

154. Lin LY, Wang RH. Effectiveness of a neck stretching intervention on nurses' primary headaches. *Work Heal Saf.* 2015;63(3):100–106. https://doi.org/10.1177/2165079915571355.

155. Wanderley D, Valença MM, de Souza Costa Neto JJ, Martins JV, MCF R, de Oliveira DA. Contract-relax technique compared to static stretching in treating migraine in women: a randomized pilot trial. *J Bodyw Mov Ther.* 2020;24(2):43–49. https://doi.org/10.1016/j.jbmt.2019.05.023.

156. Ylinen J, Nikander R, Nykänen M, Kautiainen H, Häkkinen A. Effect of neck exercises on cervicogenic headache: a randomized controlled trial. *J Rehabil Med.* 2010; 42(4):344–349. https://doi.org/10.2340/16501977-0527.

157. Jalal Y, Ahmad A, Rahman AU, Irfanullah, Daud M, Aneela. Effectiveness of muscle energy technique on cervical range of motion and pain. *J Pak Med Assoc*. 2018;68(5): 811–813.

158. Sadria G, Hosseini M, Rezasoltani A, Akbarzadeh Bagheban A, Davari A, Seifolahi A. A comparison of the effect of the active release and muscle energy techniques on the latent trigger points of the upper trapezius. *J Bodyw Mov Ther*. 2017;21(4):920–925. https:// doi.org/10.1016/j.jbmt.2016.10.005.

159. Grimshaw DN. Cervicogenic headache: manual and manipulative therapies. *Curr Pain Headache Rep*. 2001;5(4):369–375. https://doi.org/10.1007/s11916-001-0027-9.

160. Nie L, Cheng J, Wen Y, Li J. The effectiveness of acupuncture combined with Tuina therapy in patients with migraine. *Complement Med Res*. 2019;26(3):182–194. https:// doi.org/10.1159/000496032.

161. Gilbey P, Bretler S, Avraham Y, Sharabi-Nov A, Ibrgimov S, Luder A. Acupuncture for posttonsillectomy pain in children: a randomized, controlled study. *Paediatr Anaesth*. 2015;25(6):603–609. https://doi.org/10.1111/pan.12621.

162. Chokshi SK, Ladas EJ, Taromina K, et al. Predictors of acupuncture use among children and adolescents with cancer. *Pediatr Blood Cancer*. 2017;64(7):1–7. https://doi.org/ 10.1002/pbc.26424.

163. Ma YC, Peng CT, Huang YC, Lin HY, Lin JG. Safe needling depths of upper back acupoints in children: a retrospective study. *BMC Complement Altern Med*. 2016;16(1): 1–8. https://doi.org/10.1186/s12906-016-1060-x.

164. Adams D, Cheng F, Jou H, Aung S, Yasui Y, Vohra S. The safety of pediatric acupuncture: a systematic review. *Pediatrics*. 2011;128(6). https://doi.org/10.1542/peds.2011-1091.

165. Assefi NP, Sherman KJ, Jacobsen C, Goldberg J, Smith WR, Buchwald D. A randomized clinical trial of acupuncture compared with sham acupuncture in fibromyalgia. *Ann Intern Med*. 2005;143(1):10–19. https://doi.org/10.7326/0003-4819-143-1-200507050-00005.

166. Kemper KJ, Sarah R, Silver-Highfield E, Xiarhos E, Barnes L, Berde C. On pins and needles? Pediatric pain patients' experience with acupuncture. *Pediatrics*. 2000;105(4 Pt 2):941–947.

167. Gottschling S, Meyer S, Gribova I, et al. Laser acupuncture in children with headache: a double-blind, randomized, bicenter, placebo-controlled trial. *Pain*. 2008;137(2): 405–412. https://doi.org/10.1016/j.pain.2007.10.004.

168. Wang LP, Zhang XZ, Guo J, et al. Efficacy of acupuncture for acute migraine attack: a multicenter single blinded, randomized controlled trial. *Pain Med (U S)*. 2012;13(5): 623–630. https://doi.org/10.1111/j.1526-4637.2012.01376.x.

169. Linde K, Allais G, Brinkhaus B, et al. Acupuncture for the prevention of episodic migraine. *Cochrane Database Syst Rev*. 2016;2016(6):CD001218. https://doi.org/ 10.1002/14651858.CD001218.pub3.

170. Linde K, Allais G, Brinkhaus B, et al. Acupuncture for the prevention of tension-type headache. *Cochrane Database Syst Rev*. 2016;4:CD007587. https://doi.org/10.1002/ 14651858.CD007587.pub2.

171. Linde K, Allais G, Brinkhaus B, Manheimer E, Vickers A, White AR. Acupuncture for tension-type headache (Review). *Cochrane Database Syst Rev*. 2009;4:CD007587.

172. Linde K, Allais G, Brinkhaus B, Manheimer E, Vickers A, White AR. Acupuncture for migraine prophylaxis. *Sao Paulo Med J.* 2015;133(6):450. https://doi.org/10.1590/1516-3180.20151336T1.

173. Colquhoun D, Novella SP. Acupuncture is theatrical placebo. *Anesth Analg.* 2013;116(6):1360–1363. https://doi.org/10.1213/ANE.0b013e31828f2d5e.

174. Chae Y, Chang D-S, Lee S-H, et al. Inserting needles into the body: a meta-analysis of brain activity associated with acupuncture needle stimulation. *J Pain.* 2013;14(3):215–222. https://doi.org/10.1016/j.jpain.2012.11.011.

175. Chae Y, Lee I-S, Jung W-M, et al. Decreased peripheral and central responses to acupuncture stimulation following modification of body ownership. *PLoS One.* 2014;9(10):e109489. https://doi.org/10.1371/journal.pone.0109489.

176. Chae Y, Lee IS, Jung WM, Park K, Park HJ, Wallraven C. Psychophysical and neurophysiological responses to acupuncture stimulation to incorporated rubber hand. *Neurosci Lett.* 2015;591:48–52. https://doi.org/10.1016/j.neulet.2015.02.025.

177. Schedlowski M, Schedlowski M, Enck P, et al. Neuro-bio-behavioral mechanisms of placebo and nocebo responses: implications for clinical trials and clinical practice. *Pharmacol Rev.* 2015;67(3):697–730. https://doi.org/10.1124/pr.114.009423.

178. Miller FG, Colloca L. The legitimacy of placebo treatments in clinical practice: evidence and ethics. *Am J Bioeth.* 2009;9(12):39–47. https://doi.org/10.1080/15265160903316263.

179. Kam-Hansen S, Jakubowski M, Kelley JM, et al. Altered placebo and drug labeling changes the outcome of episodic migraine attacks. *Sci Transl Med.* 2014;6(218):218ra5. https://doi.org/10.1126/scitranslmed.3006175.

180. Rizzo AC, Paolucci M, Altavilla R, et al. Daith piercing in a case of chronic migraine: a possible vagal modulation. *Front Neurol.* 2017;8(NOV):1–5. https://doi.org/10.3389/fneur.2017.00624.

How can I get better? Things I can do for myself/ my child

Sleep and headache in children and adolescents ☆

21

Ana Marissa Lagman-Bartolome, MD and Kaitlin Greene, MD

For patient and family

What should you know about you/your child's sleep and headaches?

You or your child may have noticed that there is a relationship between headaches and sleep. At times, changes in sleep pattern may trigger headache. At other times, headaches themselves may make it difficult to sleep. Research has demonstrated that this is, in fact, a very complicated relationship. Children and teens with headaches are more likely to have symptoms of daytime sleepiness, difficulty falling asleep, and unusual sleep behaviors such as sleepwalking. Changes in sleep can also be a trigger for headaches or make headaches worse. For example, research has shown that there is an increase in emergency room visits for headaches in September around the start of the school year and in January after return to school from winter holidays.[1] These are times when your sleep schedule suddenly shifts from a vacation schedule to a school schedule, so perhaps the change itself is a trigger.

How much sleep is recommended?

The American Academy of Sleep Medicine (AASM) recommends that school-aged children get 9–12h of sleep a night. Teens should get 8–10h of sleep at night (Table 1).[2] It can be difficult to fit in that much sleep with school, activities, and homework. Also, teens' natural body rhythm often drives them to go to bed later and wake up later in the morning, so waking up early to get to school on time can be an additional challenge.

☆Editor's note: It is clear that sleeping well is good for one's health. Poor sleep can also exacerbate a headache. As patients move from episodic to chronic headache sleep disturbance is a common unwelcome comorbidity. The authors present the evidence for the connection between sleep and headache and offer practical suggestions for all.

Pediatric Headache. https://doi.org/10.1016/B978-0-323-83005-8.00024-0

Table 1 American Academy of Sleep Medicine recommendation for sleep duration by age group[2].

Age	Recommended hours of sleep per 24h (including naps)
Infants (4–12 months)	12–16
Children (1–2 years of age)	11–14
Children (3–5 years of age)	10–13
Children (6–12 years of age)	9–12
Teenagers (13–18 years of age)	8–10

What do you need to tell the clinician about sleep?

In order for your clinician to best help with headaches, it is important to discuss any sleep problems. Talk about bedtime and wake-up time, problems falling asleep, waking up at night, and feeling tired during the day. Also tell your clinician about snoring, teeth grinding, restless feelings in the legs, sleep walking, or frequent nightmares. All of these can be associated with headaches. Finally, it is important to tell your clinician if the headache itself wakes you up in the middle of the night or early in the morning.

What can you do to improve sleep and headache?

The good news is that there are many strategies for helping to improve sleep and headaches. The simplest way to improve sleep is to have a consistent routine around sleep. Try to go to bed at the same time every night during the week and on weekends. It can help to set aside thirty minutes to relax before the time you want to fall asleep. It is especially important to turn off screens (including TV, phone, iPad, games) because research has shown that the blue light from screens can affect your body's release of melatonin, a brain hormone that helps to regulate sleep, particularly in teens.[3]

What are the treatments available to improve sleep and headache?

Research has shown that a particular type of therapy called Cognitive Behavioral Therapy (CBT) can be helpful for treating both sleep and headache. This type of therapy focuses on identifying how thoughts and feelings affect physical symptoms like headaches and sleep problems. CBT teaches tools to help change negative thoughts and feelings. CBT is the first-line treatment for sleep problems in adults including adults with chronic migraine. It has also been shown to be a helpful treatment for adolescents with both sleep problems and migraine. Talk with your clinician about whether this would be a treatment option for your child.

For the primary care clinician

The existence of an intimate relationship between sleep and headache has been recognized for more than a century.[4] Headaches and sleep problems are common among children and adolescents, and both can be associated with significant functional impairment. While headache and sleep are intrinsically related by anatomy and physiology, the specific mechanisms that explain this complex relationship remain elusive. Evidence suggests that headache can be a symptom of disrupted nocturnal sleep and conversely that sleep disturbance can be symptom of a primary headache. Additionally, both headache and sleep disturbance can be comorbid symptoms of other conditions including primary sleep disorders, mood disorders, and anxiety.[5, 6]

Abnormal sleep behaviors and symptoms including daytime napping, problems initiating and maintaining sleep, daytime sleepiness, poor sleep hygiene, and decreased sleep quality have been found to occur with higher frequency in children and adolescents with headaches compared to heathy controls.[7–9] Specific sleep disorders like sleep apnea, bruxism, and restless leg syndrome are also common in children with headaches.[7, 10, 11]

Treatment

It is crucial to recognize and treat sleep problems in youth with headaches and migraine to potentially diminish the negative impact of headaches on daily functioning. Patient education and lifestyle modification play a significant role in overall success of the treatment. Discussion of sleep habits and sleep disturbances at each visit can facilitate intervention through behavioral changes, pharmacologic intervention, and psychological interventions including cognitive behavior therapy (CBT).

The American Academy of Sleep Medicine (AASM) has issued consensus recommendations for the optimal amount of sleep based on age to promote health and improve headaches (Table 1).[2] This can often be difficult to achieve, particularly for teenagers who naturally have a delayed sleep phase[12] but are often required to wake up early for school. In fact, a cross-sectional internet survey study found that 55% of teens whose schools started at 8:30 am or later reported getting at least 8 h of sleep as recommended by the AASM, compared to 33% of those whose school started before 8:30 am. Interestingly, the duration of sleep is not the only important factor; even after adjusting for hours of sleep, those in the schools with later start time reported lower headache frequency compared to teens with earlier school start time.[13]

Consistency of sleep schedule may also influence headache frequency or severity. This is supported by findings from a study showing peaks in the number of emergency department visits for migraine in September and January, the two times of year that sleep schedules are likely to vary the most as students transition from vacation schedule to school schedule.[1]

Counseling about healthy sleep should therefore include discussion of regularity of sleep in addition to adequate duration, appropriate timing, and good quality. The clinician should brainstorm creative ways to adjust to schedule requirements, avoiding putting blame on the patient or family. Attention to sleep-hygiene has been shown to improve frequency and duration of migraines in children and adolescents.[14]

In addition to discussion of healthy sleep habits, there is growing evidence to suggest that nonpharmacologic treatments including cognitive behavior therapy (CBT) can be helpful for both headache and insomnia. In adults, subjects who participated in CBT reported greater decrease in headache days than those treated with sham control.[15] In a pediatric population, hybrid cognitive behavior therapy (CBT) for migraine and insomnia intervention in adolescents resulted in improvement in headache days, insomnia symptoms, sleep quality, sleep hygiene, and sleep patterns at 3-month follow up.[16] The CBT protocol utilized in this study incorporated sleep hygiene education (promotion of healthy sleep habits), stimulus control (association of the bed with sleep), and sleep restriction (limiting time spent in bed to improve sleep efficiency) in addition to components of CBT pain management protocols (headache education, relaxation training, pleasant activity scheduling and positive thought tracking, and parent operant training).

While extensive review of pharmacologic interventions for sleep is beyond the scope of this chapter, it is worth noting that melatonin may have dual benefit for treatment of both headache and insomnia given its role in maintenance of circadian rhythms and potential analgesic effect in headache.[17] See chapter on nonmedication treatments for more information about melatonin.

For the headache specialist

Headaches and sleep problems are prevalent among children and adolescents and thus a thorough evaluation is essential to develop an appropriate management plan. The relationship between sleep and headache is complex and bidirectional with important implications for the treatment of both conditions. While sleep disturbance can alter pain perception and provoke headaches, headaches can also disrupt sleep. Moreover, both headaches and sleep disorders highly increase the risk for each other.[18]

Prevalence of sleep disturbance among children and adolescents with headache

A growing body of epidemiologic research has helped to identify sleep disorders that are more common among children with headache. Compared to healthy controls, children and adolescents with headaches of any type have been shown to have higher prevalence of abnormal sleep behaviors including insufficient sleep, co-sleeping, difficulty falling asleep, bedtime anxiety, restless sleep, nighttime wakening, nightmares, and daytime sleepiness.[7]

Prevalence of sleep disorders may vary by headache type. Children with migraine have been shown to have prolonged sleep onset, bedtime resistance, decreased sleep duration, daytime sleepiness, night awakenings, sleep anxiety, parasomnias, and sleep-disordered breathing compared to healthy controls.[9] Children with migraine are also more likely to report snoring, parasomnias, sweating during sleep, and day-time sleepiness than those with "nonmigraine headache" or no headache.[8] In a large population study, adolescents with migraine with aura reported more difficulty maintaining sleep, early morning awakenings, daytime fatigue, and persistent insomnia than those with migraine without aura; however, these associations were not statistically significant after adjusting for anxiety and mood disorders, suggesting that these comorbidities may mediate the relationship between headache and sleep.[6]

Other studies have also reported on the prevalence of parasomnias and other primary sleep disorders in children and adolescents with migraine. Adolescents with chronic migraine were more likely to report history of sleep terrors in childhood compared to those with episodic migraine and healthy controls,[10] while somnambulism is more common among those with migraine compared to nonmigraine headache and healthy controls and more common among those with migraine with aura compared to those without aura.[7, 11]

Headache as a symptom of primary sleep disorders

In addition to the high prevalence of sleep disorders among patients with headaches, it is also important to recognize that headache can be a symptom of primary sleep disorders including obstructive sleep apnea and sleep-disordered breathing. This relationship is well-characterized in adults, with up to 20% of patients with sleep apnea reporting morning headache[19] and up to 14% of those with nocturnal or morning headaches found to have sleep apnea on polysomnography.[20] In the pediatric population, a polysomnographic study found that children with migraine were more commonly affected by sleep-disordered breathing than those with tension headache.[21] The International Classification of Headache Disorders, 3rd Edition (ICHD-3) identifies headache attributed to sleep apnea as a discrete entity characterized by headache on waking, typically with bilateral location, pressing quality, and duration of less than four hours.[22] As this disorder can be readily diagnosed with polysomnography, and effective treatment of the underlying sleep apnea can improve headaches,[20] it is important to recognize sleep apnea as a potential underlying etiology for headache, particularly morning headache.

Bruxism and restless leg syndrome (RLS) have both been reported in association with headaches. Rates of bruxism are high among those with migraine, and children with bruxism have been shown to have higher odds of having headache than those without bruxism.[18, 23] Compared to children without headaches, children with migraine have also been shown to have higher rates of RLS[24, 25]; additionally, migraine patients with RLS had higher frequency of allodynia, vertigo/dizziness, and frequent nighttime arousals that those without RLS.[24]

Sleep disturbance as a trigger in headache and migraine

Equally important to the association between headache and various sleep disorders disturbance is the provoking role that sleep disturbance can play in headache. Up to 70% of children report sleep disturbances and insufficient sleep as triggers of migraine.[26–28]

In a population-based study of Spanish adolescents, headache was significantly more frequent among those with poor sleeping habits.[29] Specifically, in multivariate analyses, insomnia (OR 1.7 (95% CI 1.3–2.2)) and sleeping less than 8h per night (OR 1.4 (95% CI 1.1–1.8)) were significant predictors of headache.[29]

Research suggests that insomnia may contribute to the onset, maintenance, and progression of migraine and other primary headaches. Longitudinal studies of adolescents suggest that insomnia increases risk for the persistence of headache over time as well as progression from episodic to chronic headache.[30] Moreover, early onset sleep disorders have been found to predict headache persistence from infancy to childhood; in one study, 78% of children with enduring headache had early childhood sleep disturbances compared to 25% of children with headache remission.[31]

Headache as a provoking factor for poor sleep

Just as headache may be a consequence of poor sleep, poor sleep may also be driven by headaches. In fact, migraine without aura was found to be a sensitive risk factor for disorders of initiating and maintaining sleep.[32] In a study of 622 children and adolescents with pain syndromes, of which 60% were headache, sleep disturbance was among the most common complaints caused by pain.[33] Actigraphic studies of sleep quality in children and adolescents with migraine have shown mixed results. While one study found that those with headache had less time in quiet motionless sleep and earlier wake times that those without headache,[34] another study found no difference between children with migraine and controls during the interictal period, but did show decrease in nocturnal motor activity in the night preceding a migraine.[35]

Physiology and mechanism of relationship between sleep and headache

The state of sleep encompasses almost one third of a person's life, and disturbances of sleep often mirror disturbances in the physiology of body and mind. While a growing body of evidence shows the relationship between headache and sleep, potential mechanisms underlying this association have not been established.

One possibility is that headache and sleep disturbance are both manifestations of a similar underlying pathogenesis related to shared neurophysiologic and anatomic pathways.[36] Anatomic substrates for both sleep and headache overlap in the brainstem and diencephalon as do physiologic pathways involving dopamine, orexin, melatonin, and serotonin.[4, 37] These brain structures are crucial to the regulation of sleep and nociception as well migraine pathogenesis.

Primary headaches including migraine and cluster headache are characterized by a striking association with the sleep–wake cycle and other circadian biorhythms, suggesting that they may represent centrally originating chronobiological disorders. The hypothalamus, specifically the suprachiasmatic nuclei (SCN), has been considered to be the site of origin of these rhythms. While the SCN is best known for its role in driving the circadian rhythm, the hypothalamus also has important connections to nociceptive neurons in the locus ceruleus, dorsal raphe nucleus, and periaqueductal gray matter, all of which are integral to the nociceptive pathways involved in pathogenesis of headache.[4] Notably, migraine appears to occur in association with rapid eye movement (REM) sleep, as well as in association with excessive amounts of stage III and stage IV sleep,[38, 39] while chronic paroxysmal hemicrania and cluster headache also characteristically occur during REM sleep.[4]

The dorsal raphe may mediate the relationship between sleep and headache through its role in serotonin metabolism. Serotonin is known to play a role in pathogenesis of headache; pharmacologic serotonin depletion can provoke a migraine, and triptans exert their migraine abortive properties through agonism at the serotonin receptor. Interestingly, activity of the dorsal raphe nucleus is decreased during REM sleep resulting in lower systemic levels of serotonin, which has been proposed to drive the relationship between migraine and REM sleep.[4]

Finally, melatonin metabolism may influence the relationship between headache and sleep. The classic role of melatonin in the nervous system is in maintenance of the circadian rhythm, primarily by promoting sleep onset. However, additional actions include potentiation of gamma aminobutyric acid (GABA), modulation of serotonergic effects on cerebral arteries and inhibition of prostaglandin E2 synthesis, suggesting that it may have additional analgesic properties.[4] In adults, studies have shown reduction in urinary melatonin among patients with migraine including during migraine attacks,[40] and prolonged dim-light melatonin onset has been associated with more frequent migraine days per month among those with chronic migraine.[41] In a pediatric sample, there was no difference in urinary melatonin excretion between children with migraine and healthy controls; however, urinary melatonin excretion was decreased in the night preceding a migraine among those who experienced aura or premonitory symptoms with migraine.[42]

References

1. Kedia S, Ginde AA, Grubenhoff JA, Kempe A, Hershey AD, Powers SW. Monthly variation of United States pediatric headache emergency department visits. *Cephalalgia*. 2014;34:473–478.
2. Paruthi S, Brooks LJ, D'Ambrosio C, et al. Recommended amount of sleep for pediatric populations: a consensus statement of the American Academy of sleep medicine. *J Clin Sleep Med*. 2016;12:785–786.
3. Nagare R, Plitnick B, Figueiro MG. Effect of exposure duration and light spectra on nighttime melatonin suppression in adolescents and adults. *Light Res Technol*. 2019;51:530–543.
4. Dodick DW, Eross EJ, Parish JM, Silber M. Clinical, anatomical, and physiologic relationship between sleep and headache. *Headache*. 2003;43:282–292.
5. Bellini B, Arruda M, Cescut A, et al. Headache and comorbidity in children and adolescents. *J Headache Pain*. 2013;14:79.
6. Lateef T, Witonsky K, He J, Ries MK. Headaches and sleep problems in US adolescents: findings from the National Comorbidity Survey—adolescent supplement (NCS-A). *Cephalalgia*. 2019;39:1226–1235.

7. Bruni O, Fabrizi P, Ottaviano S, Cortesi F, Giannotti F, Guidetti V. Prevalence of sleep disorders in childhood and adolescence with headache: a case-control study. *Cephalalgia*. 1997;17:492–498.

8. Isik U, Ersu RH, Ay P, et al. Prevalence of headache and its association with sleep disorders in children. *Pediatr Neurol*. 2007;36:146–151.

9. Miller VA, Palermo TM, Powers SW, Scher MS, Hershey AD. Migraine headaches and sleep disturbances in children. *Headache*. 2003;43:362–368.

10. Fialho LM, Pinho RS, Lin J, et al. Sleep terrors antecedent is common in adolescents with migraine. *Arq Neuropsiquiatr*. 2013;71:83–86.

11. Casez O, Dananchet Y, Besson G. Migraine and somnambulism. *Neurology*. 2005;65:1334–1335.

12. Carskadon MA, Tarokh L. Developmental changes in sleep biology and potential effects on adolescent behavior and caffeine use. *Nutr Rev*. 2014;72(Suppl. 1):60–64.

13. Gelfand AA, Pavitt S, Ross AC, et al. Later high school start time is associated with lower migraine frequency in adolescents. *Headache*. 2021;61:343–350.

14. Bruni O, Galli F, Guidetti V. Sleep hygiene and migraine in children and adolescents. *Cephalalgia*. 1999;19(Suppl 25):57–59.

15. Smitherman TA, Kuka AJ, Calhoun AH, et al. Cognitive-behavioral therapy for insomnia to reduce chronic migraine: a sequential Bayesian analysis. *Headache*. 2018;58:1052–1059.

16. Law EF, Wan Tham S, Aaron RV, Dudeney J, Palermo TM. Hybrid cognitive-behavioral therapy intervention for adolescents with co-occurring migraine and insomnia: a single-arm pilot trial. *Headache*. 2018;58:1060–1073.

17. Gelfand AA. Melatonin in the treatment of primary headache disorders. *Headache*. 2017;57:848–849.

18. Guidetti V, Dosi C, Bruni O. The relationship between sleep and headache in children: implications for treatment. *Cephalalgia*. 2014;34:767–776.

19. Russell MB, Kristiansen HA, Kværner KJ. Headache in sleep apnea syndrome: epidemiology and pathophysiology. *Cephalalgia*. 2014;34:752–755.

20. Paiva T, Farinha A, Martins A, Batista A, Guilleminault C. Chronic headaches and sleep disorders. *Arch Intern Med*. 1997;157:1701–1705.

21. Vendrame M, Kaleyias J, Valencia I, Legido A, Kothare SV. Polysomnographic findings in children with headaches. *Pediatr Neurol*. 2008;39:6–11.

22. Headache Classification Committee of the International Headache Society (IHS) The International Classification of Headache Disorders, 3rd edition. *Cephalalgia*. 2018;38:1–211.

23. Carra MC, Bruni O, Huynh N. Topical review: sleep bruxism, headaches, and sleep-disordered breathing in children and adolescents. *J Orofac Pain*. 2012;26:267–276.

24. Sevindik MS, Demirci S, Goksan B, et al. Accompanying migrainous features in pediatric migraine patients with restless legs syndrome. *Neurol Sci*. 2017;38:1677–1681.

25. Seidel S, Bock A, Schlegel W, et al. Increased RLS prevalence in children and adolescents with migraine: a case-control study. *Cephalalgia: Int J Headache*. 2012;32:693–699.

26. Bruni O, Russo PM, Ferri R, Novelli L, Galli F, Guidetti V. Relationships between headache and sleep in a non-clinical population of children and adolescents. *Sleep Med*. 2008;9:542–548.

27. Neut D, Fily A, Cuvellier JC, Vallee L. The prevalence of triggers in paediatric migraine: a questionnaire study in 102 children and adolescents. *J Headache Pain*. 2012;13:61–65.

28. Chakravarty A, Mukherjee A, Roy D. Trigger factors in childhood migraine: a clinic-based study from eastern India. *J Headache Pain*. 2009;10:375–380.

29. Torres-Ferrus M, Vila-Sala C, Quintana M, et al. Headache, comorbidities and lifestyle in an adolescent population (The TEENs Study). *Cephalalgia*. 2019;39:91–99.

30. Boardman HF, Thomas E, Millson DS, Croft PR. The natural history of headache: predictors of onset and recovery. *Cephalalgia: Int J Headache*. 2006;26:1080–1088.

31. Balottin U, Termine C, Nicoli F, Quadrelli M, Ferrari-Ginevra O, Lanzi G. Idiopathic headache in children under six years of age: a follow-up study. *Headache*. 2005;45:705–715.

32. Carotenuto M, Guidetti V, Ruju F, Galli F, Tagliente FR, Pascotto A. Headache disorders as risk factors for sleep disturbances in school aged children. *J Headache Pain*. 2005;6:268–270.

33. Roth-Isigkeit A, Thyen U, Stöven H, Schwarzenberger J, Schmucker P. Pain among children and adolescents: restrictions in daily living and triggering factors. *Pediatrics*. 2005;115:e152–e162.

34. Bursztein C, Steinberg T, Sadeh A. Sleep, sleepiness, and behavior problems in children with headache. *J Child Neurol*. 2006;21:1012–1019.

35. Bruni O, Russo PM, Violani C, Guidetti V. Sleep and migraine: an actigraphic study. *Cephalalgia: Int J Headache*. 2004;24:134–139.

36. Paiva T, Batista A, Martins P, Martins A. The relationship between headaches and sleep disturbances. *Headache*. 1995;35:590–596.

37. Merikangas KR, Merikangas JR, Angst J. Headache syndromes and psychiatric disorders: association and familial transmission. *J Psychiatr Res*. 1993;27:197–210.

38. Dexter JD, Weitzman ED. The relationship of nocturnal headaches to sleep stage patterns. *Neurology*. 1970;20:513–518.

39. Dexter JD. The relationship between stage III + IV + REM sleep and arousals with migraine. *Headache*. 1979;19:364–369.

40. Masruha MR, de Souza Vieira DS, Minett TS, et al. Low urinary 6-sulphatoxymelatonin concentrations in acute migraine. *J Headache Pain*. 2008;9:221–224.

41. Ong JC, Taylor HL, Park M, et al. Can circadian dysregulation exacerbate migraines? *Headache*. 2018;58:1040–1051.

42. Berger A, Litwin J, Allen IE, et al. Preliminary evidence that melatonin is not a biomarker in children and adolescents with episodic migraine. *Headache*. 2019;59:1014–1023.

Meals/food/diet/caffeine/hydration☆

22

Jennifer Bickel, MD and Trevor Gerson, MD

The importance of food and water intake in pediatric headaches cannot be underestimated. Food and water intake can highly influence the disease process, from triggering a migraine to stopping it in its tracks. It can also influence whether a child has more frequent or less frequent headaches. However, even though questions about the role of nutrition and hydration in headaches are common among patients and healthcare providers alike, there is a lot of confusion regarding this subject. Hence the focus of this chapter.

Meals

Because migraines are affected by changes in routine, regular meals are a necessity. However, regular meals may be difficult in a disease such as migraine that is accompanied by significant nausea and vomiting. In a study from Ankara University with children in grades four through twelve, 52% of children with migraine, compared to 28% of those without headaches, did not regularly eat breakfast.[1] Certain comorbidities such as eating disorders, which are more frequent in kids with migraine,[2] may also make eating regular meals challenging.

Though it may be challenging to convince children, especially adolescents, to eat regular meals, there are ways to encourage this practice. Some potential options are prepreparing breakfasts to make the morning routine easier, offering regular snacking, and having backup options for meals that may be more palatable for someone who is nauseated.

☆Editor's note: Patients, parents, and doctors want to do what's right and modify things in the environment that could help. What we eat and drink are potentially modifiable. However, as presented by the authors, the evidence that these things influence headache frequency is limited. Truisms sometimes need to be challenged. "It is more important THAT you eat rather than WHAT you eat" may be sound advice.

Pediatric Headache. https://doi.org/10.1016/B978-0-323-83005-8.00010-0

Food/diet

The role of specific dietary choices in headache control is a recurrent point of controversy in the headache clinic. Since knowledge about specific diets and advice on avoiding triggers are highly publicized through the news media and social media, healthcare providers must be educated in these areas.

Questions about triggers, especially foods, are especially common in the headache clinic. Most patients believe that certain foods may trigger migraines, though they recognize that one patient's triggers may not necessarily be a problem for another. A connection between food triggers and migraines was made long ago through multiple studies employing the use of headache diaries to track activities, diet, hydration, weather, etc. and comparing this information to the frequency and intensity of headaches. A study from Belgium from 1987 found that 45% of patients with migraine reported specific foods that trigger an attack.[3] Commonly accepted triggers include monosodium glutamate (MSG), nitrite-containing foods (hot dogs, cured meats), tyramine-containing foods (such as cheese), aspartame (from diet sodas), and alcoholic beverages.

However, we are now learning that these "triggers" may not play as big of a role as we previously thought. The studies employing diaries tracked when patients had a headache, and then examined activities preceding the headache to infer a cause. The studies compared kids with headache and their food intake to kids without a headache and their intake, rather than comparing the diet of the same child with and without a headache. While possibly showing an association, this type of study is unable to prove cause and effect and is subject to "recall bias"; that is, when looking back in time certain events or behaviors may seem more or less pronounced or important than they were or may be forgotten completely. To show cause and effect, prospective studies are needed (looking forward rather than looking backward). Some small studies have been done this way. One such study found that even though children reported that certain foods would trigger a headache, the data collected in their prospective diaries did not show any trigger from food, though did show triggers from stress and lack of sleep. Instead, the data showed that a few substances (in meat and caffeine) had a small protective effect against headaches.[4] In particular, this study found that tyramine-containing foods were not associated with headaches. Also, a controlled trial studying chocolate as a trigger for migraines, found that chocolate did not provoke a headache more often than placebo (which was carob in this trial).[5] Last, in a trial of patients who described bright or flickering light or strenuous exercise as a migraine trigger, exposure to these triggers in a controlled setting rarely produced any headache or aura.[6]

One reason that people believe that triggers produce headaches may be that the body may be more sensitive to different stimuli prior to a migraine. When a migraine patient was scanned in a functional MRI every day for 30 days, and the information was correlated with a headache diary, it was found that, 24 h prior to a migraine, the signaling between the hypothalamus and the areas that act as the hub for pain sensation in the head was changed.[7] When hormones that control sleep, appetite, mood, etc. are altered, it may appear that lack of sleep may be a trigger, when in fact the inability to sleep is part of the changes prior to a headache (an effect of an oncoming headache rather than the cause).

These studies suggest a downside to judicious tracking of a child's activities and comparing them to frequency of headaches. This kind of comparison entrenches the idea of headaches as a central factor of daily activity. Headaches become a defining characteristic of every moment of the child's day, taking the focus off of being functional and happy. For this reason and those above, the use of headache diaries outside of research may not yield worthwhile results for the effort invested. Focus on keeping a diary could create a point of friction between parent and child.

Obesity

The contribution of obesity to headache is multifactorial. Besides contributing to co-morbidities such as metabolic syndrome, sleep apnea, and others, some evidence suggests that adipose tissue may itself contribute to the release of pro-inflammatory mediators that are a part of the migraine cascade. The HUNT study from Norway, which was comprised of a subjective survey as well as a physical exam of students, found that being overweight was associated with migraine and tension type headache.[8] Studies have also shown that obese children are more likely to move from episodic to chronic migraine.[9] Furthermore, weight loss is associated with decreased headache frequency and improvement in Pediatric MIDAS (Migraine Disability Assessment) scores, both of which are sustained up to a year later.[10]

Specific diets

The method of weight loss, most suitable for treating headache, has not been studied by high-quality trials at this time. Numerous diet options exist, and popular opinion holds that many of these diets will have significant benefits for all manner of conditions. One diet currently already employed in medicine for other purposes, including epilepsy, is the ketogenic diet, where instead of consuming substances such as carbohydrates to fuel the energy needs of the body, an individual consumes substances such as fat (specifically looking at a fat to protein and carbohydrate ratio) that shift the fuel source of the body to ketones (the method of how this then helps in a disease such as epilepsy is unclear). The mechanism behind the benefit of this diet is elusive, though hypotheses put forth involve restoring neuronal excitability and reducing inflammatory processes. Several small studies dating back to 1928 that recruited 18 adults showed that over 50% had some relief with their headaches while on the diet.[11] Since that time, though there have been only a handful further trials and none of which were randomized controlled trials (RCTs), these studies have demonstrated promising results. Despite this promise, this diet may be difficult to implement in practice. The difficulty in adhering to the ketogenic diet, including periods of slipping out of ketosis due to "cheating" resulting in multiple poor symptoms, may relegate this intervention to only the most treatment-refractory, dedicated patients.

Another popular diet is the elimination diet, which has varied meanings. Such diets seek to eliminate triggering foods, whether they be histamine-free, "oligoantigenic," or personalized. A number of trials have investigated the effect on migraineurs of such a diet, including RCTs, though with small numbers and few focused in the pediatric population.[12, 13] These studies have also shown promising results, but larger studies with standardized definitions will be needed to confirm efficacy. As discussed above, the role of food "triggers" may be shown to be minimal in the future after further studies.

Several studies have also investigated the role of weight loss surgery and its effect on migraine. The studies to date have been small and none have focused on pediatric patients, though the studies have consistently shown significant reduction in headache frequency, severity, as well as overall medication use and disability.[14–16]

In practical terms, counseling any patient to adhere to one diet or another is difficult, but it seems reasonable, based on available evidence, to recommend weight loss in obese patients. A screening for eating disorders is also reasonable, because of the high frequency of eating disorders in children with migraine, mentioned earlier. If a patient and his or her family are interested in following a particular diet, it is important to stress the importance of maintaining adequate nutritional content regardless of which diet they choose. Referral to a nutritionist can be invaluable.

Hydration

Dehydration is a significant trigger for migraines.[17] Especially in an era filled with sodas, juices, and other water substitutes, children today generally do not drink enough water and are more prone to dehydration.[18] In the clinic, it is common to hear parents say that their child "can't be dehydrated," since they drink what is thought of as an adequate amount. How much is enough? The only clear recommendation for children and adolescents is 2–3 L of water per day,[19] but this guideline is one source and must be individualized for the size of the child, environment (a hot day outside working compared to a relaxing day indoors), and other comorbid conditions. Conditions such as orthostatic hypotension (OH), postural orthostatic tachycardia syndrome (POTS), renal disease, and heart disease, can raise or lower the daily fluid intake (see the chapter on POTS and Dysautonomia for further information).

Caffeine

Another common topic of discussion in the headache clinic is caffeine intake. Children today consume a lot of caffeine, in the forms of coffee, tea, energy drinks, and soda.

The role of caffeine in headache and pain is unclear. Treating a headache by drinking a cup of coffee or taking over-the-counter medications caffeine is commonplace. Some small studies showing that adding caffeine (as a pill, or even as an IV medication, at doses ranging from 50 mg to over 500 mg) to other pain medicines may result in a small amount of extra pain relief.[20] However, specifically for headache, this practice may be problematic. Children with headaches have been shown to consume caffeine more regularly than children who do not have headaches,[2] though in another patient series of patients at a pediatric headache center, caffeine consumption at the initial visit was associated with lower probability of headache worsening at the second visit.[21] These types of studies may show a correlation between caffeine use and worsening headaches, but once again, correlation does not prove causation and prospective studies would be needed.

One concern related to headaches is the concept of caffeine-withdrawal headaches. Some patients who regularly drink multiple cups of coffee per day, such as at work or on the way to school, may notice they are developing headaches on the days they abstain, for example, on a weekend when they depart from their usual weekday routine. This connection is another entrenched belief that has been investigated with surprising results. In a prospective study of patients who responded on a survey that they had headaches when withdrawing from caffeine, only about one-third of patients who were then abruptly stopped from consuming caffeine developed a headache, and those who were weaned more gradually did not report any headaches.[22]

Another important consideration is the dose of caffeine and the type of food or drink that contains the drug. In the past, coffee has been the main source of caffeine used by patients, as well as what has been studied. However, a growing source of caffeine for children and adolescents today comes from various energy drinks or supplements. A typical energy drink may contain anywhere from 80 to 300 mg of caffeine (the American Academy of Pediatrics recommends children and adolescents aged 12–18 to consume no more than 100 mg of caffeine per day,[23] see Table 1), and may contain as much as 35 g of processed sugar as well as other additives such as taurine, guarana, and ginseng in just one eight ounce drink.[24] Very little data exist on how consuming energy drinks affects patients with headaches, and the data collected so far are mostly retrospective or cross-sectional. In a cross-sectional study (observing a large portion of patients across a population at one single time point) of high school age children in Canada, children who were "frequent users" of energy drinks (more than once per month) were more likely to have headaches, to seek medical care for headaches in the past 6 months, and to have difficulties with sleep as well as with anger.[25] In another large population-based study in Korea, frequent (>3 times per week) consumption of energy drinks was found to be associated with a three times higher chance of attempting suicide.[26] Side effects such as these, as well as the lack of FDA regulation (as these drinks are marketed as "supplements"), were some of the reasons that the American Academy of Pediatrics stated that "caffeine and other stimulant substances contained in energy drinks have no place in the diet of children and adolescents".[23]

Healthcare providers may experience situations related to beneficial effects of caffeine in the setting of postdural puncture headache (PDPH, also known as post LP headache). One such situation is a lumbar puncture, or even an epidural, where

Table 1 Caffeine content of popular drinks.

Caffeine Content of Popular Drinks

Drink	Caffeine Content (mg)
Dunkin Donuts Iced Coffee, Original (12 oz)	297
Starbucks Blonde Roast (Tall)	270
5 Hour Energy (2 oz)	200
Starbucks Dark Roast (Tall)	193
Jolt Cola (473mL bottle)	160
Red Bull (12 oz can)	111
Starbucks Cafe Mocha (Tall)	95
Starbucks Esspresso (1 shot)	75
Mountain Dew (12 oz can)	54
Diet Coke (12 oz can)	46
Coca Cola (12 oz can)	34
Starbucks Iced Black Tea (Tall)	25
Barqs Root Beer (12 oz can)	22
Gold Peak Tea Unsweetened (16.9 oz)	21
Starbucks Decaf Pike Place Roast (Tall)	20
Starbucks Hot Chocolate (Tall)	20
Sprite (12 oz can)	0

Data regarding caffeine content taken directly from manufacturer websites.

the patient exhibits a headache that is positional (worse with upright position). Here, caffeine has been investigated as a potential treatment with strong initial data (though more study is needed). Caffeine in an oral or IV form (the dose is unclear) is generally recommended to treat or prevent this kind of headache, and studies have shown that it may resolve PDPH in as little as 1–2 hours.[27] This effect is thought to be due to the action of caffeine causing increased cerebrospinal fluid production, though in rat studies this increased CSF has been seen with chronic caffeine use; in acute use, CSF production is decreased.[28]

Conclusion

Counseling patients regarding nutrition and hydration may be difficult for healthcare providers when time with patients is already short; however, this is a topic that is often front and center in the minds of the patient and his or her family. These issues can help or hinder a patient's progress in his or her migraine journey and should thus be deliberately investigated by patient and provider alike. However, it is important to critically view beliefs regarding issues such as triggers that have been commonly accepted in the past but may not play as much of a role as we have previously thought. Time and effort previously focused on these subjects may be better served working on other more impactful interventions, such as those discussed in the other chapters of this book.

References

1. Bektaş Ö, Uğur C, Gençtürk ZB, Aysev A, Sireli Ö, Deda G. Relationship of childhood headaches with preferences in leisure time activities, depression, anxiety and eating habits: a population-based, cross-sectional study. *Cephalalgia*. 2015;35(6):527–537.
2. Kandemir G, Hesapcioglu ST, Kurt ANC. What are the psychosocial factors associated with migraine in the child? Comorbid psychiatric disorders, family functioning, parenting style, or Mom's psychiatric symptoms? *J Child Neurol*. 2018;33(2):174–181.
3. Van den bergh V, Amery WK, Waelkens J. Trigger factors in migraine: a study conducted by the Belgian migraine society. *Headache*. 1987;27(4):191–196.
4. Connelly M, Bickel J. An electronic daily diary process study of stress and health behavior triggers of primary headaches in children. *J Pediatr Psychol*. 2011;36(8):852–862.
5. Marcus DA, Scharff L, Turk D, Gourley LM. A double-blind provocative study of chocolate as a trigger of headache. *Cephalalgia*. 1997;17(8):855–862.
6. Hougaard A, Amin FM, Amin F, Hauge AW, Ashina M, Olesen J. Provocation of migraine with aura using natural trigger factors. *Neurology*. 2013;80(5):428–431.
7. Schulte LH, May A. The migraine generator revisited: continuous scanning of the migraine cycle over 30 days and three spontaneous attacks. *Brain*. 2016;139(Pt 7):1987–1993.
8. Robberstad L, Dyb G, Hagen K, Stovner LJ, Holmen TL, Zwart JA. An unfavorable lifestyle and recurrent headaches among adolescents: the HUNT study. *Neurology*. 2010;75 (8):712–717.
9. Scher AI, Lipton RB, Stewart W. Risk factors for chronic daily headache. *Curr Pain Headache Rep*. 2002;6:486–491.
10. Verrotti A, Agostinelli S, D'Egidio C, et al. Impact of a weight loss program on migraine in obese adolescents. *Eur J Neurol*. 2013;20:394–397.
11. Schnabel T. An experience with a ketogenic dietary in migraine. *Ann Intern Med*. 1928;2:341–347.
12. Mitchell N, Hewitt CE, Jayakody S, et al. Randomised controlled trial of food elimination diet based on IgG antibodies for the prevention of migraine like headaches. *Nutr J*. 2011;10:85.
13. Egger J, Carter CM, Wilson J, Turner MW, Soothill JF. Is migraine food allergy? A double-blind controlled trial of oligoantigenic diet treatment. *Lancet*. 1983;2 (8355):865–869.
14. Bond DS, Vithiananthan S, Nash JM, Thomas JG, Wing RR. Improvement of migraine headaches in severely obese patients after bariatric surgery. *Neurology*. 2011;76 (13):1135–1138.

15. Novack V, Fuchs L, Lantsberg L, et al. Changes in headache frequency in premenopausal obese women with migraine after bariatric surgery: a case series. *Cephalalgia.* 2011;31 (13):1336–1342.
16. Razeghi jahromi S, Abolhasani M, Ghorbani Z, et al. Bariatric surgery promising in migraine control: a controlled trial on weight loss and its effect on migraine headache. *Obes Surg.* 2018;28(1):87–96.
17. Blau JN. Water deprivation: a new migraine precipitant. *Headache.* 2005;45(6):757–759.
18. D'Anci KE, Constant F, Rosenberg IH. Hydration and cognitive function in children. *Nutr Rev.* 2006;64:457–464.
19. Medicine IO, Board FA, Intakes SC, et al. *Dietary Reference Intakes for Water, Potassium, Sodium, Chloride, and Sulfate.* National Academies Press; 2005.
20. Derry CJ, Derry S, Moore RA. Caffeine as an analgesic adjuvant for acute pain in adults. *Cochrane Database Syst Rev.* 2014;12:CD009281.
21. Orr SL, Turner A, Kabbouche MA, et al. Predictors of short-term prognosis while in pediatric headache care: an observational study. *Headache.* 2019;59(4):543–555.
22. Dews PB, Curtis GL, Hanford KJ, O'brien CP. The frequency of caffeine withdrawal in a population-based survey and in a controlled, blinded pilot experiment. *J Clin Pharmacol.* 1999;39(12):1221–1232.
23. Committee on Nutrition and the Council on Sports Medicine and Fitness. Sports drinks and energy drinks for children and adolescents: are they appropriate? *Pediatrics.* 2011;127(6):1182–1189.
24. Clauson KA, Shields KM, Mcqueen CE, Persad N. Safety issues associated with commercially available energy drinks. *J Am Pharm Assoc.* 2008;48(3):e55–e63.
25. Bashir D, Reed-schrader E, Olympia RP, et al. Clinical symptoms and adverse effects associated with energy drink consumption in adolescents. *Pediatr Emerg Care.* 2016;32(11):751–755.
26. Kim SY, Sim S, Choi HG. High stress, lack of sleep, low school performance, and suicide attempts are associated with high energy drink intake in adolescents. *PLoS One.* 2017;12 (11):e0187759.
27. Basurto ona X, Osorio D, Bonfill cosp X. Drug therapy for treating post-dural puncture headache. *Cochrane Database Syst Rev.* 2015;7:CD007887.
28. Han ME, Kim HJ, Lee YS, et al. Regulation of cerebrospinal fluid production by caffeine consumption. *BMC Neurosci.* 2009;10:110.

Activity/exercise including yoga ☆

23

Samantha Lee Irwin, MB BCh, MS

Exercise and headache

Management of migraine is complex, and involves both lifestyle modification measures, and pharmacotherapy options to manage acute attacks and prevent future attacks. As part of the multidisciplinary treatment approach for migraine, exercise is frequently recommended.[1–4] In a critical review published in 2008, exercise as a therapy for migraine was graded as evidence level B-C.[1]

Individuals with migraine have been shown to be less physically active. In a large study ($n=48,713$) physical inactivity was noted in 68.4%–68.7% of patients with migraine, compared to 63.6% of patients without migraine.[5] Patients with migraine also seem to have a reduced aerobic capacity. A survey-based study looking at patients with headache versus control patients ($n=58$) found a significant reduction in aerobic endurance in migraine patients and significantly higher body fat in female migraineurs compared to controls.[6]

Obesity is associated with headache and migraine and is felt to be a negative prognostic marker in the development of chronic migraine.[7] In a prospective cross-sectional study in adolescents ($n=273$), overweight females had a 4-fold greater risk of headache when compared to normal weight females.[8] A further study in pediatrics ($n=913$) showed that body mass index (BMI) was associated with both headache frequency and disability and that weight loss was associated with a reduction in headache frequency.[9] The association between obesity and chronic headache was duplicated in two further adolescent studies, a retrospective cross-sectional study ($n=925$)[10] and a prospective study ($n=3342$).[11] A retrospective cross-sectional trial in adults ($n=181$) noted that obesity was specifically a risk factor for migraine, not tension type headache, and that obesity seemed to be related to both the frequency and disability of headache.[12] In a small trial of adolescents with migraine on the ketogenic diet and with weight loss, a significant 50-point reduction in PedMIDAS scores, a measure of disability, was observed.[13] A further prospective cross-sectional study in adolescents ($n=135$) found that weight loss led to improvement of migraine. In obese adolescents with migraine who participated in a 12-month

---

☆ Editor's note: Exercise is another potentially modifiable behavior that may help headache frequency. Certainly regular exercise is good for overall health.

Pediatric Headache. https://doi.org/10.1016/B978-0-323-83005-8.00008-2

long intervention for weight loss, a significant reduction in both adiposity and head-ache was noted at the 6-month mark and maintained throughout the second 6 months. Better migraine outcomes appeared to be associated with the percent change in BMI. In this trial, the exercise 'prescribed' included 60 min of moderate intensity activity, preferably daily, in addition to a balanced diet and cognitive behavioral therapy (CBT). In addition to the significant changes in adiposity, BMI, and headaches fre-quency, there were also improvements noted in headache intensity, PedMIDAS scores and the use of acute medications.[14]

Physical inactivity has been shown to be associated with an increased prevalence of future migraine. In a large longitudinal trial ($n=22,397$) over an 11-year period, low physical activity was associated with higher prevalence of migraine and nonmi-graine headache, and there was also a linear trend showing that higher prevalence of 'low physical activity' was associated with increased headache frequency.[5] A more recent study ($n=3,124$) noted that, in women only, those with <30 min of exercise per week had a 60% higher risk of later developing migraine.[15] A further study ($n=148$) noted that the risk of migraine was 4.4-fold higher in those with low physical activity (defined as <30 min of moderate intensity exercise on most days) versus those with high levels of physical activity (1 h per day or more).[16] When looking at VO2-peak by ergospirometry as an index of physical fitness in adults ($n=3899$), an inverse relationship was observed whereby a higher level of phys-ical fitness was associated with reduced migraine prevalence.[17] Interestingly, in the same study, those with the lowest VO2-peak quintile had the strongest asso-ciation for experiencing migraine aggravated by physical activity. This might sug-gest that exercise is a trigger for migraine only in those with low baseline physical fitness levels. In a more recent study by the same group, a sample of 15,276 adults were followed over an 11-year period. During this study, those with 1–3 h of "low intensity" physical exercise per week had a 22% lower risk of developing migraine compared to inactivity. Those with 1–2 h of "hard intensity" physical exercise per week had a 29% lower risk of developing migraine.[18] Finally, in ado-lescents ($n=1260$), a prospective study noted that in those with a low-level met-abolic exercise, there was a 4.2-fold higher risk of migraine when compared to those with a higher level of metabolic exercise. Using a different study popula-tion, a 2002 study was completed in 791 division one (D1) basketball players in the USA and found that the prevalence of migraine (2.9% overall, 0.9% of men, 4.4% of women) in this very active cohort was less than that of the general population.[19]

Multiple studies have shown that the regular practice of exercise is associated with a reduction in headache frequency, duration, intensity, and improvement in overall wellbeing, quality of life, cognitive outcomes, and improved mood. A few early trials noted that migraines decreased as VO2 max, a measure of fitness, increased,[20] that pain severity improved as VO2 max increased[21] and that all of fre-quency, intensity, and duration of headaches improved as cardiovascular fitness increased.[21] Using chemiluminescence to analyze plasma nitric oxide, adult women with migraine ($n=40$) were nonrandomly placed in the exercise group (1 h of aerobic exercise three times weekly) or the standard of care group. Those in the exercise group showed a significant reduction in pain severity scores (measured using the Visual Analogue Score, VAS), migraine frequency, duration, and improved quality of life. The authors postulated that the improvement might be mediated by the increased production of nitric oxide with regular exercise.[22] Further work looking at beta endorphin levels in patients with migraine ($n=40$) found a reduction in migraine frequency, duration, and intensity in association with an increase beta endorphin levels both acutely and after 6 weeks of exercise. The correlation between beta endorphins and the headache parameters was difficult to ascertain from the data, but the authors note that, curiously, those with low preexercise beta endorphin levels appeared to have the greatest improvement in headache parameters post exercise, and also that those with lower beta endorphin levels seem to have longer duration of headaches.[23] In adults with episodic migraine ($n=48$) randomized into either high intensity training (HIT), moderate continuous exercise training (MCT) or usual activities (control group) for a 12-week program, it was shown that both types of exercise lead to a reduction of migraines. HIT seemed to be most effective (-63% of attacks) vs MCT (-26% of attacks). HIT also seemed to be more beneficial for retinal vasculature outcomes, which was used as a measure of cerebrovascular health.[24]

Other trials have emphasized improvement in measures beyond headache parameters. In adult patients ($n=30$) randomized to aerobic exercise in addition to standard medical care or standard medical care only, a significant reduction in migraine pain intensity was noted after the 6-week intervention and also a trend towards improved depression-related symptoms was found with the use of exercise.[25] Others have noted that in adult patients with migraine ($n=26$), an exercise program consisting of aerobic exercise for 40 min, 3 times a week for 12 weeks not only led to a reduction in migraine days (7.5 at baseline to 5.4 days per month in month 3), migraine intensity and the use of acute medications, but also to an increase in quality of life.[26] Most importantly, in this specific trial, the exercise program was well tolerated, and no patients noted deterioration in their migraine status after commencing the exercise program. In medical students ($n=480$), a survey study noted that those who were physically active had less functional disability, as measured by the PedMIDAS, from their migraine headaches.[27] In migraineurs with coexisting tension type headache (TTH) and/or neck pain ($n=52$) randomized into aerobic exercise (45 min 3 days a week for 3 months) versus controls, the within group outcomes at 6 months revealed a reduction in migraine days in the exercise group in those with migraine. More specifically, in those with chronic migraine, headache frequency reduced from 16 to 9 days and in those with episodic migraine, from 7 to 5 days. There was also a within group reduction for migraine duration, pain intensity and neck pain. Quality of life and ability to engage in activities also improved between groups leading to a significant reduction in 'migraine burden' in the exercise group.[28] Finally, in addition, to migraine frequency reduction, a further trial showed that exercise therapy also led to improved cognitive function (information processing and attention) in migraineurs versus controls.[29]

When compared to standard of care therapeutics for migraine, exercise appears to be at least noninferior to pharmaceutical treatments and potentially additive. In a 3-arm trial looking at adults with episodic migraine ($n=91$), submaximal exercise (3 times a week for 3 months) was compared to topiramate (to the highest tolerated dose, with a maximum dose of 200 mg/day) or relaxation. All interventions were found to be equivalent with regards to their ability to reduce headache frequency, but adverse events only occurred in the topiramate group.[30] In a subsequent treatment trial in adults with chronic migraine ($n=60$), amitriptyline (25 mg/day) used in combination with aerobic exercise therapy lead to a superior reduction in headache frequency, duration, intensity, and depression and anxiety scores when compared to amitriptyline used alone.[31]

There are, however, some studies that either have shown negative or nonconclusive results with regards to the interaction between exercise and migraine and have also noted that exercise may trigger pain in some patients. The lifetime prevalence of exercise triggering a migraine in patients with migraine was 38% in one study ($n=108$)[32] and 22% in another large prospective study ($n=1207$).[33] Interestingly, a further study seemed to find an association between the baseline attack frequency of migraine and the risk of developing an attack post exercise in patients with migraine ($n=14$).[34] It also appears that migraine may co-exist with primary exertional headache (PEH) in 6.2% 30% of patients with migraine.[35–37] Importantly, despite the possible triggering of attacks in patients with migraine doing exercise initially, this effect appears to lessen with time, and one author has noted that a 'tolerance' to the possible pain-inducing effects of moderate exercise may develop with time.[38]

When looking at large scale reviews, systematic reviews, and metanalyses, it appears, however, that the overall effect of exercise in migraine is favorable. In a recent review paper looking at exercise and migraine, the conclusion was given that "*although exercise can trigger migraines, regular exercise may have a prophylactic effect on migraine frequency.*"[39] Furthermore, a systematic review concluded that there was strong evidence for the absence of adverse events following exercise and strong evidence that exercise can lower headache intensity, frequency, and duration of pain in those with tension type headache.[40] A further systematic review and meta- analysis concluded that despite having a "low" level of evidence, aerobic exercise had a significant effect on reducing migraine intensity and frequency after removal of studies with so called "high risk of bias domains."[41] The grade of evidence given for exercise as a therapy in migraine was B—C in an earlier critical review.[1] But, in a recent 2018 review, aerobic exercise of moderate intensity for >40 min, 3 times a week for use in migraine prevention was recommended, as it can lead to considerable improvement in migraine frequency, severity, duration, and improvement of quality of life.[42] Finally, a systematic review and meta-analysis from 2019 found moderate quality evidence that aerobic exercise treatment in migraine leads to on average a reduction of 0.6 ± 0.3 migraine days/month.[43]

How exercise improves headache is poorly understood, but postulated mechanisms include decreased peripheral sensitization and activation of the descending inhibitory pain pathway;[44] increased production of beta-endorphins,[23,45] which is known to be lower in those with migraine,[46] specifically chronic migraine;[47] changes in blood nitric oxide (NO) levels;[22] modulation of the endocannabinoid system,[48–51] known to be dysfunctional in migraine patients;[52,53] and finally through up-regulation brain-derived neurotrophic factor (BDNF) after exercise.[54] Likewise, the mechanisms for why pain may be triggered by exercise in migraine are also poorly understood, but might include the release of hypocretin from the hypothalamus post exercise,[32] the increase in lactate with intense exercise[55] or the possible release of CGRP with exercise.[56]

Yoga and headache

Yoga has been shown to be an effective therapy for headache and migraine. In a randomized control trial in adults ($n=72$) assigned to 1 h of yoga 5 days a week versus self-care, a significant reduction in migraine frequency was noted in those practicing yoga (10.22 ± 2.59 to 4.56 ± 1.79 days per month) vs controls (9.82 ± 2.31 to 10.18 ± 2.14, $P < 0.001$). There is also a significant reduction in pain intensity and duration.[57] In a trial in adults with migraine ($n=60$) looking at the combination of a bio-purification process known as "Ayurvedic" followed by yoga for 3 months compared to standard symptomatic treatment, it was noted that both quality of life and headache intensity significantly improved.[58] In a further randomized control trial in adults with chronic tension type headache (CTTH) ($n=23$), temporalis EMG muscle recordings were analyzed 4 weeks after a 7 week therapeutic course of yoga versus symptomatic acute treatment with NSAIDs and versus botulinum toxin treatment (50–60 unites divided into 10–12 equal doses over "tender points"). Pain score were noted to be reduced using the VAS in those using NSAID acute treatment and yoga, but not in the Botox group. Temporalis EMG recordings, that were noted to be higher at rest in those with CTTH versus controls, showed a significant reduction after the yoga intervention.[59] In a trial of female migraineurs ($n=32$), a 12-week program of yoga (3 sessions a week for 75 min each) was compared to medication only. Headache frequency, severity, and functional impact decreased in the yoga group as compared to the medication only group.[60] There is limited data for the use of yoga in pediatrics, but a pilot program of 8 weekly 75-min yoga sessions was performed and importantly concluded feasibility and acceptability of such a paradigm in this age group.[61] Finally, in a meta-analysis on yoga for pain, a moderate effect was noted for reducing chronic pain intensity.[62]

Other trials have looked to assess both efficacy and the possible mechanism for why yoga might be effective in migraine and headache. In adult patients with and without migraine aura ($n=60$), yoga therapy (5 days a week for 6 weeks) versus conventional care not only reduced headache frequency, intensity, and disability (using the HIT-6 score), but it also led to enhanced vagal tone and decreased sympathetic tone. Regulation of autonomic tone is postulated to be one of the reasons by yoga is effective in patients with migraine.[63] In a further trial, of adults with migraine ($n = 42$), practicing yoga was associated with a significant decrease in plasma vascular cell adhesion molecule (VCAM), which is possibly a marker of improved cerebrovascular health.[64]

In conclusion, both aerobic exercise and yoga seem be well tolerated for headache, specifically migraine. Data supports that both may offer preventive benefit with regards to headache frequency, intensity, and duration and may improve measures of quality of life. Data also supports that there is limited evidence to suggest that headache will worsen with the commencement of a regular exercise program and if it does, this worsening may habituate over time.

References

1. Busch V, Gaul C. Exercise in migraine therapy- is there any evidence for efficacy? A critical review. *Headache*. 2008;48(6):890–899.
2. Linde M. Migraine: a review and future directions for treatment. *Acta Neurol Scand*. 2006;114:71–83.
3. Mathew N, Tfelt-Hansen P. General and pharmacologic approach to migraine management. In: Olesen J, Tfelt-Hansen P, Welch KMA, eds. *The Headaches*. Philadelphia, PA: Lippincott Williams & Wilkins; 2006:433–440.
4. Silberstein SD. Considerations for management of migraine symptoms in the primary care setting. *Postgrad Med*. 2016;128:523–537.
5. Varkey E, Hagen K, Zwart JA, Linde M. Physical activity and headache: results from the Nord-Trondelag health study (HUNT). *Cephalalgia*. 2008;28:1292–1297.
6. Neususs K, Neumann B, Steinhoff BJ, Thegeder H, Bauer A, Reimers D. Physical activity and fitness in patients with headache disorders. *Int J Sports Med*. 1997;18:607–611.
7. Bigal ME, Lipton RB, Holland PR, Goadsby PJ. Obesity, migraine, and chronic migraine: possible mechanisms of interaction. *Neurology*. 2007;68(21):1851–1861.
8. Pinhas-Hamiel O, Frumin K, Gabis L, et al. Headache in overweight children and adolescents referred to a tertiary-care center in Israel. *Obesity*. 2008;16(3):659–663.
9. Hershey AD, Powers SW, Nelson TD, et al. Obesity in the pediatric headache population: a multicenter study. *Headache*. 2009;49:170–177.
10. Pakalnis A, Kring D. Chronic daily headache, medication overuse, and obesity in children and adolescents. *J Child Neurol*. 2012;27(5):577–580.
11. Lu SR, Fuh JL, Wang SJ, et al. Incidence and risk factors of chronic daily headache in young adolescents: a school cohort study. *Pediatrics*. 2013;132(1):e9–e16.
12. Ravid S, Shahar E, Schiff A, Gordon S. Obesity in children with headaches: association with headache type, frequency and disability. *Headache*. 2013;53(6):954–961.
13. Kossoff ED, Huffman J, Turner Z, Gladstein J. Use of the modified Atkins diet for adolescents with chronic daily headache. *Cephalalgia*. 2010;30(8):1014–1016.
14. Verrotti A, Agostinelli S, D'Egigio C, et al. Impact of a weight loss program on migraine in obese adolescents. *Eur J Neurol*. 2013;20:394–397.
15. Lebedeva ER, Kobzeva NR, Gilev DV, et al. Factors associated with primary headache according to diagnosis, sex, and social group. *Headache*. 2016;56:341–356.

16. Krøll LS, Hammarlund CS, Westergaard ML, et al. Level of physical activity, well-being, stress and self-rated health in persons with migraine and co-existing tension-type headache and neck pain. *J Headache Pain*. 2017;18:46.

17. Hagen K, Wisloff U, Ellingsen O, et al. Headache and peak oxygen uptake: the HUNT3 study. *Cephalalgia*. 2016;36:437–444.

18. Hagen K, Asberg AN, Stovner L, et al. Lifestyle factors and risk of migraine and tension-type headache. Follow-up data from the Nord-Trondelag Health Surveys 1995–1997 and 2006–2008. *Cephalalgia*. 2018;333102418764888 [Epub ahead of print].

19. Kinart CM, Cuppett MM, Berg K. Prevalence of migraines in NCAA division I male and female basketball players. National Collegiate Athletic Association. *Headache*. 2002;42:620–629.

20. Grimm L, Douglas D, Hanson P. Aerobic training in the prophylaxis of migraine. *Med Sci Sports Exerc*. 1981;13:98.

21. Lockett DM, Campbell JF. The effects of aerobic exercise on migraine. *Headache*. 1992;32(1):50–54.

22. Narin SO, Pinar L, Erbas D, Oztürk V, Idman F. The effects of exercise and exercise-related changes in blood nitric oxide level on migraine headache. *Clin Rehabil*. 2003;17(6):624–630.

23. Köseoglu E, Akboyraz A, Soyuer A, Ersoy AO. Aerobic exercise and plasma beta endorphin levels in patients with migrainous headache without aura. *Cephalalgia*. 2003;23 (10):972–976.

24. Hanssen H, Minghetti A, Magon S, et al. Superior effects of high-intensity interval training vs. moderate continuous training on arterial stiffness in episodic migraine: a randomized controlled trial. *Front Physiol*. 2017;8:1086.

25. Dittrich SM, Gunther V, Franz G, Burtscher M, Holzner B, Kopp M. Aerobic exercise with relaxation: influence on pain and psychological well-being in female migraine patients. *Clin J Sport Med*. 2008;18(4):363–365.

26. Varkey E, Sider A, Carlsson J, Linde M. A study to evaluate the feasibility of an aerobic exercise program in patients with migraine. *Headache*. 2009;49(4):563–570.

27. Domingues RB, Teixeira AL, Domingues SA. Physical practice is associated with functional disability in medical students with migraine. *Arq Neuropsiquiatr*. 2011;69(1):39–43.

28. Kroll LS, et al. The effects of aerobic exercise for persons with migraine and co-existing TTH and neck pain. A randomized, controlled, clinical trial. *Cephalalgia*. 2018;1–12.

29. Overath CH, Darabaneanu S, Evers MC, et al. Does an aerobic endurance programme have an influence on information processing in migraineurs? *J Headache Pain*. 2014;15:11.

30. Varkey E, Cider A, Carlsson J, et al. Exercise as migraine prophylaxis: a randomized study using relaxation and topiramate as controls. *Cephalalgia*. 2011;31:1428–1438.

31. Santiago MD, Carvalho DS, Gabbai AA, et al. Amitriptyline and aerobic exercise or amitriptyline alone in the treatment of chronic migraine: a randomized comparative study. *Arq Neuropsiquiatr*. 2014;72:851–855.

32. Koppen H, van Veldhoven PLJ. Migraineurs with exercise triggered attacks have a distinct migraine. *J Headache Pain*. 2013;14:99.

33. Kelman L. The triggers or precipitants of the acute migraine attack. *Cephalalgia*. 2007;27:394–402.

34. Varkey E, Gruner Svealv B, Edin F, et al. Provocation of migraine after maximal exercise: a test-retest study. *Eur Neurol*. 2017;78:22–27.

35. Chen SP, Fuh JL, Lu SR, Wang SJ. Exertional headache - a survey of 1963 adolescents. *Cephalalgia.* 2009;29:401–407.

36. Hanashiro S, Takazawa T, Kawase Y, Ikeda K. Prevalence and clinicalhallmarks of primary exercise headache in middle-aged Japanese on health check-up. *Intern Med.* 2015;54:2577–2581.

37. Van Der Ende-Kastelijn K, Oerlemans W, Goedegebuure S. An online survey of exercise-related headaches among cyclists. *Headache.* 2012;52:1566–1573.

38. Hindiyeh NA, Krusz JC, Cowan RP. Does exercise make migraines worse and tension type headaches better? *Curr Pain Headache Rep.* 2013;17:380.

39. Amin FM, Aristeidou S, Baraldi C, et al. The association between migraine and physical exercise. *J Headache Pain.* 2018;19:83.

40. Gil-Martínez A, Kindelan-Calvo P, et al. Therapeutic exercise as treatment for migraine and tension-type headaches: a systematic review of randomised clinical trials. *Rev Neurol.* 2013;57(10):433–443.

41. Luedtke K, Allers A, Schulte LH, et al. Efficacy of interventions used by physiotherapists for patients with headache and migraine-systematic review and meta-analysis. *Cephalalgia.* 2016;36:474–492.

42. Lippi G, Mattiuzzi C, Sanchis-Gomar. Physical Exercise and Migraine: for or against? *Ann Transl Med.* 2018;6(10):181.

43. Lemmens J, De Pauw J, Van Soom T, et al. The effect of aerobic exercise on the number of migraine days, duration and pain intensity in migraine: a systematic literature review and meta-analysis. *J Headache Pain.* 2019;20:16.

44. Fernandes-de-las-Peñas C. Physical therapy and exercise in headache. *Cephalalgia.* 2008;28(1 Suppl):S36–S38.

45. Schwarz L, Kindermann W. Beta-endorphin, adrenocorticotropic hormone, cortisol and catecholamines during aerobic and anaerobic exercise. *Eur J Appl Physiol Occup Physiol.* 1990;61:165–171.

46. Sicuteri F. Endorphins, opiate receptors and migraine headache. *Headache.* 1978;17:253–257.

47. Misra UK, Kalita J, Tripathi GM, Bhoi SK. Is β endorphin related to migraine headache and its relief? *Cephalalgia.* 2013;33:316–322.

48. Boecker H, Sprenger T, Spilker ME, et al. The runner's high: Opioidergic mechanisms in the human brain. *Cereb Cortex.* 2008;18:2523–2531.

49. Buse DC, Manack A, Serrano D, Turkel C, Lipton RB. Sociodemographic and comorbidity profiles of chronic migraine and episodic migraine sufferers. *J Neurol Neurosurg Psychiatry.* 2010;81:428–432.

50. Dietrich A, McDaniel WF. Endocannabinoids and exercise. *Br J Sports Med.* 2004;38:536–541.

51. Sparling PB, Giuffrida A, Piomelli D, Rosskopf L, Dietrich A. Exercise activates the endocannabinoid system. *Neuroreport.* 2003;14:2209–2211.

52. Perrotta A, Arce-Leal N, Tassorelli C, et al. Acute reduction of anandamide-hydrolase (FAAH) activity is coupled with a reduction of nociceptive pathways facilitation in medication-overuse headache subjects after withdrawal treatment. *Headache.* 2012;52:1350–1361.

53. Sarchielli P, Pini LA, Coppola F, et al. Endocannabinoids in chronic migraine: CSF findings suggest a system failure. *Neuropsychopharmacology.* 2007;32:1384–1390.

54. Dinoff A, Herrmann N, Swardfager W, et al. The effect of exercise training on resting concentrations of peripheral brain-derived neurotrophic factor (BDNF): a meta-analysis. *PLoS One.* 2016;11:e0163037.

55. Watanabe H, Kuwabara T, Ohkubo M, Tsuji S, Yuasa T. Elevation of cerebral lactate detected by localized 1H-magnetic resonance spectroscopy in migraine during the inter-ictal period. *Neurology*. 1996;47:1093–1095.

56. Jonhagen S, Ackermann P, Saartok T, Renstrom PA. Calcitonin gene related peptide and neuropeptide Y in skeletal muscle after eccentric exercise: a micro-dialysis study. *Br J Sports Med*. 2006;40:264–267.

57. John PJ, Sharma N, Sharma CM, Kankane A. Effectiveness of yoga therapy in the treatment of migraine without aura: a randomized controlled trial. *Headache*. 2007; 47:654–661.

58. Sharma VM, Manjunath NK, Nagendra HR, Ertsey C. Combination of ayurveda and yoga therapy reduces pain intensity and improves quality of life in patients with migraine headache. *Complement Ther Clin Pract*. 2018;32:85–91.

59. Bhatia R, Dureja GP, Tripathi M, Bhattacharjee M, Bijlani RL, Mathur R. Role of temporalis muscle over activity in chronic tension type headache: effect of yoga-based management. *Indian J Physiol Pharmacol*. 2007;357:333–344.

60. Boroujeni MZ, Marandi SM, Esfarjani F, Sattar M, Shaygannejad V, Javanmard SH. Yoga intervention on blood NO in female migraineurs. *Adv Biomed Res*. 2015;4:259.

61. Hainsworth KR, Salamon KS, Khan KA, et al. A pilot study of yoga for chronic headaches in youth: promise amidst challenges. *Pain Manag Nurs*. 2014;15(2):490–498.

62. Bussing A, Ostermann T, Ludtke R, Michalsen A. Effects of yoga interventions on pain and pain-associated disability: a meta-analysis. *J Pain*. 2012;357:1–9.

63. Kisan R, Sujan M, Adoor M, et al. Effect of yoga on migraine: a comprehensive study using clinical profile and cardiac autonomic functions. *Int J Yoga*. 2014;357:126–132.

64. Naji-Esfahani H, Zamani M, Marandi SM, Shaygannejad V, Javanmard SH. Preventive effects of a three-month yoga intervention on endothelial function in patients with migraine. *Int J Prev Med*. 2014;5(4):424–429.

Managing migraine at school

24

Elizabeth K. Rende, DNP, FAANP and Scott B. Turner, DNP, FNP-C

Myth busters

Though the myth that "children don't get migraine" was debunked many years ago, it remains a common misperception among the general public, in many schools, and even with healthcare providers. The truth is that migraine in children and adolescents is even more common than asthma, yet a lack of understanding often leads to a delay in diagnosis, ineffective treatment, and needless disability.[1] It is important to teach yourself, your child, and your child's teachers and coaches about migraine, and help them learn how to prevent and manage your child's headaches.

Here are some suggestions to help your child or teen:

- Share your child's migraine diagnosis with the school nurse. The nurse may have you complete special forms to allow staff to give your child headache medicine while at school.
- Share your child's migraine diagnosis with their teacher(s). This can be done at the beginning of the school year when you first meet their teacher(s) or after a visit to your health provider. Make sure their teacher(s) know the importance of prompt migraine treatment and ask them to allow your child to drink water and use the restroom periodically throughout the day.
- Share your child's migraine diagnosis with all those who will be working with your child after school. This might include their coach, band director, and afterschool care provider.
- Make sure your child has a written action plan to tell caregivers what to do to treat their headaches at home, school, and at afterschool activities.
- Encourage your child to tell their teacher right when a headache begins.

☆Editor's note: One of the tasks of childhood is to be successful at school. Having migraines poses a challenge in the school setting. Setting expectations with teacher, coach, nurse, and family will help the youngster be successful. This chapter offers practical ways to help families negotiate the school setting to optimize outcomes for their child with migraines. It includes self-efficacy and words to use to get the job done.

Pediatric Headache. https://doi.org/10.1016/B978-0-323-83005-8.00001-X

After the school bell rings...

Parents rely on school staff to be watchful and to care for their children while they are at school. It is the goal of all school nurses to keep students healthy and "ready to learn." A migraine headache that goes untreated can certainly be a hindrance to learning. Unfortunately, children with migraine miss twice as many school days each year as their healthy peers.[2]

When a migraine strikes, your child needs to take their medication right away. While laws will vary, all states have strict regulations about how medications are to be dispensed to children while attending a public school. Medication administration policies are also created by local school districts or county education boards. The school nurse, school staff, parents, and providers must follow these rules to make sure your child has quick access to their medication when needed. Afterschool programs housed in schools or at other organizations will often require the same written permission to administer medications to your child.

Key players at school include your child's teacher(s), school nurse, unlicensed assistive personnel (UAP), and other staff such as coaches, trainers, administrative staff, food workers, and bus drivers. Remember these individuals form a team of caring people who want what's best for your child.

- The school nurse practices under a license issued by their state's Board of Nursing. Since the school nurse must often cover more than one school, they may "delegate" the responsibility to treat your child's headache to a UAP.
- UAPs are school staff members who have received some additional training to allow them to give medications and other health-related treatments when the nurse is not physically in the building. The UAP cannot make a diagnosis or medical decision; they are only allowed to follow the instructions the nurse has written in a child's health plan.
- Coaches, extracurricular teachers and support staff should also be aware of the health needs of a child with migraine.

Your child's health history is considered private, so the information shared with school personnel and extracurricular staff can be limited to the information *you* want shared. These same individuals are required to keep your child's health information private, except when that information is necessary to properly care for your child.

Empowering your child

Your child or teen needs to learn how to manage their headaches when you are not around. Teach your child to advocate for themselves. Starting with their first headache, your child should be encouraged to alert a parent, teacher, or coach at the very beginning of their headache symptoms. For the younger child who may be shy, a special hand signal or "hall pass" might be a good way for your child to tell their teacher they are getting a headache.

Next, your child will need a plan for treating headaches that start at school or during afterschool activities. This plan needs to be age and developmentally appropriate and tailored to their specific symptoms and individual needs. We recommend using the Pediatric Migraine Action Plan (PedMAP) as a template to create a customized plan for managing your child's headaches.[3] This tool was designed by pediatric headache specialists from the U.S. and Canada to guide you, your child, their healthcare provider, coaches, and school caregivers in preventing and responding to headaches both within and outside the home. The plan was designed to match the stoplight format of an asthma action plan with a green zone that tells your child what to do to prevent their headaches, a yellow zone that tells them what actions to take when a headache starts and what to do next if that isn't working, and a red zone with next steps if the treatment plan isn't working.

Your child should learn more about migraine and what she can do to prevent them. One of our favorite websites for learning about headaches is www.head achereliefguide.com.[4] This website was developed by a multidisciplinary team of headache specialists to help children and their families learn about what causes headaches, what actions can be taken to prevent them, and how to treat headaches more effectively.

The perfect scenario...

Your child reports their headache right away to their teacher, who sends them to the health office. The school nurse or their delegated UAP reviews the PedMAP on file and gives your child their quick-relief medication (that you have provided in a container labeled by the pharmacy). They are allowed some time to rest in a quiet place for 30–45 min (allowing time for the medication to work). Your child soon feels better, their headache has resolved, and they return to the classroom ready to learn.

A word about homebound, home-schooled, and online education

If your child has been or will be unable to attend school for an extended period of time, school officials may recommend a homebound education program. Homebound programs are temporary measures to try to ensure that a child does not fall too far behind while recovering from a single period of illness. This is not the scenario for children and adolescents with migraine who will likely experience recurrent headaches for several years. Students on homebound education usually receive instruction from a licensed teacher for about 5–10 h a week.[5] A homebound teacher can only cover a few lessons from a small number of core subjects. High school students using this program for more than a few weeks may find it difficult to earn the credits they need to graduate on time. These short-term solutions are simply insufficient to allow them to keep up with their schoolwork.

Some families consider home-schooling or online education when their child is struggling to attend school. Both options offer some advantages over the traditional school setting (e.g., flexible scheduling, self-pacing, and individualized curriculum). It is important to consider your child's personality and level of motivation. Parents of highly motivated children often report that online schooling works well for their family; however, other parents describe an ongoing struggle to keep their child engaged and on task. Children in pain can find it hard to find the motivation to get out of bed in the morning and get to work. They may struggle to wake up at their usual time and may find themselves napping throughout the day, staying up later at night, and unintentionally changing their body's sleep-wake cycle. They often let their pain level dictate their activity level; they become less active, their bodies become deconditioned, and they begin to feel bad every time they try to move. They begin to avoid moving, avoid working, and avoid thinking because all of this makes them feel worse. Obviously, this becomes counterproductive and can produce a downward spiral of increasing disability.

School health plans and 504 accommodations

In a nutshell, students with migraine must learn how to function in spite of their pain. So how are they going to survive and make the best of it? Attending school with some strategic accommodations may be a better answer. For most children and teens with migraine or recurrent headaches, the Pediatric Migraine Action Plan (PedMAP) should be sufficient to assure your child receives their acute medication(s) promptly and that school staff provide some reasonable allowances to keep them functioning at school despite their pain and other symptoms. The PedMAP provides some specific strategies you can review with school officials to tailor an individual health plan that works well for your child and all involved in their care. For example, a health plan for a student with migraine may allow them to eat a snack or drink from a water bottle periodically to prevent migraines. Light- and sound-sensitive students might be allowed to wear dark glasses or work in a quiet spot when their headaches are severe. A student managing a severe headache might be allowed to work in the library or media center for part of the school day or given an alternative PE activity such as yoga, stretching, progressive muscle relaxation, deep breathing, or other relaxation exercises while their headache is severe.

Students whose frequent headaches "substantially limit" their ability to receive an appropriate education may qualify for specific accommodations under Section 504 of the Rehabilitation Act of 1973.[6] A 504 Plan is a formal process that adjusts school services to meet the needs of a child with a mental or physical impairment that is limiting them from full participation at school. Students whose headaches severely limit their ability to concentrate may be given additional time to complete assignments. Students who miss school for doctor appointments or CBT (Cognitive Behavioral Therapy) sessions might be allowed extended time to turn in their assignments. Sometimes, severely affected students who are falling behind can be given a reduced workload or abbreviated schedule to allow them some time to recover. Students returning to school after a prolonged absence might be allowed to turn in a smaller number of key assignments to show that they have mastered the content. Here is how the 504 process works:

- Any concerned person (e.g., a parent, counselor, or healthcare provider) can refer a student for evaluation
- If the school shares their concern, a review committee (often called a 504 team) is assembled
- The 504 team will consider information from a variety of sources (e.g., medical diagnosis, school performance, attendance records, teachers' reports, etc.)
- The 504 team will determine which accommodations your child needs in order to have an equal opportunity to compete successfully when compared with their nondisabled peers
- If the school refuses to provide a 504 plan or if you disagree with the team's recommendations, you can request a due process hearing or file a complaint with the Office of Civil Rights
- You can learn more about your rights under Section 504 by visiting http://www2. ed.gov/about/offices/list/ocr/index.html.

Private schools are not required to create 504 Plans but may follow a similar process to grant accommodations.

Pace yourself

We have found that many teens with migraines are high-achievers. With so much pressure from school, sports, and extracurricular activities, their busy schedules can lead to late nights with not enough sleep. Lack of sleep can be a potent stressor on the brain and trigger headaches. Daytime headaches can make it more difficult for them to concentrate and take longer to complete their work. With little flexibility in their schedules and a low tolerance for a dip in performance, the high-achiever can quickly become overwhelmed. This added stress makes it even harder for them to sleep, harder to concentrate, and harder to maintain their high level of performance. All of this can trigger even more headaches and lead to more stress. It becomes a vicious cycle. Here is some advice to guide them:

- Consider scaling back on academic and extracurricular activities
- Encourage your child to strive for fulfilling goals, not perfection
- Create a realistic schedule and build in some down time
- Think about ways to advocate for these changes on a group rather than individual scale—does every teen at your school need to take 8 AP classes and play on multiple travel teams?

A message to kids about returning to school...

This is hard, but you can do it. Because you have been brave, you will find that you will be stronger and better-equipped for handling hard things that come up in the future. Pace yourself. Don't let how you feel dictate your schedule; but be realistic about the limitations your headaches impose on you. Going to school for part of the day is better than not going at all. Reduce your workload. Build in break periods. Wear sunglasses or polarized lenses when light is bothering you. You may be able to use ear plugs or wear headphones when noise is really bothering you. Find quiet areas to eat and to work. Sometimes the school library or media center is a good option for quiet self-paced study. Though being overly active can worsen your headaches, a lack of activity will decondition your body and make you feel even worse. Try to find a balance in rest, school, work, friends, and activities. Be sure you are doing something in each of these areas of your life. Don't let your headaches define you. They aren't the boss of you—you are. Be a fair boss. Be kind to yourself. Don't expect more than you can do, but don't accept anything less than your best from you. This is hard, but you can do it. You are brave.

Summary

Migraines are common in children and adolescents and it should not be surprising that children commonly experience migraines at school. The Pediatric Migraine Action Plan (PedMAP) is a great tool to give school nurses, teachers, and coaches the instructions they need to help your child properly manage their headaches at school and on the ball field. Homebound programs cannot provide an adequate education for students with recurrent headaches. Online programs can offer more flexibility, but parents should be careful not to let how their child feels dictate their schedule. Creating a health plan with your child's school nurse is usually the best option to reduce some of the headache-related challenges they face at school. A 504 plan may be needed when frequent migraines "severely limit" your child's ability to function properly at school. With a good plan and reasonable accommodations, your child can learn to manage their headaches outside your home and be better prepared to handle other challenges in life.

For primary care and specialty providers

Migraine is among the world's most disabling conditions, and youth with migraine are at risk for developing lifelong disability.[7] A primary goal of headache care is to enable youth with migraine to attend school regularly and to function optimally despite their headaches and associated symptoms. While fewer than 50% of youth with headache report having seen a primary care provider or specialist in the past year, children with headaches commonly visit the school nurse or health office.[8]

In fact, data collected from a large suburban school district found that 33% of all students had at least one visit to the school nurse for headache, and 7% of students made at least eight headache-related visits during the school year.[9] Students lacking a management plan are often sent back to class with a lowered ability to function or sent home from school. Students who miss as few as two days of school a month are at risk for chronic absenteeism which has been linked to poor school performance, high school dropout, and adverse economic and health outcomes in adulthood.[10]

As such, it is essential that youth with migraine are identified quickly and given the necessary tools to effectively manage their headaches at school. School nurses are well-positioned to identify and refer students with migraine before they become disabled by the condition. The Pediatric and Adolescent Migraine Screen (PAMS) is a three-item screening tool with excellent sensitivity that can be used in school settings to identify students with migraine.[11,12,a] Once identified, youth with migraine need an effective action plan and permission to take acute medication(s) while at school. We recommend the Pediatric Migraine Action Plan (PedMAP) as an efficient way to communicate this plan to parents, teachers, coaches, school nurses, and health aides.[3]

Students with recurring headaches should be counseled to avoid missing school as this leads directly to increased disability. Instead, they should be equipped and encouraged to manage their headaches at school. An Individualized Health Plan or a 504 Plan can be used to allow a student with migraine the accommodations needed to enable them to stay at school while managing their headaches. Not only is an acute medication strategy essential, but nonmedical interventions can also increase their functional capacity. Relaxation strategies such as mindfulness, diaphragmatic breathing, and progressive muscle relaxation can improve their ability to cope with pain. Permitting a child experiencing migraine to wear dark glasses or work in a quiet room might enable them to continue their schoolwork. Allowing an alternative PE activity or additional time to make up missed work may mitigate some of the physical and psychological stress that can perpetuate headaches. Prevention strategies such as increased water intake, scheduled snack breaks, and wearing light-filtering lenses in brightly lit classrooms or while working on a computer can also be included in such a plan. A sample 504 plan request letter is included in the appendix.

Appendix: Supplementary material

Supplementary material related to this chapter can be found on the accompanying CD or online at https://doi.org/10.1016/B978-0-323-83005-8.00001-X.

---

[a]The Pediatric and Adolescent Migraine Screen (PAMS) is available to download at https:/www.cincinnatichildrens.org/service/h/headache-center/pams.

References

1. American Migraine Foundation. *Why Migraine in Children Is Oftentimes Overlooked, Misdiagnosed and Left Untreated*; 2018 [Retrieved 9/15/19 at:] https://americanmigrainefoundation.org/resource-library/understanding-pediatric-migraine/.
2. Migraine Research Foundation. About Migraine Migraine Facts; 2021. Retrieved at: https://migraineresearchfoundation.org/about-migraine/migraine-facts/ (15 June 2021).
3. Turner S, Rende E, Pezzuto T, et al. Pediatric migraine action plan (PedMAP). *Headache.* 2019;59:1871–1873.
4. Bickel J, Connelly M. *Headache Relief Guide website*; 2021. http://www.headachereliefguide.com/. Accessed 21 June 2021.
5. South Bend Community School Corporation Special Education Services. *Homebound Students*; 2018 [Retrieved 9/15/19 at] http://www.sped.sbcsc.k12.in.us/ppm/homebound.html#medical.
6. GreatSchools.org. *A Parent's Guide to Section 504 in Public Schools*; 2019 [Retrieved 9/28/19 at] https://www.greatschools.org/gk/articles/section-504-2/.
7. GBD 2015 Neurological Disorders Collaborators Group. Global, regional, and national burden of neurological disorders during 1990–2015: a systematic analysis for the Global Burden of Disease Study 2015. *Lancet Neurol.* 2017;16(11):877–897.
8. Lipton RB, Serrano D, Holland S, Fanning KM, Reed ML, Buse DC. Barriers to the diagnosis and treatment of migraine: effects of sex, income, and headache features. *Headache.* 2013;53(1):81–92. https://doi.org/10.1111/j.1526-4610.2012.02265.x.
9. Connelly M, Bickel J, Wingert T, Galemore C. The headache action plan project for youth (HAPPY): school nurses as facilitators of system change in pediatric migraine care. *NASN Sch Nurse.* 2018;33(1):40–47.
10. Allison MA, Attisha E, Council on School Health. The link between school attendance and good health. *Pediatrics.* 2019;143(2).
11. DiSabella MT, Somers MM, Chmelik EA, et al. PAMS (Pediatric and Adolescent Migraine Screen): an effective tool to identify pediatric migraine by school nurses. Abstract S54. In: *49th Annual Scientific Meeting American Headache Society June 7–11, 2007, Chicago, IL. Headache.* vol. 47; 2007:741–812. [Available at] https://www.cincinnatichildrens.org/service/h/headache-center/pams.
12. The Pediatric Migraine Assessment Screen (PAMS) Tool. Accessed 21 June 2021.

Advocacy for children with migraine ☆

25

William Young, MD and Shirley Kessel, BS

Headache expert perspective

Migraine is the most common neurological disease and, in adults, it has the largest overall impact after stroke, and the largest effect on disability.[1] Relative to its huge impact, society allocates to migraine only a small fraction of the resources it should be getting from the research community and the treatment infrastructure.[2, 3] This is in part due to the stigmatization of the headache patient and the doctors who treat them. This stigma results in low levels of advocacy relative to disease burden. Advocacy drives access to resources and policy changes that favor those with larger, more vibrant advocacy efforts.[4]

Stigma is an attitude by society that undercuts the value of the individual with a condition or disease, poisons their identity and leads to social sanction or discrimination.[5] *Social stigma* affects many diseases. *Enacted stigma* from public policies, and individual statements and attitudes become internalized and lead to a decreased sense of self-worth and eventually this can have profound mental health consequences.[6] *Disease related stigma* impairs quality of life in several ways (Table 1). It impedes the seeking of health care for the stigmatized condition, increases mental health burden, and may increase pain itself.[3,7] Many diseases and conditions have been shown to be stigmatized, for example obesity, HIV, and mental illness. Stigma is intertwined with bullying.[8]

In adults with migraine, stigma can be severe. As might be predicted for an invisible disease, stigma relates to the degree of disease-induced disability, and not to visible signs of disease.[9] In other words, migraine becomes very stigmatized when it affects functioning in performing a social responsibility, such as work in adults, and school in children. Men stigmatize people with migraine more than women, and nonwhites stigmatize more than whites.[10] Unfortunately, there is little data about

---

☆Editor's note: In this eye-opening chapter, we see why migraine has not gotten the attention it deserves. It is not enough for the good headache physician to just treat patients. (S)he must also advocate to reduce stigma and enhance awareness. Particularly moving was a multigenerational plea to get out there and make a difference. We hope that Ms. Kessel's impassioned words will empower patients and families to help change migraine from an overlooked disease to one that receives the attention and research funding it deserves.

Pediatric Headache. https://doi.org/10.1016/B978-0-323-83005-8.00005-7

Table 1 Three types of stigma.

Type of stigma	Definition	Migraine specific examples
Structural	Prejudice and discrimination by policies, laws, and constitutional practice	Lack of accommodations— leaving class, access to medication, making up tests, lack of quiet environment for learning
Public = enacted	Stereotypes, prejudice, and discrimination	"It's just a headache" from a parent, teacher, or friend "I get migraine, and I can do that" bullying
Self-stigma = internalized	Shame, low self-esteem, lack of engagement in treatment	Not seeking a diagnosis, or treatment Negative self-talk

the sources of stigmatizing attitudes encountered by children. Anecdotally many adults with migraine recall their first stigmatizing experiences in childhood. Statements from their parents, teachers and to a lesser extent their friends are recalled as hurtful and impactful in their lives.

Advocacy is public support for a cause or policy and is necessary to reverse the effects of public stigma. Parents need to advocate for their children and teach their children to advocate for themselves. Advocacy begins by educating the child and their friends and siblings about migraine, its' impacts and treatments. Then the parent advocate should consider what advocacy activities for their kids would be helpful in school, such as talking to their teachers, a 504 plan, or an individualized education plan (IEP). Efforts to educate children generically about migraine through classroom lesson plans and teaching materials may be helpful.

Successfully changing negative reactions toward a disease takes careful thought. This process, called *reframing*, requires that people with a disease, or their family members, make themselves visible, and mobilize. Successful efforts include: HIV, autism, breast cancer, and multiple sclerosis. For migraine, such efforts have not succeeded at a societal level because migraine re-branding has not mobilized the migraine community to act.

A more realistic goal is to reframe migraine for the child, the family, friends, and school. In children, there have been successful efforts to educate the community through art programs and through adolescent camps.

Minen developed, piloted, and tested the Headache and Arts Program. This 2-week Headache and Arts Program with lesson plans and art assignments for high school visual arts classes included an age-appropriate assessment to assess students' knowledge of migraine and concussion. The program improved the learners' knowledge, which they retained over 3 months. The use of a visual arts-based curriculum may be effective for migraine and concussion education among high school students.[11]

Table 2 Advocacy plan of action.

For health care providers	For caregivers/parents and kids
Turn patients and family members into migraine warriors	Learn how to become a migraine warrior
Reduce self-stigma	Reduce self-stigma through education and support groups
Advocacy in the community	Advocate at patient-participatory events
Self-advocacy	Join a support group and access education
Educate schools	Speak to school administrators, nurses, teachers, school board
Offer hope	Find like-minded support

As an outgrowth of clinical care, we developed the Miles for Migraine Youth Camp, a recurring 1-day event for adolescents with chronic headache and their parents. Migraine Camp was developed to provide expanded headache education, teach coping strategies for living with chronic pain, and encourage development of a supportive community for adolescents living with chronic headache disorders and their families. The creation and curriculum of the Camps at the University of California San Francisco and Children's Hospital of Philadelphia are described in our manuscript, along with patient and caregiver feedback. Overall, feedback was positive. Teens reported feeling less isolated and more prepared to cope with headaches using new strategies. Both patients and caregivers consistently described benefit from connecting with others who experience similar challenges. The Migraine Camp teams at both institutions found it feasible to conduct the Camps 1–2 times per year using existing resources, but noted that to scale it to a more regular event additional administrative and/or volunteer support would be needed. In summary, the experience has been positive for patients, caregivers, and staff, and we hope that this manuscript can serve as a "how to" model for similar events at other institutions.[12]

In the office setting, clinicians should make advocacy part of the treatment plan. Turning the patient's self-image from migraine sufferer or victim, to migraine warrior can improve self-efficacy. Self-advocacy involves getting the accommodations that maximizes their ability to learn, or participate in other important activities, and educating schools as well as family and friends. In some cases, directly discussing stigma and self-stigma may be helpful in reducing negative self-talk and improving self-esteem (Table 2).

Family perspective

In 1985 at age 24, I was diagnosed with chronic migraine. No one—not my doctor or any other healthcare professional—sat me down to explain the reason they were prescribing me an antiseizure medication, even though I had migraine, was because there was so little research being done in this field and there weren't any medicines specifically designed to treat this disabling disease. Over the course of a year my doctor prescribed 12 different medications—none of which worked.

Fast forward to 2013, when my daughter Sydney was diagnosed at age 16 with chronic migraine, and her doctor prescribed the same antiseizure medication I had received back in 1985. When I questioned her on this she replied, "There is nothing new for migraine." Incredulous, my daughter turned to me and said, "Mom we have to do something about this! Why am I getting the same old medication you received so long ago?"

At that moment I realized how unfairly the medical system was treating my child. Why wasn't there a medication that was derived from research specifically for migraine? The reason there are so few treatment options developed specifically for migraine is because it receives little funding for research relative to the disability it causes. Furthermore, diseases like breast cancer and HIV/AIDS received more research funding when patients began to advocate, but there were only a few options for migraine advocacy up until several years ago.

On the drive home we discussed options and decided to find a race for migraine, but to our dismay we only found one in the entire country and it was in San Francisco. When I contacted the founder of Miles For Migraine—Eileen Jones, a nurse—I asked her if I could bring the race to Philadelphia. She told me I had no idea what I was getting into and she was right. Putting a race together has more intricate moving parts than I realized and I soon understood that I was in way over my head. However, watching my daughter spend day after day in a dark room while missing school, made me fight all the harder, to bring this race to Philadelphia which we succeeded in doing in the fall of 2013.

As time prevailed, I came to realize that I would need to educate everyone I encountered since the only way to a cure is by reducing stigma, and the only way to reduce stigma was to open my mouth and make a lot of noise. Advocating requires effort yet the plus side is that advocacy made me feel more connected to others experiencing the shame, stigma, and isolation I was feeling. My daughter also felt empowered when she spoke up about her needs to school administrators.

Advocacy is a vital part of helping to find a cure for migraine and other headaches. You don't need to begin your own nonprofit to be an effective advocate, as there are plenty of ideas and resources available. Discover what works for you and your family, and then educate and enlist friends and co-workers to join you.

Advocacy plan of action

- **Share your story well**—It's vital to talk to friends, family and schools about migraine. However, speaking up about an invisible disease is often fraught with fear due to the pervasive stigma migraine receives. Do it anyway. You can learn more on how to speak about migraine by visiting the websites outlined below.

- **Get on social media**—Posting about your actions and educating others on social media is a low effort act of advocacy.
- **Attend live events**—All of the organizations in the next section offer live, patient—participatory events. It's vital to attend these because we need to make more noise and knock on the world's door so the perception of migraine changes. This is the same plan of action other stigmatized diseases took, such as HIV/AIDS, and breast cancer. Have you heard of those diseases? Yes! They began as "whisper diseases" but now they are diseases that have become the leaders in research and NIH funding. This could not have happened without advocates in the public eye.
- **Volunteer**—Every nonprofit needs help.
- **Join a support group**—As a caregiver, you need to remember to put your own oxygen mask on first. Practice self-care and serve as a role model for your child to emulate you. The organizations below offer links to online support groups and other information for helping you and your child.
- **Education**—Your time with the health care practitioner is limited, so come prepared with questions that you cannot find answers to on your own.
- **Donate**—Nonprofits are dedicated to education, research, and advocacy. They are the forces that will continue to work with patients and caregivers to help find a cure.

In summary, addressing stigma and the need for advocacy are intricately connected in migraine. Advocacy is necessary to gain necessary accommodations at the individual level, but is also important locally, in school, in the family, in the community, and nationally. Advocacy should be considered an essential part of the treatment plan. One can reasonably expect that teaching advocacy and reducing stigma can improve the child's health and prevent a life-time of self-stigmatization and the complications that follow.

Advocacy organizations
Alliance for headaches advocacy
http://allianceforheadacheadvocacy.org/what-we-can-do/

The alliance is a group of nonprofits focused on headaches, including migraine. Sign up for their email and look at their advocacy page to see if there are any "actionable" items that you may want to do such as attend the annual Headache on the Hill event.

American migraine foundation
https://americanmigrainefoundation.org/migraine-stories/

The American Migraine Foundation provides education, support, and resources for the millions of men, women, and children living with migraine. Its mission is to advance migraine research, promote patient advocacy, and expand access to care for patients worldwide. Migraine, and other disabling diseases that cause severe head pain, impact more than 37 million people in the United States alone. By educating caregivers and giving patients the tools to advocate for themselves, the American Migraine Foundation has cultivated a movement that gives a collective voice to the migraine community.

Association of migraines

www.migrainedisorders.org/get-involved

The Association of Migraine Disorders (AMD) is devoted to improving the understanding of migraine. Because migraine is a full body condition with a broad spectrum of symptoms, AMD incorporates the experience of many medical specialties in managing this disease. It has produced a comprehensive online course to accelerate the training of a broader range of medical professionals in the management of migraine. AMD supports Shades for Migraine, a playful public awareness campaign. It strives to connect and grow an integrated migraine research community. And it shares the opinions of experts in our Shades of Migraine podcasts. Buy "team" migraine merchandise to start a conversation, start a migraine club, fundraise, speak out about migraine!

CHAMP (coalition for headache and migraine patients)

https://headachemigraine.org

The Coalition for Headache and Migraine Patients (CHAMP) is an organization that provides support to people with headache, migraine, and cluster diseases who are often stigmatized and underserved. CHAMP brings together organizations and leaders in this disease area to enhance communication, coordination, and collaboration to more effectively help people wherever they are on their patient journey. CHAMP is working to identify unmet needs of those with headache, migraine, and cluster diseases, and will work to better support patients and their caregivers.

Chronic migraine awareness

https://chronicmigraineawareness.org/

Chronic Migraine Awareness, Inc. is a 501 (c) 3 nonprofit, with a mission to be the voice of the chronic migraine community by offering support, information, and education to empower individuals to advocate for their own health.

Global healthy living foundation

https://www.50statenetwork.org

The Global Healthy Living Foundation (GHLF) is a 501(c)(3) nonprofit organization whose mission is to improve the quality of life for people living with chronic illnesses (such as arthritis, osteoporosis, migraine, diabetes, psoriasis, and cardiovascular disease) by advocating for improved access to health care at the community, state, and federal levels, and amplifying education and awareness efforts within its social media framework. Become an advocate with them via the link above and you will receive a call—tell them your specific interest is migraine.

Headache relief guide

http://www.headachereliefguide.com/

Headache doctors created this website to help teens and their families to gain better control of headaches, get appropriate medical care, and limit the disability caused by headaches.

Migraine research foundation

www.migraineresearchfoundation.org

This foundation raises money to fund innovative migraine research grants to further the understanding of the causes of migraine, develop better treatments, and ultimately, to cure and prevent migraine. Since all of their costs are underwritten, all donations go directly to fund migraine research.

Miles for migraine

www.milesformigraine.org

Miles for Migraine creates live, patient-participatory events that reduce the burden of isolation and stigma for people with migraine and headaches, and their caregivers. It builds community by bringing people together at fun walk/runs and through educational and support programs. Miles for Migraine also has programs specifically focused on engaging and supporting adolescents. All of their programs foster empowerment, increase disease awareness, teach skills to advocate for better access to treatments and raise funds for headache fellowship programs. Get involved with Miles for Migraine by showing up, volunteering or fundraising, or contact them about writing a blog article: info@milesformigraine.org.

The migraine world summit

www.migraineworldsummit.com

The Migraine World Summit is the largest patient event in the world for those with chronic headache and migraine. Its mission is to reduce the global burden of migraine through world-class education. Each year the event brings together tens of thousands of people to learn from world leading doctors, experts, and specialists. It is available free and online. They look for volunteers every year in November/ December in preparation for their March event.

National headache foundation

https://headaches.org/

Founded in 1970, the National Headache Foundation is the oldest and largest foundation for patients with headaches. Its mission is "To cure headache and end its pain and suffering." Its vision is "A World Without Headache." The Foundation is the premier educational and informational resource for those with headache, health care providers, and the public. The work of the Foundation is through education, raising awareness, advocacy, and research. The Foundation established the Certificate of Added Qualification in Headache Medicine for physicians, nurse practitioners, physician assistants, dentists, and clinical psychologists who treat headache patients. The NHF publishes *HeadWise* magazine, and *NHF News to Know*. If you like to write, consider sharing your story by clicking the link above!

US pain foundation

www.uspainfoundation.org/get-involved

The US Pain Foundation is the leading advocacy organization for people with pain. Its mission is to empower, educate, connect, and advocate for individuals living with chronic illness that causes pain, as well as their caregivers and clinicians. Through multiple programs and services, the US Pain Foundation works to enhance the quality of life for people with pain, improve patient outcomes, address access and affordability issues, and increase public awareness, and empathy for the issue of pain. Sign up for their emails and consider sharing your story, becoming a pain ambassador or advocating through them.

References

1. Global, regional, and national burden of migraine and tension-type headache, 1990–2016: a systematic analysis for the Global Burden of Disease Study 2016. *Lancet Neurol.* 2018;17(11):954–976.
2. Schwedt TJ, Shapiro RE. Funding of research on headache disorders by the National Institutes of Health. *Headache.* 2009;49(2):162–169.
3. Parikh SK, Young WB. Migraine: stigma in society. *Curr Pain Headache Rep.* 2019;23 (8).
4. Best RK. Disease campaigns and the decline of treatment advocacy. *J Health Polit Policy Law.* 2017;42(3):425–457.
5. Goffman E. *Stigma: Notes on the Management of Spoiled Identity.* Englewood Cliffs, NJ: Prentice-Hall; 1963.
6. Rao D, Choi SW, Victorson D, et al. Measuring stigma across neurological conditions: the development of the stigma scale for chronic illness (SSCI). *Qual Life Res.* 2009;18 (5):585–595.
7. Burgess DJ, Grill J, Noorbaloochi S, et al. The effect of perceived racial discrimination on bodily pain among older African American men. *Pain Med.* 2009;10(8):1341–1352.

8. Thornberg R. School bullying as a collective action: stigma processes and identity struggling. *Child Soc*. 2015;29:310–320.

9. Young WB, Park JE, Tian IX, Kempner J. The stigma of migraine. *PLoS One*. 2013;8(1): e54074. https://doi.org/10.1371/journal.pone.0054074.

10. Shapiro RE, Araujo AB, Nicholson RA, et al. Stigmatiing attitudes about migraine by people without migraine: results of the OVERCOME study. *Headache*. 2019;59(Suppl. 1):14–16.

11. Minen MT, Boubour A. A pilot educational intervention for headache and concussion. The headache and arts program. *Neurology*. 2018;90:e1799–e1804.

12. Hall AL, Karvounides D, Gelfand AA, et al. Improving the patient experience with migraine camp, a one-day group intervention for adolescents with chronic headache and their parents. *Headache*. 2019;59(8):1392–1400. https://doi.org/10.1111/head.13570.

Growing up: Transitioning to adult care ☆

26

Maggie Waung, MD, PhD, Ana Marissa Lagman-Bartolome, MD, Jennifer Hranilovich, MD, and Hope O'Brien, MD

Health-care transition from a child-centered to an adult-oriented health system is a planned process aimed at ensuring continuity of care and patients' adherence to medical care, with an emphasis on promoting active involvement of the patients, whenever possible.[1] The lack of a structured transition plan can lead to disruption of health care,[2–4] higher emergency room and hospital visits,[5] higher health-care costs,[6, 7] and poor medical compliance.[8] Similar to all pediatric patients with special needs, goals for transitioning the care of headache patients include development of self-care skills by the patient, efficient communication of medical history between providers, engaging patients and parents in decision making, setting expectations, and informing patients about practice differences.

Transitioning to adult care can be very challenging for youngsters with migraine and other headache disorders. The timing of transition occurs at a vulnerable time of development for the patient, when the triggers, features, and severity of headache are often in flux.[9, 10] Early diagnosis, treatment, and anticipatory guidance in this headache population, with a directed understanding of their unique needs and concerns, are crucial in facilitating the transition of patients into the adult health system. Since aggressive treatment of new-onset headache in adolescence may lead to disease modification,[11] a successful transition of care may improve patient outcomes, although more directed studies are needed to fully understand this transition period specifically in patients with challenging headache disorders.

Headache specialist

For the headache specialist, gaining knowledge about commonly occurring changes in the adolescent headache condition and overall health will help inform best clinical

---

☆Editor's note: In this chapter, the authors aim to help bridge a common gap in headache care. When a youngster switches from pediatric to adult providers, the culture is different and expectations change. Empowering a teenager with headache to take charge of his/her care ideally starts at the age of 12 years, so that when the transition occurs the young adult is ready for it. Solid advice is given to the generalist, specialist, and family.

Pediatric Headache. https://doi.org/10.1016/B978-0-323-83005-8.00022-7

practices. Long-term prognostic indicators of increased headache frequency in adolescents include female gender, decreases in social interaction, and depressive symptoms.[10] Furthermore, the onset of sexual activity and gynecologic conditions may prompt usage of oral contraceptives in female headache patients and necessitate conversations about the risks and benefits of estrogen-containing medications in patients with migraine with aura or in those who smoke.[12] Therefore, incorporating a comprehensive social history and screening for depression along with other migraine comorbidities (such as anxiety and substance use disorder) during care visits is crucial to understanding prognostic factors, guiding headache treatment, and providing a more comprehensive management of headache patients.

In addition to understanding the clinical changes affecting adolescent patients with headache disorders, education on the process of transition for headache specialists helps prevent common pitfalls and gaps in care. Common barriers to a successful transition include (1) communication gaps between providers, (2) a lack of health-care resources to support care coordination, (3) a lack of patient engagement or uneasiness with adult care, and (4) the inability to access appropriate providers with the capacity to provide comprehensive services.[12] Although there is an increased recognition of the importance of transition to adult care, there is limited evidence on the needs of migraine and headache patients as they transition into adults; however, many of the same principles can be drawn from studies on transitional care for children with special needs. To overcome these barriers, we recommend the adoption of the six core elements of transition developed by the Maternal and Child Health Bureau and The National Alliance to Advance Adolescent Health.

Six T's of transitioning health care of headache patients

Clinical recommendations for transition of health care of headache patients based on the six core elements of transition are as follows[13]:

- *Transition policy*
  - Formalize the transition criteria (i.e., setting the ideal and ceiling ages for transfer, emotional maturity, and independence). Develop pipelines and criteria to transition patients either to specialty clinics, local neurologist, or back to primary care providers. Identify adult providers who are comfortable with providing transitional care or who are receptive to learning about this unique patient population.
  - Identify patients ready for transition and introduce the topic of transition early, around 12 years of age, or soon after diagnosis. Provide patients with formal transition policies.

- o Anticipate insurance gaps and legal issues including privacy changes occurring on the day a patient turns 18 years old, which requires obtaining consent from patients for release of health information to parents and caregivers.
- *Tracking and monitoring:*
  - o Develop a mechanism for tracking progress through the six core elements of transition to monitor progress at individual and institution levels using electronic health records and standard documentation or flowsheets.
- *Transition readiness:*
  - o Formal assessment of transition readiness, or formally using the transition readiness assessment questionnaire (TRAQ),[14] or youth and young adult assessment tools (https://www.gottransition.org/resources/index.cfm).
  - o Informal assessment of independence by observation of parent–child interactions and by communication with other care providers, including psychiatrists and therapists.
  - o Discussion and implementation of self-care skill development, including calling in prescriptions, feeling comfortable speaking to the physician regarding symptoms, maintaining a headache diary, taking medications without prompts from parents, scheduling appointments, and handling electronic communication.
- *Transition planning:*
  - o Reach out to the patients, their caregivers, and other providers to identify the patient's strengths and weaknesses.
  - o Submit transfer packages to adult providers with a medical summary, emergency plan, legal documents, psychosocial concerns, and final readiness assessment. See a sample headache medical transfer packet (Fig. 1) created by the consensus of pediatric headache neurologists across North America.[15]
    - ■ A medical summary includes past providers, past medication trials, relevant past medical history, headache history "road map", and completed diagnostic tests
  - o Emphasize strengths as well as skills/tasks requiring assistance.
  - o Discuss complicated cases by telephone or in person including a joint agreement about emergency care prior to adult care visit. Patients, caregivers, and providers should know where to go in an emergency.
  - o Develop a plan for managing health care of college students who are away during the year, but are back home during holidays and school breaks.
  - o Before the visit, contact from the adult team should ideally address insurance changes, self-care practices, and psychosocial needs before the visit.
- *Transfer of care:*
  - o Welcome patients and orient them to adult care, focusing on concerns and similarities/differences between pediatric and adult care

HEALTHY HEADACHE TRANSITIONS: MEDICAL TRANSFER PACKET

Purpose: *To facilitate transition of care for adolescents and young adults with headache disorders and an ongoing need for neurological care by standardizing communication of the medical plan.*

Patient name:	Date of birth:
Referring provider:	Accepting provider:

Primary headache diagnosis:

Other headache diagnoses:

- Current headache frequency:
- Last PedMIDAS grade: 0 - Little to none as of _____ (date)
- Active work/school accommodations: ☐ No ☐ Yes:

Reason for transfer *(i.e. ongoing neurological care needs)*:

CURRENT HEADACHE INTERVENTIONS

Current headache interventions *(including non-pharmacologic interventions)*

Type	Name	Dose	Initiation Date	Response* *(if known)*	Side Effects
Acute (used at home)				Response	☐ No ☐ Yes:
				Response	☐ No ☐ Yes:
				Response	☐ No ☐ Yes:
Preventive				Response	☐ No ☐ Yes:
				Response	☐ No ☐ Yes:
				Response	☐ No ☐ Yes:

HEADACHE INVESTIGATIONS

Completed *(see attached results)*:
☐ Blood work ☐ Lumbar puncture ☐ Neuroimaging ☐ Vision assessment ☐ Cardiology/autonomic testing ☐
Other:

PAST HEADACHE INTERVENTIONS

Past acute headache interventions *(used at home)*

Intervention	Max dose	Duration/dates	Response* *(if known)*	Side Effects
			Response	☐ No ☐ Yes:
			Response	☐ No ☐ Yes:
			Response	☐ No ☐ Yes:
			Response	☐ No ☐ Yes:
			Response	☐ No ☐ Yes:

FIG. 1

Sample headache medical transfer packet.

From Orr SL, et al. The development of the medical transfer packet for transition of care of the pediatric patient with headache. Headache 2020;60:2589–2591, https://doi.org/10.1111/head.13948.

(Continued)

Past preventive headache interventions *(pharmacological or nutraceutical)*

Intervention	Dose	Duration/dates	Response* *(if known)*	Side Effects
			Response	☐ No ☐ Yes:
			Response	☐ No ☐ Yes:
			Response	☐ No ☐ Yes:
			Response	☐ No ☐ Yes:
			Response	☐ No ☐ Yes:

Past non-pharmacologic headache interventions *(e.g. psychological, injections, manual, neuromodulation)*

Intervention	Provider	Duration/dates	Response* *(if known)*	Side Effects
			Response	☐ No ☐ Yes:
			Response	☐ No ☐ Yes:
			Response	☐ No ☐ Yes:
			Response	☐ No ☐ Yes:
			Response	☐ No ☐ Yes:

Past emergency department or infusion center visits for headache:

☐ No ☐ Yes:

- *(last visit date)*
- Interventions with response *(if known)*:
- Interventions with incomplete or no response *(if known)*:

Past admissions to hospital for headache:

☐ No ☐ Yes:

- *(last admission date)*
- Interventions with response *(if known)*:
- Interventions with incomplete or no response *(if known)*:

***Response Definitions Legend*:**

Setting / Efficacy	Acute at home treatment	In-hospital acute treatment	Preventive treatment
Response	Pain-free within 2 hours, 9-10 times out of 10	Pain-free at discharge	≤4 headache days/month OR ≥50% reduction in headache days/month
Incomplete response	Some improvement within 2 hours, not meeting response criteria	Some improvement at discharge, not meeting response criteria	Some reduction in headache days/month or disability, not meeting response criteria
No response	No improvement in pain intensity within 2 hours	No improvement in pain intensity at discharge	No improvement in headache days/month or disability
Unclear	Unable to assess		

FIG.1, CONT'D

- Discuss confidentiality, access to information, shared decision making, and best routes for communication.
- Subsequent visits should work on gaps in self-care noted from the pediatric team.
- *Transition completion:*
  - Follow-up evaluation with patients to ensure completion of transfer, and review short-term outcomes and transition experience within 6 months of transfer.
  - Self-management and self-advocacy skills and behaviors often continue to develop after the initial 6 months after transfer.

Implementation of a planned and well-considered transition process leads to improvements in adherence to medical care and patient experience,[16] and is thus crucial for the ongoing care of these patients.

Primary care providers

Pediatrician

The unique role of a pediatrician in health-care transitions arises from the longitudinal relationship pediatricians have with patients and their caretakers. Starting discussions early about anticipated transitions and life goals with patients and their caretakers fosters a family-centered approach. The American Academy of Pediatrics/American Academy of Family Physicians/American College of Physicians (AAP/AAFP/ACP) guidelines recommend starting the transition process by notifying patients of the transition policy as early as age 12 years.[13] Asking parents about their thoughts on their child's future and initiating discussions with children about their own life goals and plans can be instrumental in providing a framework and in guiding expectations for transitions.[17] As withdrawal from social activities can be a risk factor for poor long-term headache prognosis,[10] encouraging engagement in the community may be beneficial for transitioning patients and their families.

Pediatricians may learn more about options and opportunities for their patients by reaching out to academic headache centers and patient advocacy groups. A few academic centers have established transition programs for headache patients, although more are needed. In addition, partnering with adult primary care providers is critical for a successful transition.

Adult care provider

Adult primary care providers play an instrumental role in the well-being of their patients by providing health care for patients with chronic medical conditions, including those with primary headache disorders. However, the median age of many adult care practices is over 40 years of age. Young adults often represent only a small

Table 1 Steps to implement the six core elements of pediatric to adult transition.

Transition intervention: "Six core elements for health-care transition"	
Pediatric health	**Adult health**
1. Transition policy	1. Privacy and consent policy (adult-centered care)
2. Transitioning youth registry	2. Young adult patient registry
3. Transition preparation (use of transition readiness assessment)	3. Transition preparation (continuation of transition readiness assessment)
4. Transition planning (use of portable medical summary with transition action plan)	4. Transition planning (continuation of transition action plan and updating of portable medical summary)
5. Transition and transfer of care (transition or transfer to adult model of care, transfer checklist, communication with adult provider, and, if needed, shared care with adult provider)	5. Transition and transfer of care (review of transfer of care package and consultation with pediatric provider as needed)
6. Transition completion (documentation of transfer)	6. Transition completion (documentation of transfer and initiation of care)

From McManus M, et al. Pediatric to adult transition: a quality improvement model for primary care. J Adolesc Health 2015;56:73–78, https://doi.org/10.1016/j.jadohealth.2014.08.006.

proportion of adult patient panels, making it challenging for adult providers to learn and take into account the unique needs of adolescents and young adults.

On the basis of the AAP/AAFP/ACP guidelines, we recommend that adult providers develop a plan to implement the six core elements of transition (Table 1). Materials to aid with plan development and implementation are available at https://www.gottransition.org. As a corollary to the transition readiness assessment skill tool for youth, a transition readiness assessment for young adults is available for adult providers. Given the clinical and financial challenges for adult primary care providers and lack of care coordination infrastructure, it may be useful to have a self-selected group of physicians in a practice to care for young adults and to coordinate care with pediatric providers.[18]

Patient and families

Why do you need to know about this stuff? We want the best care for our patients, and we are worried about this time when lots of changes are happening all at once. Whether your headaches are in or out of control, we want to make sure you are plugged in to get help when you need it. There are a lot of teens and young adults who stop seeing their doctor because they are healthy, have to pay for their own insurance for the first time, or because they have moved. As you might know from your own condition, if you ignore your headache, it often gets a lot worse. Then, it is even more stressful to find a new doctor, get in to see them right away, and get treated when you are already in trouble.

Why do I need to transition care? Sometimes, it is an insurance thing or the policy of the hospital where you are seen. Other times, you may have adult health problems, such as high cholesterol, high blood pressure, or pregnancy, which should be treated by an adult doctor.

When should I switch to an adult provider? It depends on your situation. Providers will generally want you to change over between 18 years and sometime in your early 20s. If you are heading to college, some providers will keep seeing you on your breaks when you come home.

How can I prepare for this transition? Learn about how and when your insurance will change. If your parents have private insurance, you might lose coverage when you are 26 years old. If you have Medicaid or other public insurance, you might be on your own for insurance sooner – it varies from state to state.

Choosing a new provider: First of all, talk with your headache doctor about whether you need a headache specialist or a general neurologist. It is easier to find a general neurologist. If you have other conditions that your headache provider is prescribing medicines for (such as depression, postural orthostatic tachycardia syndrome (POTS), anxiety, attention-deficit hyperactivity disorder (ADHD), etc.), then you may have to find a separate doctor to treat those conditions. Not all headache providers and neurologists are able to treat those conditions. In addition, if you were seen in a "multidisciplinary" or "comprehensive" clinic where you saw multiple providers (such as physical therapists, psychologists, social workers, etc.) at the same visit, there may not be an adult clinic that does the same. Again, you may have to find separate providers for those other conditions. Moreover, know that as your insurance changes, you may need a referral from your primary care provider to see a specialist, or there may be only some specialists covered by your new insurance.

Preventing a gap in your care: Think about the timing of when you will need your next visit. Will you need a new prescription soon? Another Botox treatment? It sometimes takes a while to get in for that first appointment. During the first visit with a new provider, a lot of time will be spent getting to know you, and you may not be able to get your prescription or treatment the same day as that first appointment. Think ahead about the timeline for signing up for insurance at your new job – it may take time for you to get a new insurance card.

How your care might change: There are medications and treatments that we know are helpful in adults, but have not been proven to work in kids. Your adult provider might recommend new therapies. Your insurance may cover new therapies for this reason as well. Another difference is that the style of adult headache care may be different from that of pediatric care. In many cases, providers assume adults are "tougher", and so you may not be offered treatments before or during procedures to deal with pain or anxiety. If this happens, speak up and let your new doctor know what would help you be more comfortable. Finally, you may start seeing your new provider on your own, so you will need to remember what to ask, what to tell them, and make it through procedures alone. Jotting things down before your appointment might be helpful. Some adult patients bring a relative or friend to help with this.

Managing your own care: Learn how to manage your own medical record. What is your login to see your doctor's notes and prescriptions online? How do you contact your new provider if you need help over the weekend? Parents and their children should have a verbal and written agreement about if, when, or how the parents can access children's medical records after the transition. Know your pharmacy, the names of your medication, and their doses. Get in the habit of remembering to take them on your own. If a headache diary is part of your care, get in the habit of remembering to maintain it on your own.

Advocating for yourself: If you are going to college or starting a new job, you should know if you had accommodations in high school (longer time to take tests, a dark room to recover). If you need things like that for the next stage in your life, you will have to get these set up. Some colleges allow you to make specific housing requests, but they may also ask for a doctor's note. A few employers are experimenting with programs to accommodate patients with migraine. Ask your pediatric provider how your care will be transferred to your adult provider. Ask how you can get a copy of your records, so that you can bring it with you to your new provider or send them to your new provider ahead of time.

Educating yourself: Be aware that things some adults do in college, in the military, or while living on their own, such as drinking alcohol, can have negative effects on your headaches. Find out more about migraines from patient advocacy sites – search for the American Migraine Foundation site (https://americanmigrainefoundation.org) or about transitioning to adult care from the National Alliance to Advance Adolescent Health website "Got Transition" (https://www.gottransition.org/youthfamilies/index.cfm).

References

1. Blum RW, et al. Transition from child-centered to adult health-care systems for adolescents with chronic conditions: A position paper of the Society for Adolescent Medicine. *J Adolesc Health*. 1993;14:570–576.
2. Wojciechowski EA, Hurtig A, Dorn L. A natural history study of adolescents and young adults with sickle cell disease as they transfer to adult care: a need for case management services. *J Pediatr Nurs*. 2002;17:18–27.
3. Montano CB, Young J. Discontinuity in the transition from pediatric to adult health care for patients with attention-deficit/hyperactivity disorder. *Postgrad Med*. 2012;124:23–32. https://doi.org/10.3810/pgm.2012.09.2591.
4. Luque Ramos A, et al. Transition to adult rheumatology care is necessary to maintain DMARD therapy in young people with juvenile idiopathic arthritis. *Semin Arthritis Rheum*. 2017;47:269–275. https://doi.org/10.1016/j.semarthrit.2017.05.003.

5. Shepard CL, et al. Ambulatory care use among patients with Spina Bifida: Change in care from childhood to adulthood. *J Urol.* 2018;199:1050–1055. https://doi.org/10.1016/j.juro.2017.10.040.

6. Cohen E, et al. Health care use during transfer to adult care among youth with chronic conditions. *Pediatrics.* 2016;137. https://doi.org/10.1542/peds.2015-2734, e20152734.

7. Mosquera RA, et al. Effect of an enhanced medical home on serious illness and cost of care among high-risk children with chronic illness: a randomized clinical trial. *JAMA.* 2014;312:2640–2648. https://doi.org/10.1001/jama.2014.16419.

8. Annunziato RA, et al. Strangers headed to a strange land? A pilot study of using a transition coordinator to improve transfer from pediatric to adult services. *J Pediatr.* 2013;163:1628–1633. https://doi.org/10.1016/j.jpeds.2013.07.031.

9. Antonaci F, et al. The evolution of headache from childhood to adulthood: a review of the literature. *J Headache Pain.* 2014;15:15. https://doi.org/10.1186/1129-2377-15-15.

10. Larsson B, Sigurdson JF, Sund AM. Long-term follow-up of a community sample of adolescents with frequent headaches. *J Headache Pain.* 2018;19:79. https://doi.org/10.1186/s10194-018-0908-5.

11. Mazzotta G, et al. Outcome of juvenile headache in outpatients attending 23 Italian headache clinics. Italian Collaborative Study Group on Juvenile Headache (Societa Italiana Neuropsichiatria Infantile [SINPI]). *Headache.* 1999;39:737–746. https://doi.org/10.1046/j.1526-4610.1999.3910737.x.

12. O'Brien HL, Cohen JM. Young adults with headaches: the transition from adolescents to adults. *Headache.* 2015;55:1404–1409. https://doi.org/10.1111/head.12706.

13. White PH, et al. Supporting the health care transition from adolescence to adulthood in the medical home. *Pediatrics.* 2018;142. https://doi.org/10.1542/peds.2018-2587.

14. Wood DL, et al. The transition readiness assessment questionnaire (TRAQ): its factor structure, reliability, and validity. *Acad Pediatr.* 2014;14:415–422. https://doi.org/10.1016/j.acap.2014.03.008.

15. Orr SL, et al. The development of the medical transfer packet for transition of care of the pediatric patient with headache. *Headache.* 2020;60:2589–2591. https://doi.org/10.1111/head.13948.

16. Gabriel P, McManus M, Rogers K, White P. Outcome evidence for structured pediatric to adult health care transition interventions: a systematic review. *J Pediatr.* 2017;188. https://doi.org/10.1016/j.jpeds.2017.05.066. 263–269e215.

17. Olsen DG, Swigonski NL. Transition to adulthood: the important role of the pediatrician. *Pediatrics.* 2004;113. https://doi.org/10.1542/peds.113.3.e159. e159–162.

18. McManus M, et al. Pediatric to adult transition: a quality improvement model for primary care. *J Adolesc Health.* 2015;56:73–78. https://doi.org/10.1016/j.jadohealth.2014.08.006.

Next steps

VI

How to set up a headache clinic ☆

27

Serena L. Orr, MD, MSc and Marcy Yonker, MD

Introduction

Although the majority of children and adolescents with headaches can be cared for outside of the tertiary care setting, pediatric headache clinics play an important role, not only in the provision of care to this underserviced population, but also in educating the community and other providers in the standard of care for pediatric headaches. In this chapter, we will describe the rationale for pediatric headache clinics, proposed models for both acute and outpatient headache care, the evidence for multidisciplinary headache clinics and finally, we will outline some ideas on how to advocate for the resources necessary to implement the proposed care models in a multidisciplinary pediatric headache clinic. We aim to structure our recommendations around the best available evidence, and where evidence is lacking, we have made recommendations based on expert opinion.

The societal impact of pediatric headache

Headache occurs in the majority of children and adolescents: according to a recent systematic review, the worldwide prevalence of headache in the pediatric population is 58.4%[1] and the prevalence of migraine in the pediatric age group is 7.7%.[1] Across the lifespan, headaches are the second most prevalent of all chronic diseases worldwide.[2]

Not only are primary headaches common, but they cause a great amount of disability. In the most recent iteration of the Global Burden of Disease Study, headaches were the second most important cause of years lived with disability amongst all diseases and injuries.[2] Pediatric patients with migraine have higher levels of disability as compared to controls due to impaired educational, social, and extra-curricular

---

☆Editor's note: In this chapter the authors share how to set up a headache clinic that is multidisciplinary and comprehensive. They show the data that these clinics work to improve outcome for patients and families. They give advice on how to convince skeptics that such an approach is helpful. I would add that in addition to sharing data, bringing a patient and family to such meetings to discuss how the clinic has dramatically affected a young life is best of all!

Pediatric Headache. https://doi.org/10.1016/B978-0-323-83005-8.00011-2

functioning.[3,4] Quality of life is also significantly lower in children and adolescents with migraine as compared to controls,[5] and quality of life scores are lower than those of patients with other chronic diseases, such as diabetes and chronic rheumatologic diseases.[6] It has also been shown that children with migraine have problems in school with inferior academic performance as compared to their peers.[7,8] Therefore, primary headaches have an important impact on children and adolescents and on the community through their effects on social, occupational, and educational functioning.

The importance of evidence-based pediatric headache care

The provision of evidence-based headache care is important not only due to its impact on short-term patient outcomes, but also because appropriate headache care in childhood may alter the long-term course of disease in primary headaches.

First, when patients are given a diagnosis, the door to receiving evidence-based, effective intervention opens, and long-term outcomes may be improved. In case of migraine, a longer lag between the time of disease onset and presentation to a multi-disciplinary pediatric headache clinic predicts a poorer long-term outcome characterized by a higher risk of chronic migraine at 10-year follow-up.[9] It is likely that a delay in presentation results in a delayed diagnosis, which in turn delays appropriate care. In fact, it has been proposed that there may be a window of opportunity in pediatric migraine, whereby early, targeted, and effective intervention may result in long term disease modification.[10] If this is correct, then the existence of pediatric headache clinics and their role in modeling and providing evidence-based care may have a significant public health impact on the community at large.

Second, multidisciplinary headache clinics not only provide a diagnosis and intervention for headache, but also support patients in the development of effective self-management and pain coping strategies. Given that migraine is a lifelong disease that persists through adulthood in approximately 50% of pediatric patients,[9, 11-14] it is critical that patients learn effective self-management and pain coping strategies early in their disease course. Teaching patients self-management skills may improve self-efficacy,[15] and this in turn may be associated with better long-term outcomes.[16]

The societal and health care costs of chronic migraine are significant[17-20] and several modifiable factors may mediate the risk of episodic migraine progressing to chronic migraine.[21,22] Longitudinal studies have shown that depression, high baseline headache frequency, and overuse of acute medications contribute to the risk of developing chronic migraine in adolescents.[23,24] In addition to the effect of depression on the risk of progression to chronic migraine, negative emotional states, including symptoms of depression and anxiety, appears to contribute to the risk of headache persistence,[25] and depression may also predict a poorer short-term prognosis in children and adolescents with migraine.[26] All of these modifiable risk factors can be addressed through the provision of evidence-based multidisciplinary headache care, thereby underscoring the importance of access to care.

Thus, for patients whose primary headaches are onset in childhood and adolescence, access to evidence-based pediatric headache care may significantly alter their life through the reduction of disability, improved self-management, and pain coping skills and the prevention of both chronic migraine and the long-term socioeconomic impairment associated with this condition.

The structure of multidisciplinary headache care in the clinic setting

There is substantial evidence to support the efficacy of multidisciplinary headache care in reducing disability and improving patient outcomes, as is reviewed below. In addition, multidisciplinary headache care appears to yield significant cost savings for the healthcare system as compared to care in other settings.[27] In this model, a multidisciplinary team works together to provide integrated headache care, similar to the model used in many chronic pain clinics, but tailored to the unique needs of patients experiencing headache.[27,28]

The core of a multidisciplinary headache clinic comprises expertise from a headache specialist, with input from Psychology, Nursing, and Physiotherapy. Fig. 1 illustrates the essential elements of multidisciplinary headache care. The headache specialist's role is to diagnose the headache, exclude secondary headaches, order appropriate investigations, make referrals to other disciplines as needed and tailor pharmacologic management with appropriately chosen acute and preventive medications.

Psychological care is another vital component in the multidisciplinary approach to pediatric headache management due to the high prevalence of internalizing symptoms[29–31] and of poor pain coping strategies[6] in pediatric migraine. Pain coping and quality of life are correlated in children and adolescents with migraine[32] and, as above, internalizing symptoms have an influence on headache prognosis. Psychologists provide a vital service in multidisciplinary headache clinics through the diagnosis and management of psychiatric symptoms and disorders, which, when untreated, are associated with a higher risk of migraine chronification.[21] In addition, psychologists teach patients pain coping skills, an essential component of headache management. There is robust meta-analysis level evidence to support the efficacy of psychological therapies for the treatment of pediatric headache,[33] and there is high quality randomized controlled trial evidence to support the efficacy of cognitive behavioral therapy for pediatric chronic migraine.[34,35]

In the multidisciplinary headache clinic, the headache nurse assists in communication between disciplines, provides headache education to the patient and provides regular follow-up to outpatients in the community. The role of the headache nurse may be more extensive in certain clinics, as nurses may be involved with monitoring

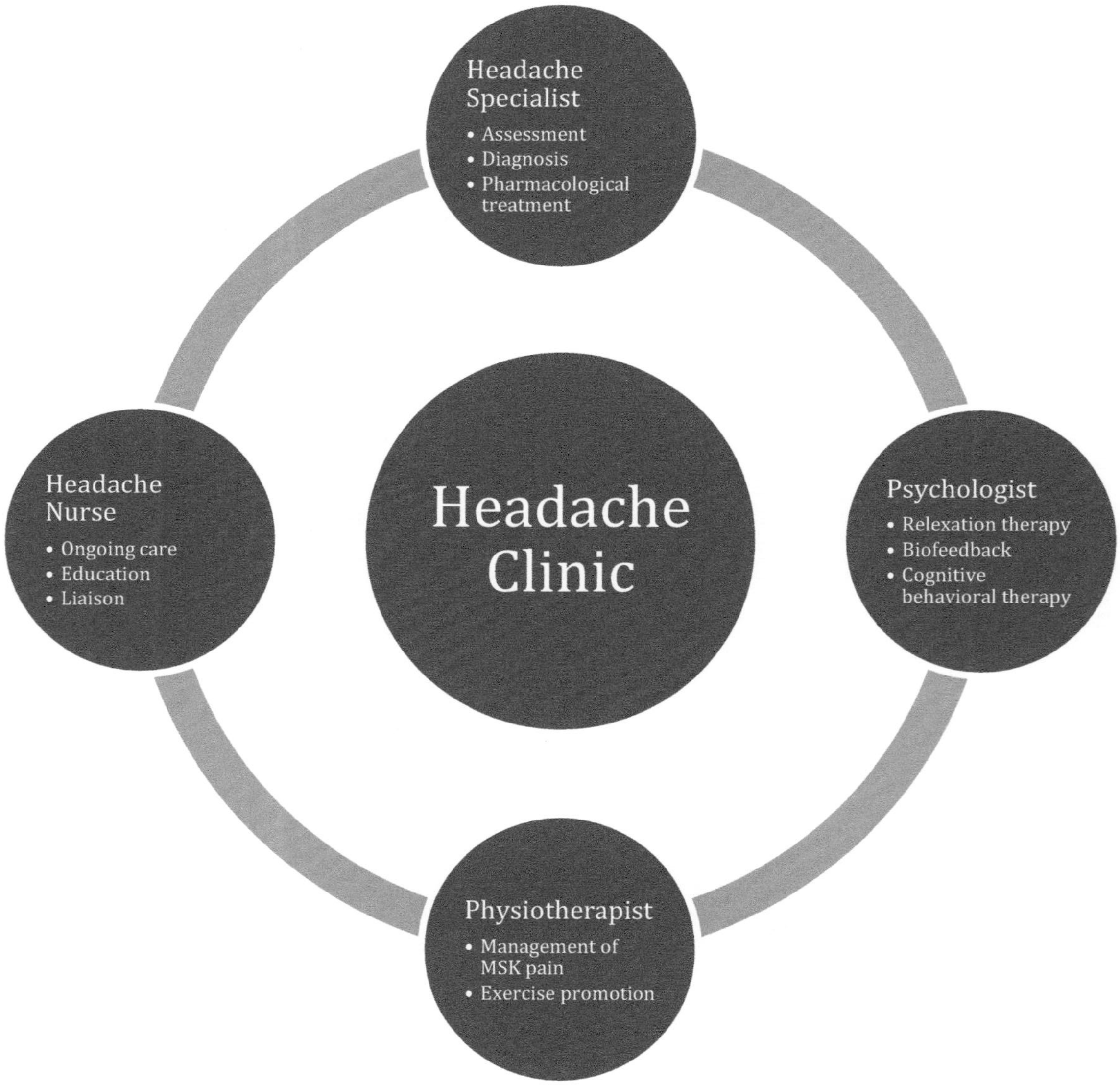

FIG. 1

Core multidisciplinary headache clinic components.

Adapted from J Headache Pain 2011;12:511–19.

medication side effects, assisting in research studies, and in other tasks such as programming neurostimulation devices.[28]

Physiotherapy might be an effective part of the treatment plan for certain patients with headache.[28] A recent systematic review supports the use of physiotherapy for migraine, tension-type headache, and cervicogenic headache in adults.[36] Though the extent and quality of the evidence is limited, select patients, especially those with cervicogenic headache and myofascial pain, might benefit significantly from physiotherapy interventions as part of their management plan.

Thus, the ideal structure for a pediatric multidisciplinary headache clinic would involve: (1) care by a headache specialist focused on diagnosis and pharmacologic management, (2) involvement of a psychologist for teaching pain coping skills and for patients with comorbid internalizing or other psychological symptoms, (3) involvement of a nurse for coordination of care, headache education, and ongoing follow-up, and (4) physiotherapy for select patients who may benefit from manual interventions and exercise training. In addition to the above core components of multidisciplinary pediatric headache care, additional elements that can be beneficial include the involvement of a social worker and a dietician. Given that a proportion of children and adolescents with headaches have problems with school absenteeism, in some cases it is beneficial to involve a social worker to assist the patient, their family, and the school in developing and communicating an individualized school reintegration plan and/or an individualized education plan. Although evidence for the efficacy of dietary interventions in headache management is limited,[37] it may also be beneficial, in certain cases, to involve a dietician to assist in establishing a healthy diet in order to optimize outcomes. If available, experts in complementary medicines such as herbs, yoga, and acupuncture can be incorporated.

In practical terms, delivering multidisciplinary services in a headache clinic can take on different forms. In some settings, what is most feasible is a "traditional" model where the headache specialist initially assesses the patient, and then makes referrals as needed to the other care providers (i.e., psychologist, physical therapist, etc.). Where resources permit, it can be useful to adopt the model of having multiple providers in clinic at the initial visit. This enriches the initial assessment and alleviates some of the travel burden for families. For example, at the Cincinnati Children's Hospital, all patients who complete an initial assessment in the Headache Clinic are seen by both a headache neurologist and a pain psychologist at their initial visit. Having a headache nurse meet with the patient and their family immediately following the headache specialist visit can be a useful way of enhancing patient education and allowing patients additional time for their questions and concerns to be addressed by a care team provider. In some clinics, a physician carries out the initial consultation assessment and follow-up visits are led by nurse practitioners. A variety of clinic structures can be employed contingent on available resources, though maximizing access and contact with multidisciplinary care teams allows patients to choose from a greater breadth of intervention options and appears to yield favorable treatment outcomes (see Section 7: The Evidence for Multidisciplinary Headache Care).

The structure of headache care in the acute setting

Given that migraine is a multigenic disorder with multiple associated comorbidities, headache patients may not fit the same mold as other neurology patients and may bring with them other health conditions that may influence their trajectory. It is thus important to have a variety of options for treatment built into multidisciplinary care for when things go awry. Generally, after an evaluation, a patient is given a concrete written plan of care including a preventive plan and an acute treatment plan (Headache Action Plan) in addition to advice regarding stress management and lifestyle changes they can implement to improve health. In the pediatric population, the Headache Action Plan (HAP) and medication needs to be provided to the school so that if a headache begins in school, the plan can be initiated early in order to maximize efficacy.[38] When the HAP does not result in resolution of headache, other interventions can be offered and it is important to have pathways in place to facilitate accessing these treatments.

Acute interventions that can be offered to headache patients include nerve blocks, sphenopalatine ganglion (SPG) blocks, and infusions. These interventions can be delivered either in an infusion center or in the Emergency Department (ED).

In order for patients to be able to access nerve blocks and SPG blocks, there needs to be an adequate number of providers trained to perform these procedures. If local expertise in administering these procedures is lacking, training can be accessed through the American Headache Society (AHS) and American Academy of Neurology (AAN); these societies provide excellent hands-on training courses on headache procedures. Appointments for blocks that are available on a same day or next day basis can improve patients' access to care. Most headache centers are scheduled many months in advance for appointments so flexibility must be built into the schedule to accommodate urgent requests. In the US, different insurance plans have different policies regarding coverage, so a system that includes the ability for urgent prior authorization including staff and appropriate documentation should be in place so that patients do not need to pay out of pocket unnecessarily for covered services. Discussion with payors at the outset of program development should occur in order to avoid service delays.

In addition to nerve and SPG blocks, infusions are an essential component of the acute treatment armamentarium that can often "break" or lower headache pain to a level where the patient can function. There are numerous ED studies on the efficacy of different medications or combinations of medications that have been reviewed elsewhere in detail.[39,40] Because the quality and quantity of the evidence in this area is limited, at present, different centers have different pathways based on their interpretation of the evidence and their clinical experience. Infusion medication options comprise many of the same medications used in the ED and inpatient setting including ketorolac, neuroleptic antiemetics (e.g., prochlorperazine or metoclopramide), and dihydroergotamine (DHE).

In the pediatric ED setting, treatment protocols for the acute management of migraine have been shown to be effective,[41,42] and it is likely that this evidence would extend to support the use of protocols in the infusion center setting. In fact, an infusion center offers the benefit of a quiet environment without the possibility of being bumped by other ED patients with more pressing needs. Although there is practice variation around how to intervene in acute pediatric migraine that has not responded to the at-home HAP, all headache centers should have an acute protocol established, that: (1) avoids administration of narcotics, as per published adult acute migraine guidelines[43] and the AAN's Choosing Wisely campaign,[44] (2) is based on evidence, and (3) is consistently followed with some flexibility for individuals patients in case a particular part of the pathway is not tolerated, or is contraindicated due to allergy or comorbidity. It is highly unlikely that there will ever be one medication or combination of medications that is universally effective; however, having a set pathway clearly improves patient outcomes.[42]

Infusions centers can provide a number of benefits to patients as opposed to ED care. When considering appropriate use of the infusion center, it is important to ensure patients referred to this setting are stable, established patients of the headache center. First, an appointment can be made for the patient, and generally infusion centers offer a less chaotic, less overstimulating environment for a child or adolescent with headache. Second, generally, the patient's regular provider would make the determination as to which intervention(s) would be used and what the appropriate goal for treatment would be based on their knowledge of the patient. For example, for some patients with chronic migraine refractory to multiple therapies, the treatment goal may be reduction of pain to their baseline intensity, whereas for patients with episodic migraine who have failed their HAP, headache freedom is likely a more appropriate goal as their baseline is no headache and failure to achieve pain freedom may be associated with a significant risk of headache recurrence.[45–47] Third, the infusion center keeps migraine patients out of the ED, which lowers costs,[48] allows ED providers to take care of life-threatening emergencies, and presumably helps to provide more personalized and standardized care.

When the patient does not experience significant relief in the ED or infusion center, inpatient admission for IV DHE or other therapies should be considered on a case-by-case basis. Again, there are numerous pathways to guide IV DHE administration, however, having a set plan with all team members (inpatient providers, nursing, pharmacy etc.) on board can facilitate treatment and improve outcomes. In most pediatric centers, treatment paradigms are based on the Cincinnati Children's Hospital pathway.[49]

Chronic headache care

As indicated in the introduction, patients with migraine, in particular those with chronic migraine, often require more headache specialist visits and medication(s). Ideally, headache clinics are multidisciplinary and comprise additional resources for those with more difficult and complex problems. Two examples of additional resources are included below for illustrative purposes.

Biofeedback/CBT

In a randomized controlled trial of adolescents with chronic migraine, amitriptyline combined with cognitive behavioral therapy (which included biofeedback-assisted relaxation instruction) was shown to be superior to amitriptyline plus sham therapy.[34] Additionally, biofeedback alone has shown promise in the treatment of migraine in children.[50] Therapist-led cognitive behavioral therapy requires licensed psychotherapists to administer a series of interventions over the course of 8–10 sessions. This resource is unfortunately difficult to access and frequently not available even in tertiary centers. Thus, depending on local resource availability and expertise, a variety of models for psychological headache care can be considered, though, ideally, they should be evidence-based. In order to improve access to psychological resources, it is important to present the extensive evidence for its efficacy in managing pediatric headaches[33,50,51] to local decision-makers and stakeholders. In addition, forming local partnerships with psychologists who have experience or interest in treating children and adolescents with headache is essential.[52] Where no such providers are available, the headache specialist should consider advocating for headache-specific training for local psychologist(s).

Chemodenervation for chronic migraine

Although there is currently no FDA indication for this treatment in the pediatric population, in a dose-finding study for onabotulinumtoxinA prophylaxis in adolescents with chronic migraine, no safety concerns were identified. The study was not adequately designed to rigorously assess efficacy.[53] A number of retrospective studies have suggested that onabotulinumtoxinA might be an effective prophylactic intervention for chronic migraine in adolescents.[54–58] Procedure training is available from the AHS, the AAN and from the manufacturers. Generally, as the injections are provided every 3 months, it is important to set up a system of prior authorization and scheduling so that patients are kept on track, as delay in treatment results in wearing off of the therapy results.

In addition to direct support for the patients in providing clinical care, support outside of clinic visits is vital. Having a provider (e.g., nurse) who can take patient phone calls outside of clinic visits to provide ongoing support to families helps to optimize care in the community setting. In addition, support groups for patients and parents can provide a welcome outlet for sharing of experience and knowledge amongst migraine sufferers and their families. Miles for Migraine, a nonprofit organization, raises money for headache fellowship training and teen/family education camps that occur at Pediatric Headache Centers across the United States. Coalition for Migraine and Headache Patients (CHAMP) sponsors patient symposia under the auspices of the American Headache Society. Migraine Canada is an educational and advocacy resource for Canadians suffering from chronic headaches. There are numerous other headache advocacy organizations globally and headache specialists should become familiar with their local patient advocacy resources.

The evidence for multidisciplinary headache care

Numerous studies support the multidisciplinary clinic model for headache care and this model has been formally endorsed in European[59] and Canadian[60] guidelines.

Prospective studies amongst adult headache patients have found that multidisciplinary clinics composed of neurologists, psychologists, physiotherapists, and headache nurses yield high treatment response rates and favorable outcomes amongst patients with a variety of primary headaches.[61–64] In addition, a randomized controlled trial in adult patients with chronic migraine found that a multidisciplinary headache program was significantly more effective as compared with routine care, involving predominantly specialist referrals and pharmacologic management. The intervention group not only had improved pain-related outcomes, but also had lower depression scores, higher functional and health status scores, and lower disability after multidisciplinary care. The benefits of multidisciplinary care were sustained at postintervention follow-up.[65]

Interestingly, it appears that younger patients may be most likely to have a favorable treatment response in multidisciplinary headache clinics.[61,62] Two studies specifically carried out amongst pediatric headache patients also support the efficacy of multidisciplinary care for headache management.[66,67] One prospective study of 169 children and adolescents with a variety of headaches found that multidisciplinary care provided by a neurologist, headache nurse, psychologist, and a physiotherapist resulted in 70% of the patients improving at follow-up, with the majority also having a significant increase in quality of life, and this was sustained at 12 months follow-up. Half of the patients had a 50% or greater reduction in headache frequency, which is a highly desirable treatment outcome for pediatric headache.[66,68] In another prospective study amongst 96 pediatric headache patients, multidisciplinary care resulted in headache improvement in 93% of patients, and this was sustained as far as at 5-year follow-up. In addition, patients missed an average of 3 days less of school per month at 5-year follow-up as compared to baseline.[67]

How to advocate for resources in a multidisciplinary headache clinic

Ease of access to allied health resources will vary considerably from center-to-center and from country-to-country. In addition, depending on the setting, the stakeholders who will execute the decisions about access to resources will vary. Depending on the country and center, one may be presenting their proposal for resource access to hospital administrators, to leaders within the Department or Division, to government officials (e.g., in a publicly funded health care system) or even to the board of a hospital's charitable foundation. When preparing for these discussions, it is important to consider one's audience and target the presentation according to their background and frame of reference. In general, when presenting proposals to decision-makers and stakeholders, arguments for multidisciplinary care can be made based on the evidence presented above, both from the clinical studies and guidelines that support this type of care model. For example, when advocating for access to psychology, one should present the data both from systematic reviews that support the efficacy of psychological interventions in the treatment of pediatric migraine,[33,50,51] and from the recent AAN guidelines that stipulate that there is Class I evidence to support cognitive behavioral therapy plus amitriptyline for chronic pediatric migraine and that this evidence should be discussed with patients.[35] In the case of psychological interventions for pediatric migraine, decision-makers and stakeholders should be made aware that these interventions are part of the standard of care, based on the evidence described above.

In addition to using data to advocate for resources, financial considerations can also be used to persuade decision-makers to fund programs. For example, if one is aiming to establish an infusion center for acute migraine management, data on the cost savings resulting from diverting patients away from the ED can be presented.[48] Another way of highlighting the importance of multidisciplinary care is to include patients and families in these discussions with decision-makers. Adding the patient experience lens to the available data and financial considerations can strengthen the arguments for funding multidisciplinary care.

Although some data are available that can assist clinicians in advocating for resources for headache clinics, more work needs to be done. If we are to effectively advocate for better access to multidisciplinary pediatric headache care as a clinical and research community, we must carry out more studies on the efficacy and cost-benefit profile of pediatric headache care models. Having more data on the efficacy and relative costs associated with both outpatient headache clinics and acute infusion centers will render the task of convincing decision-makers to increase access to resources less arduous and ultimately result in better access to care for our patients.

Summary and recommendations

In summary, pediatric headache is very common and poses a great burden to the individual and to society through associated disability and socioeconomic impairment, which persists into adulthood if proper treatment is not accessed. The best available care model for pediatric headache is through a multidisciplinary clinic model, whereby care is integrated across the disciplines of neurology, psychology, nursing, and physiotherapy. This multidisciplinary clinic model is supported by evidence and endorsed by expert guidelines.

References

1. Abu-Arafeh I, Razak S, Sivaraman B, Graham C. Prevalence of headache and migraine in children and adolescents: a systematic review of population-based studies. *Dev Med Child Neurol.* 2010;52(12):1088–1097.
2. James SL, Abate D, Abate KH, et al. Global, regional, and national incidence, prevalence, and years lived with disability for 354 diseases and injuries for 195 countries and territories, 1990–2017: a systematic analysis for the Global Burden of Disease Study 2017. *Lancet.* 2018;392:1789–1858.
3. Kröner-Herwig B, Heinrich M, Vath N. The assessment of disability in children and adolescents with headache: adopting PedMIDAS in an epidemiological study. *Eur J Pain.* 2010;14(9):951–958.
4. Hershey AD, Powers SW, Lecates S, Kabbouche MA, Maynard MK. PedMIDAS: development of a questionnaire to assess disability of migraines in children. *Neurology.* 2001;57:2034–2039.
5. Powers SW, Patton SR, Hommel KA, Hershey AD. Quality of life in childhood migraines: clinical impact and comparison to other chronic illnesses. *Pediatrics.* 2003;112(1 Pt 1):e1–e5.
6. Orr SL, Christie SN, Akiki S, McMillan HJ. Disability, quality of life, and pain coping in pediatric migraine: an observational study. *J Child Neurol.* 2017;32(8):717–724.
7. Rocha-Filho PA, Santos PV. Headaches, quality of life, and academic performance in schoolchildren and adolescents. *Headache.* 2014;54(7):1194–1202.
8. Arruda MA, Bigal ME. Migraine and migraine subtypes in preadolescent children: association with school performance. *Neurology.* 2012;79(18):1881–1888.
9. Galinski M, Sidhoum S, Cimerman P, Perrin O, Annequin D, Tourniaire B. Early diagnosis of migraine necessary in children: 10-year follow-up. *Pediatr Neurol.* 2015;53(4):319–323.
10. Charles JA, Peterlin BL, Rapoport AM, Linder SL, Kabbouche MA, Sheftell FD. Favorable outcome of early treatment of new onset child and adolescent migraine-implications for disease modification. *J Headache Pain.* 2009;10(4):227–233.
11. Bille B. A 40-year follow-up of school children with migraine. *Cephalalgia.* 1997;17:488–491.
12. Guidetti V, Galli F. Evolution of headache in childhood and adolescence: an 8-year follow-up. *Cephalalgia.* 1998;18(7):449–454.
13. Virtanen R, Aromaa M, Rautava P, et al. Changing headache from preschool age to puberty. A controlled study. *Cephalalgia.* 2007;27(4):294–303.
14. Monastero R, Camarda C, Pipia C, Camarda R. Prognosis of migraine headaches in adolescents: a 10-year follow-up study. *Neurology.* 2006;67(8):1353–1356.
15. Leroux E, Beaudet L, Boudreau G, et al. A nursing intervention increases quality of life and self-efficacy in migraine: a 1-year prospective controlled trial. *Headache.* 2018;58(2):260–274.
16. Probyn K, Bowers H, Caldwell F, et al. Prognostic factors for chronic headache: a systematic review. *Neurology.* 2017;89(3):291–301.
17. Osumili B, McCrone P, Cousins S, Ridsdale L. The economic cost of patients with migraine headache referred to specialist clinics. *Headache.* 2018;58(2):287–294.
18. Stewart WF, Wood GC, Manack A, Varon SF, Buse DC, Lipton RB. Employment and work impact of chronic migraine and episodic migraine. *J Occup Environ Med.* 2010;52(1):8–14.

19. Stokes M, Becker WJ, Lipton RB, et al. Cost of health care among patients with chronic and episodic migraine in Canada and the USA: results from the international burden of migraine study (IBMS). *Headache*. 2011;51(7):1058–1077.

20. Munakata J, Hazard E, Serrano D, et al. Economic burden of transformed migraine: results from the American Migraine Prevalence and Prevention (AMPP) Study. *Headache*. 2009;49:498–508.

21. Buse DC, Greisman JD, Baigi K, Lipton RB. Migraine progression: a systematic review. *Headache*. 2019;59:306–338.

22. May A, Schulte LH. Chronic migraine: risk factors, mechanisms and treatment. *Nat Rev Neurol*. 2016;12(8):455–464.

23. Lu SR, Fuh JL, Wang SJ, et al. Incidence and risk factors of chronic daily headache in young adolescents: a school cohort study. *Pediatrics*. 2013;132(1):e9–16.

24. Wang S, Fuh J, Lu S, Juang K. Outcomes and predictors of chronic daily headache in adolescents: a 2-year longitudinal study. *Neurology*. 2007;68(8):591–596.

25. Huguet A, Tougas ME, Hayden J, et al. Systematic review of childhood and adolescent risk and prognostic factors for recurrent headaches. *J Pain*. 2016;17(8):855–873.

26. Orr SL, Turner A, Kabbouche MA, et al. Predictors of short-term prognosis while in pediatric headache care: an observational study. *Headache*. 2019;59(4):543–555.

27. Diener HC, Gaul C, Jensen R, Göbel H, Heinze A, Silberstein SD. Integrated headache care. *Cephalalgia*. 2011;31(9):1039–1047.

28. Gaul C, Liesering-Latta E, Schäfer B, Fritsche G, Holle D. Integrated multidisciplinary care of headache disorders: a narrative review. *Cephalalgia*. 2016;36(12):1181–1191.

29. Balottin U, Poli PF, Termine C, Molteni S, Galli F. Psychopathological symptoms in child and adolescent migraine and tension-type headache: a meta-analysis. *Cephalalgia*. 2012;33(2):112–122.

30. Bruijn J, Locher H, Passchier J, Dijkstra N, Arts WF. Psychopathology in children and adolescents with migraine in clinical studies: a systematic review. *Pediatrics*. 2010;126(2):323–332.

31. Amouroux R, Rousseau-Salvador C. Anxiété et dépression chez l'enfant et l'adolescent migraineux: revue de la littérature. *Encephale*. 2008;34(5):504–510.

32. Frare M, Axia G, Battistella PA. Quality of life, coping strategies, and family routines in children with headache. *Headache*. 2002;42(10):953–962.

33. Fisher E, Law E, Dudeney J, Palermo T, Stewart G, Eccleston C. Psychological therapies for the management of chronic and recurrent pain in children and adolescents. *Cochrane Database Syst Rev*. 2018;1–123.

34. Powers SW, Kashikar-Zuck SM, Allen JR, et al. Cognitive behavioral therapy plus amitriptyline for chronic migraine in children and adolescents: a randomized clinical trial. *JAMA*. 2013;310(24):2622–2630.

35. Oskoui M, Pringsheim T, Billinghurst L, et al. Practice guideline update summary: pharmacologic treatment for pediatric migraine prevention: report of the Guideline Development, Dissemination, and Implementation Subcommittee of the American Academy of Neurology and the American Headache Society. *Neurology*. 2019;93:1–10.

36. Luedtke K, Allers A, Schulte L, May A. Efficacy of interventions used by physiotherapists for patients with headache and migraine—a systematic review and meta-analysis. *Cephalalgia*. 2016;36(5):4749–4792.

37. Orr SL. Diet and nutraceutical interventions for headache management: a review of the evidence. *Cephalalgia*. 2016;36(12):1112–1133.

38. Turner SB. Pediatric migraine action plan (PedMAP). *Headache*. 2019;59:1871–1873 [in press].

39. Patniyot IR, Gelfand AA. Acute treatment therapies for pediatric migraine: a qualitative systematic review. *Headache*. 2016;56(1):49–70.
40. Richer L, Billinghurst L, Linsdell M, et al. Drugs for the acute treatment of migraine in children and adolescents (review). *Cochrane Database Syst Rev*. 2016;4(4), CD005220.
41. Kaar CRJ, Gerard JM, Nakanishi AK. The use of a pediatric migraine practice guideline in an emergency department setting. *Pediatr Emerg Care*. 2016;32(7):435–439.
42. Leung S, Bulloch B, Young C, Yonker M, Hostetler M. Effectiveness of standardized combination therapy for migraine treatment in the pediatric emergency department. *Headache*. 2013;53(3):491–497.
43. Orr SL, Friedman BW, Christie S, et al. Management of adults with acute migraine in the emergency department: the American Headache Society evidence assessment of parenteral pharmacotherapies. *Headache*. 2016;56(6).
44. Callaghan BC, De Lott LB, Kerber KA, Burke JF, Skolarus LE. Neurology choosing wisely recommendations: 74 and growing. *Neurol Clin Pr*. 2015;5(5):439–447.
45. Richer L, Craig W, Rowe B. Randomized controlled trial of treatment expectation and intravenous fluid in pediatric migraine. *Headache*. 2014;54(9):1496–1505.
46. Trottier ED, Bailey B, Lucas N, Lortie A. Prochlorperazine in children with migraine: a look at its effectiveness and rate of akathisia. *Am J Emerg Med*. 2012;30(3):456–463.
47. Brousseau DC, Duffy SJ, Anderson AC, Linakis JG. Treatment of pediatric migraine headaches: a randomized, double-blind trial of prochlorperazine versus ketorolac. *Ann Emerg Med*. 2004;43(2):256–262.
48. Foss A, Brammer E. Cocktails for kids: coordinating outpatient care for the refractory headache. In: *Child Neurology Society Meeting*; 2016.
49. Kabbouche MA, Powers SW, Segers A, et al. Inpatient treatment of status migraine with dihydroergotamine in children and adolescents. *Headache*. 2009;49(1):106–109.
50. Stubberud A, Varkey E, McCrory DC, Pedersen SA, Linde M. Biofeedback as prophylaxis for pediatric migraine: a meta-analysis. *Pediatrics*. 2016;138(2):e20160675.
51. Ng QX, Venkatanarayanan N, Kumar L. A systematic review and meta-analysis of the efficacy of cognitive behavioral therapy for the management of pediatric migraine. *Headache*. 2017;57(3):349–362.
52. Ernst M, O'Brien H, Powers S. Cognitive-behavioral therapy: how medical providers can increase patient and family openness and access to evidence- based multimodal therapy for pediatric migraine. *Headache*. 2015;55(10):1382–1396.
53. Allergan. *A Study Using Botulinum Toxin Type A as Headache Prophylaxis in Adolescents with Chronic Migraine [Internet]*; 2019. clinicaltrials.gov. Available from: https://clinicaltrials.gov/ct2/show/NCT01662492?term=botulinum+toxin+adolescents&cond=migraine&rank=1.
54. Chan VW, McCabe EJ, MacGregor DL. Botox treatment for migraine and chronic daily headache in adolescents. *J Neurosci Nurs*. 2009;41(5):235–243.
55. Kabbouche M, O'Brien H, Hershey AD. Onabotulinumtoxin A in pediatric chronic daily headache. *Curr Neurol Neurosci Rep*. 2012;12(2):114–117.
56. Shah S, Calderon MD, Der Wu W, Grant J, Rinehart J. Onabotulinumtoxin A (BOTOX®) for prophylactic treatment of pediatric migraine: a retrospective longitudinal analysis. *J Child Neurol*. 2018;33(9):580–586.
57. Ahmed K, Oas KH, MacK KJ, Garza I. Experience with botulinum toxin type a in medically intractable pediatric chronic daily headache. *Pediatr Neurol*. 2010;43(5):316–319.
58. Ali SS, Bragin I, Rende E, Mejico L, Werner KE. Further evidence that onabotulinum toxin is a viable treatment option for pediatric chronic migraine patients. *Cureus*. 2019;11(3):e4343.

59. Steiner TJ, Antonaci F, Jensen R, Lainez MJA, Lanteri-Minet M, Valade D. Recommendations for headache service organisation and delivery in Europe. *J Headache Pain*. 2011;12(4):419–426.
60. Pringsheim T, Davenport WJ, Mackie G, et al. Canadian headache society guideline for migraine prophylaxis. *Can J Neurol Sci*. 2012;39(2 Suppl. 2):S1–S59.
61. Wallasch TM, Angeli A, Kropp P. Outcomes of a headache-specific cross-sectional multidisciplinary treatment program. *Headache*. 2012;52(7):1094–1105.
62. Gaul C, Brömstrup J, Fritsche G, Diener HC, Katsarava Z. Evaluating integrated headache care: a one-year follow-up observational study in patients treated at the Essen headache centre. *BMC Neurol*. 2011;11:124.
63. Zeeberg P, Olesen J, Jensen R. Efficacy of multidisciplinary treatment in a tertiary referral headache centre. *Cephalalgia*. 2005;25(12):1159–1167.
64. Barton PM, Schultz GR, Jarrell JF, Becker WJ. A flexible format interdisciplinary treatment and rehabilitation program for chronic daily headache: patient clinical features, resource utilization and outcomes. *Headache*. 2014;54(8):1320–1336.
65. Lemstra M, Stewart B, Olszynski WP. Effectiveness of multidisciplinary intervention in the treatment of migraine: a randomized clinical trial. *Headache*. 2002;42(9):845–854.
66. Soee ABL, Skov L, Skovgaard LT, Thomsen LL. Headache in children: effectiveness of multidisciplinary treatment in a tertiary paediatric headache clinic. *Cephalalgia*. 2013;33(15):1218–1228.
67. Kabbouche MA, Powers SW, Vockell ALB, et al. Outcome of a multidisciplinary approach to pediatric migraine at 1, 2, and 5 years. *Headache*. 2005;45(10):1298–1303.
68. Abu-Arafeh I, Hershey AD, Diener HC, Tassorelli C. Guidelines of the international headache society for controlled trials of preventive treatment of migraine in children and adolescents, 1st edition. *Cephalalgia*. 2019;39(7):803–816.

Where can I learn more? A listing of resources☆ 28

Meghan S. Candee, MD, Jessica R. Gautreaux, MD, and Carrie O. Dougherty, MD

Multiple studies have shown that educating patients about their disease state and treatment plans can improve patient outcomes, yet every provider struggles with the ability to provide adequate education and counseling to patients and their families within the time constraints of clinic visits. Educational resources for further reading can supplement and reinforce in-office discussions. While many families do extensive online research prior to and following their clinic visits, a web-engine search for "migraine in children" generates an overwhelming list of sources, many of which are focused upon an individual child or family's journey, may challenge the established treatment plan and can undermine patient-provider rapport by recommending unnecessary imaging, anecdotal interventions, or controversial procedures. The resources and references below have been selected as reliable and up-to-date, many having been developed in conjunction with headaches specialists. These websites focus on the need to address lifestyle factors which can, and often do, contribute to headache perpetuation. They highlight strategies for headache prevention and management with the ultimate goal of reducing migraine-related disability and optimizing function.

Websites

American Headache Society
https://americanheadachesociety.org/news/?tag=pediatric-headache
The American Headache Society is dedicated to improving the care and lives of headache sufferers by encouraging scientific research and educating patients and healthcare professionals.
American Migraine Foundation
https://americanmigrainefoundation.org/

☆Editor's note: We spend a lot of time during visits, dispelling misleading information gleaned from websites or chat groups. The authors give their opinions about reputable websites to guide families into getting helpful information.

Pediatric Headache. https://doi.org/10.1016/B978-0-323-83005-8.00028-8

The American Migraine Foundation is the patient advocacy organization affiliated with the American Headache Society. AMF is dedicated to the advancement of research and awareness surrounding migraine. This website includes patient guides and a library of articles about topics related to headache.

Migraine Research Foundation

https://migraineresearchfoundation.org/resources/find-a-doctor/childrens-headache-doctors/

The Migraine Research Foundation is dedicated to raising financial support for migraine research. The website includes a specific section on migraine in teens and kids which includes proprietary list of headache specialists.

National Headache Foundation

https://headaches.org/resources/pediatric-headache/

The National Headache Foundation is an organization dedicated to migraine advocacy, awareness, research, and education. This website includes numerous resources, tools, and current research information.

Headache Relief Guide

http://headachereliefguide.com/

The Headache Relief Guide is a website designed by headache specialists to help teenagers and their families gain better control of headaches, find appropriate medical care with the ultimate goal of reducing disability caused by headaches.

Global Healthy Living Foundation: Migraine Patient Guidelines

https://www.ghlf.org/migraine-patient-guidelines/

Global Healthy Living Foundation is a non-profit organization whose mission is to improve the quality of life for people living with chronic illness. This downloadable PDF guide provides a comprehensive overview of migraine diagnosis and current treatment options, written by both providers and patients.

CHAMP: Coalition for headache and migraine patients

https://headachemigraine.org/

CHAMP is a patient support organization involved with education, community, advocacy, and increased awareness of headache and migraine.

Miles for Migraine

https://www.milesformigraine.org/

Miles for Migraine is a nonprofit charity dedicated to improving the lives of people with migraine and headaches. Miles for Migraine produces run/walk events, patient education seminars, and support groups. They also host day camps for teenagers with migraine and their caregivers.

Seminal articles

Gelfand AA. Episodic syndromes of childhood associated with migraine. *Curr Opin Neurol*. 2018;31(3):281–285. https://www.ncbi.nlm.nih.gov/pubmed/29601304.

Gelfand AA. Pediatric and adolescent headache. *Continuum (Minneap Minn)*. 2018;24(4, Headache):1108–1136. https://www.ncbi.nlm.nih.gov/pubmed/30074552.

Patterson-Gentile C, Szperka CL. The changing landscape of pediatric migraine therapy: a review. *JAMA Neurol*. 2018;75(7):881–887. https://jamanetwork.com/journals/jamaneurology/article-abstract/2674283.

Powers SW, Coffey CS, et al. Trial of amitriptyline, toiramate and placebo for pediatric migraine. *N Engl J Med*. 2017;376(2):115–124. https://www.ncbi.nlm.nih.gov/pubmed/27788026.

Szperka CL, VanderPluym J et al. Recommendations on the Use of Anti-CGRP Monoclonal Antibodies in Children and Adolescents. *Headache*. 2018;58(10):1658–1669. https://www.ncbi.nlm.nih.gov/pubmed/30324723.

Oskoui M, Pringsheim T, et al. Practice guidelines update summary: pharmacologic treatment for pediatric migraine prevention. *Headache*. 2019;59(8):1144–1157. https://www.ncbi.nlm.nih.gov/pubmed/31529477.

Oskoui M, Pringsheim T, et al. Practice guidelines update summary: acute treatment of migraine in children and adolescents. *Headache*. 2019;59(8):1158–1173. https://www.ncbi.nlm.nih.gov/pubmed/31529481.

AAN/AHS pediatric migraine treatment guidelines

Practice Guideline Update: Acute Treatment of Migraine in Children and Adolescents. Published August 2019. https://www.aan.com/Guidelines/home/GuidelineDetail/966.

Practice Guideline Update: Pharmacologic Treatment for Pediatric Migraine Prevention. Published August 2019. https://www.aan.com/Guidelines/home/GuidelineDetail/967.

Index

Note: Page numbers followed by *f* indicate figures, *t* indicate tables, and *b* indicate boxes.

A

AAN/AHS pediatric migraine treatment guidelines, 343
Abdominal migraine, 47–48
  headache specialist, 48
  parents, 48
  primary care provider, 48
Abnormal sleep behaviors. *See* Sleep disturbance
Active headache coping skills
  clinical hypnosis, 155–156
  cognitive reframing, 156–157
  distraction, 153–155
  parent education, 157
  relaxation and mindfulness strategies, 156
Acupuncture
  headache specialists, 251–254
  patients and families, 247–250
  primary care providers, 251–254
Acute medication treatments
  headache specialist, 146–149
  parents, 143–144
  primary care providers, 144–145
Adult care provider, 320
Adverse childhood experiences (ACEs), 14
Advocacy, 306
  organizations, 309–312
  plan of action, 307*t*, 308–309
Aerobic exercise, 289–290
Alexithymia, 86
Alliance for headaches advocacy, 309
American Academy of Neurology (AAN), 171–172
American Academy of Pediatrics, 269, 270*t*, 271, 283
American Headache Society (AHS), 148, 171–172, 187, 341
American Migraine Foundation, 309–310, 323, 341
Amitriptyline, 175
Antidepressants, 175
Antiepileptic medications, 174–175
Antihistamine, 176–177
Antihypertensives, 175–176
Anxiety, 85, 154, 185
Association of Migraine Disorders (AMD), 310

Atogepant, 219–220
Atopic disorders, 88
Attention deficit hyperactivity disorder (ADHD), 88
Auditory processing, 89
Autoimmune mechanism, 126
Autonomic dysfunction, 119
Ayurvedic, 291

B

Behavioral CBT strategies, 195
Behavioral headache management
  families, 192–193
  parental role, 201–202
Benign paroxysmal torticollis (BPT), 45–46
  families, 46
  headache specialist, 46
  primary care provider, 46
Benign paroxysmal Vertigo (BPV), 46–47
  families, 47
  headache specialist, 47
  primary care provider, 47
Beta blockers, 175–176
Beta endorphins, 288–289
Biobehavioral referrals, 90–91
Biofeedback, 156, 199–200, 334
Body mass index (BMI), 287–288
Boswellia serrata, 233
Botox. *See* Onabotulinum toxin A
Brain tumor, 3, 5
Bruxism, 89–90, 273
Bupivacaine, 105–106
Butterbur *(Petasites hybridus)*, 230
Butyrophenones, 148

C

Caffeine, 282–284
Calcitonin gene-related peptide (CGRP) pathway
  monoclonal antibodies, 27, 47–48, 115–116, 163
  adolescents, 218*b*
  dosing, routes and half-lives, 218, 218*t*
  headache specialists, 216–218, 217*t*
  patients and families, 215–216
  primary care providers, 216

Calcium channel blockers, 176
Cannabinoid hyperemesis syndrome (CHS), 49
Capsaicin, 231
Cefaly. *See* Transcranial supraorbital nerve stimulation (tSNS)
Celiac disease, 90–91
Cervicogenic headaches, 114–115, 119–120
Childhood Brain Tumor Consortium, 16
Chinese Medicine (CM), 247–248
Chlorpromazine, 148
Chronic daily headache (CDH), 6, 61, 72–73
Chronic migraine (CM), 62–63, 72–74
  burden of disease associated with, 64–65
  chemodenervation, 334–335
  epidemiology, 62–63
  general practitioners, 24
  headache care, 333–335
  headache specialists, 28
  patients and families, 22
  risk factors, 65–66
Chronic tension-type headache (CTTH), 67–68, 72–73, 291
Cinnarizine, 176
Clinical hypnosis, 155
  efficacy, 155
Cluster headache (CH), 15, 68–70, 274–275
Coalition for Headache and Migraine Patients (CHAMP), 175, 310, 334–335, 342
Co-enzyme Q10, 226
Cognitive behavioral therapy (CBT), 154, 194–196, 270, 272, 287–288, 334
Cognitive CBT strategies, 195
Cognitive reframing, 156–157
Combined oral contraceptives (COCs), 55–56
Community, 3, 5–6
Comorbidity, 118, 279
  definition, 79
  general providers, 85–91
  headache specialists, 85–91
Complementary and Alternative Medicine (CAM), 224
Concussion, 111–113, 115, 118, 120–121
Conditioned pain modulation (CPM), 211
Connective tissue disorders, 127
Cortical spreading depression (CSD), 23–24, 26, 28, 207
Crying. *See* Infant colic
Cyclical vomiting syndrome (CVS), 48–50
  headache specialists, 50
  parents, 49
  primary care provider, 50
Cyproheptadine, 176–177

D
Daith piercing, 254
Danish Central Persons Registry, 36
Dehydration, 282
Depression, 14–15, 55–56, 85
Diaphragmatic breathing, 197–198
Diet, 280–282
Dietary Supplement Health and Education Act (DSHEA) of 1994, 224
Dihydroergotamine (DHE), 162
Diphenhydramine, 148–149
Disability, 233–237
Discomfort, 21, 23, 25–26
Disease related stigma, 305
Distraction, 153–155
Divalproex sodium, 174
Dopamine receptor antagonists, 148–149, 162
Dynamic stretching, 246–247

E
Educational resources, 341
Ehlers-Danlos syndrome (EDS), 127
Electrolyte solution, 161
Electronic resources, 196
Elimination diet, 282
Endogenous dietary supplements, 225–229
Energy drinks, 283
Environmental influences, 36–37
Epidemiology
  for families, 11–12
  for headache specialists, 12–13
  for primary care providers, 12–13
Epilepsy, 87
Epstein-Barr virus (EBV) infection, 104
Eptinezumab, 163
Erenumab, 215–217
Estrogen, 22–24, 28, 55–58
European Headache Federation (EHF), 56
European Society of Contraception and Reproductive Health (ESCRH), 56
Evidence-based headache care, 328–329
Exercise, 287–291

F
Familial hemiplegic migraine (FHM), 37
Feverfew (*Tanacetum parthenium*), 229–230
Flunarizine, 176
Folic acid, 228
Food, 280–282
Food and Drug Administration (FDA), 145–146, 207, 224

Fremanezumab, 217
Frovatriptan, 57
Functional disorders, 86

G

Gabapentin, 174
Galcanezumab, 217
Generalized Anxiety Disorder Scale, 7-item
    (GAD-7), 85
Genetics, of migraine
    general practitioners, 38
    headache specialists, 38–39
    patients and families, 39
Genome-wide association studies, 14
Gepants, 149
    headache specialists, 219–220
    patients and families, 219
    primary care providers, 219
Global Burden of Disease Study, 12, 327–328
Global Healthy Living Foundation (GHLF),
    310–311, 342
Guided imagery, 198

H

Headache Action Plan (HAP), 332–333
Headache and Arts Program, 306
Headache care
    acute setting, 332–333
    chronic migraine, 333–335
    evidence-based, 328–329
Headache disorders, 13
Headache phase, 21–22, 24, 26
Headache Relief Guide, 311, 342
Headache visits, barriers to, 6–7
Hemicrania continua (HC), 71–72
Hepatotoxicity, 219
Herbal supplements, 229–233
High intensity training (HIT), 288–289
Homebound education program, 299
Homeopathy, 233
Home-schooling, 300
Hormones
    families, 57–58
    headache specialist, 55–57
Hydration, 282
Hyperadrenergic state, 126
Hypnosis. *See* Clinical hypnosis
Hypovolemic state, 126

I

ICHD-3, 61–62, 63–64*f*, 66–68, 69–70*t*
Infant colic, 44–45

headache specialist, 45
    parents, 44
    primary care provider, 45
Infant Toddler Quality of Life scale scores,
    45–46
Inflammation, 162
Infusions centers, 333
Inter-ictal period, 21, 23, 25
International Classification of Headache Disorders,
    3rd Edition (ICHD-3), 13, 37, 39, 43,
    47–48, 55–56, 102, 114, 273
Intravenous hydration, 161

J

Joint hypermobility, 127

K

Ketogenic diet, 281
Ketorolac, 162

L

Lavender, 231–232
Leukotriene, 105–106
Levetiracetam, 175

M

Magnesium, 226–227
Magnetic resonance spectroscopy (MRS), 25
Manipulation, 244–245
Manual therapies
    headache specialists, 243–247
    patients and families, 243
    primary care providers, 243–247
Marijuana, 232
Massage, 246
Mast cell disorders, 126
Meals, 279
Medical therapy, for postural orthostatic
    tachycardia syndrome (POTS),
    134–135
Medication overuse headache (MOH), 66–67, 73,
    144–145, 147*t*, 219
Medications, 22, 27, 73, 74*t*, 118, 120, 161, 239
Melatonin, 228, 275
Metoclopramide, 148
Migraine cycle
    general practitioners, 23–24
    headache specialists, 25–27
    patients and families, 21–22
Migraine Disability Assessment (MIDAS) scores,
    106, 281
Migraine Research Foundation, 311, 342

Migraine World Summit, 311
Miles for Migraine, 311, 334–335, 342
Miles for Migraine Youth Camp, 307
Mindfulness, 156, 200–201
Moderate continuous exercise training (MCT), 288–289
Molecular genetics, 37
Mood disorders, 103
Multidisciplinary headache care
    clinic components, 329, 330f
    evidence, 335
    resources, advocate for, 335–336
    structure, 329–331
Muscle energy technique (MET), 247

N

N-acetylcysteine (NAC), 229
Naproxen, 57, 145
Naratriptan, 57
Narcolepsy, 89
National Alliance to Advance Adolescent Health, 323
National Headache Foundation, 312, 342
Nerivio. See Remote electrical neuromodulation (REN) device
Nerve blocks, 163, 184–188
Neurobehavioral issues, 88–89
Neurodevelopmental issues, 88–89
Neuromodulation, 143, 207
New daily persistent headache (NDPH), 16, 101
    child/parents, 106–107
    diagnostic workup, 104–105
    epidemiology, 103
    pathogenesis, 103–104
    prognosis, 106
    treatment, 105–106
Nimodipine, 176
Nitric oxide (NO), 288–289, 291
Nocturnal disorders, 89–90
Non-hormonal treatments, 57
Noninvasive vagal nerve stimulation (nVNS)
    patients and families, 210
    providers, 210–211
Nonpharmaceutical options, 143
    acupuncture, 247–254
    manual therapies, 243–247
    nutraceuticals, 223–242
Nonsteroidal anti-inflammatory drugs (NSAIDs), 145, 162
Nutraceuticals
    headache specialist, 224–242
    patients and families, 223–224

O

Obesity, 86–87, 281, 287–288
Occipital nerve blocks, 186
Omega-3 polyunsaturated fatty acids, 227
Onabotulinum toxin A, 334
    families, 181–182
    headache specialists, 183–184
    primary care clinicians, 182–183
Online education, 299–300

P

Parent education, 157
Paroxysmal hemicrania (pH), 71
Patient Health Questionnaire, 9-item (PHQ-9), 85
Pediatric and Adolescent Migraine Screen (PAMS), 303
Pediatric Migraine Action Plan (PedMAP), 299–300, 303
Pediatric Migraine Disability Assessment (Ped-MIDAS) scores, 171–172, 179, 287–290
Peppermint, 231
Peripheral nerve blocks, 163, 184–187
Phase III Research Evaluating Migraine Prophylaxis Therapy (PREEMPT) trial, 182–184
Physical activity, 133
Physical inactivity, 288
Physiotherapy, 331
Placebo, 253–254
Population studies, 14, 36
Population twin studies, 36
Postdromal period, 21–22, 24, 27
Postdural puncture headache (PDPH), 283–284
Posttraumatic headaches (PTH)
    evaluation, 116
    families, 111–114
    headache specialist, 118–121
    management, 116–117
    medications, 118
    pathophysiology, 115–118
    primary care clinicians, 114–118
    prognosis, 114
    red flags, 115
    risk factors, 116
Postural orthostatic tachycardia syndrome (POTS)
    clinical features, 127–128, 127–128t
    epidemiology, 126
    evaluation, 128–131, 129–132t
    medical therapy, 134–135
    pathophysiology, 126–127
    physical activity, 133

prognosis, 135
sleep, 134
symptoms, 125
triggers, 134
volume expansion, 133
PREMICE trial, 209
Premonitory period, 21–23, 25–26
PRESTO trial, 210
Preventive therapy
    clinical setting, 177–179
    goals, 172
    indications, 171–172
    pharmacologic treatment, 172–177
Primary exertional headache (PEH), 290
Primary headaches, 11–12, 233
Primary stabbing headache, 15
Probiotics, 229
Prochlorperazine, 148, 162
Progressive muscle relaxation (PMR), 198
Promethazine, 148
Propranolol, 175–176
Psychological care, 329
Psychological disorders, 85–86
Psychosocial Assessment Tool 2.0 (PAT), 85
Pterygopalatine, 187
Puberty, 22–23

R

Rapid eye movement (REM) sleep, 274–275
Recurrent vomiting, 45–46, 48–50
Reframing, 306
Relaxation strategies, 156, 196–199, 303
Remote electrical neuromodulation (REN) device
    patients and families, 211
    providers, 211–212
Restless leg syndrome (RLS), 90, 273
Riboflavin, 225–226
Rimegepant, 219–220

S

School health plans, 300–301
School nurse, 298–299, 302–303
Section 504 of the Rehabilitation Act of 1973,
        300–301, 303
Selective serotonin reuptake inhibitors (SSRIs),
        148
Seminal articles, 342–343
Serotonin, 275
Sex hormones
    general practitioners, 24
    headache specialists, 28
    patients and families, 22–23

Short-lasting unilateral neuralgiform headaches
        with conjunctival injection and tearing
        (SUNCT), 71
Short-lasting unilateral neuralgiform headaches
        with cranial autonomic symptoms
        (SUNA), 71
Single pulse transcranial magnetic stimulation
        (sTMS)
    patients and families, 208
    providers, 208
Sleep
    headache specialist, 272–275
    patient and family, 269–270
    postural orthostatic tachycardia syndrome
        (POTS), 134
    primary care clinician, 271–272
Sleep disturbance, 89–90
    prevalence, 272–273
    treatment, 271–272
    trigger in headache, 273–274
Social stigma, 305
Specialist visit, 5–6
Specific diets, 280–282
Sphenopalatine ganglion (SPG) blocks
    families, 184–186
    headache specialists, 187–188
    primary care clinicians, 186–187
Static stretching, 246–247
Steroids, 162
Stigma, 305
Subthreshold exercise training, 112
Sumatriptan, 147

T

Tension type headache (TTH), 12, 15, 252
Testosterone, 55–57
TNF alpha, 104
Topiramate, 120, 174
Traditional Chinese Medicine (TCM), 247–248,
        251–252
Transcranial supraorbital nerve stimulation (tSNS)
    patients and families, 209
    providers, 209–210
Transformed migraine (TM), 66
Transition intervention, 321, 321*t*
Transition of adult health care, 315–320
Transmagnetic stimulation (TMS), 207–208
Traumatic brain injury (TBI), 111, 114–116, 118,
        120
Trigeminal autonomic cephalalgias (TACs), 6, 15,
        68, 69–70*t*, 72
Trigeminal nucleus caudalis (TNC), 187

Trigeminovascular nucleus, 209
Triptans, 27, 57, 144–148, 150*t*
Twin studies, 14

U

Ubrogepant, 219–220
Urinary melatonin excretion, 275
US Pain Foundation, 312

V

Vagal nerve stimulation. *See* Noninvasive vagal
    nerve stimulation (nVNS)
Valproic acid, 162–163
Vertigo. *See* Benign paroxysmal Vertigo (BPV)
Vestibular therapy, 118–119
Visual attention, 88–89
Visual oculomotor screen (VOMS), 118–119
Visual therapy, 118–119

Vitamin B6, 228
Vitamin B12, 228
Vitamin C, 229
Vitamin D3, 227–228
Vitamin E, 229
Vomiting. *See* Cyclical vomiting syndrome (CVS)

W

Websites, 341–342
Wrap around care, 120

Y

Yoga, 291–292

Z

Zolmitriptan, 57
Zonisamide, 175